SANFORD GUIDE

Thirtieth Edition

THE SANFORD

GUIDE TO ANTIMICROBIAL THERAPY

2000

David N. Gilbert, MD
Robert C. Moellering, Jr, MD
Merle A. Sande, MD

THE SANFORD GUIDE TO ANTIMICROBIAL THERAPY 2000 (30TH EDITION)

Jay P. Sanford, M.D.
1923-1996

EDITORS

David N. Gilbert, M.D.
*Director of Medical Education and
Earl A. Chiles Research Institute
Providence Portland Medical Center
Professor of Medicine
Oregon Health Sciences University
Portland, Oregon*

Robert C. Moellering, Jr., M.D.
*Physician-in-Chief
Beth Israel Deaconess Medical Center
Herrman L. Blumgart Professor of Medicine
Harvard Medical School
Boston, Massachusetts*

Merle A. Sande, M.D.
*Clarence M. and Ruth N. Birrer Professor of Medicine
University of Utah School of Medicine
Salt Lake City, Utah*

The Sanford Guide to Antimicrobial Therapy is published annually by:

ANTIMICROBIAL THERAPY, INC.
P.O. Box 70, 229 Main Street
Hyde Park, VT 05655 USA
Tel 802-888-2855   Fax 802-888-2874
Email: info@sanfordguide.com

PUBLISHER'S NOTE

You, the reader, should know that the SANFORD GUIDE is not prepared for any single pharmaceutical company or distributor. Though copies are distributed by multiple companies in the health care field, the SANFORD GUIDE has been independently prepared and published since its inception in 1969. Decisions regarding the content of the SANFORD GUIDE are solely those of the editors and the publisher. Please feel free to contact us.Your comments and questions are encouraged and appreciated.

Our thanks to the Editorial Board, Carolyn Wickwire for her continued dedication to preparation of this complex manuscript, Gateway Graphics for printing of this edition of the SANFORD GUIDE.

Jeb C. Sanford, Publisher

— TABLE OF CONTENTS —

TABLE 1
CLINICAL APPROACH TO INITIAL CHOICE OF ANTIMICROBIAL THERAPY
Treatment based on presumed site or type of infection. In selected instances, treatment based on identification of pathogens.

ANATOMIC SITE/DIAGNOSIS/ MODIFYING CIRCUMSTANCES	ETIOLOGIES (usual)	SUGGESTED REGIMENS* PRIMARY	SUGGESTED REGIMENS* ALTERNATIVE§	ADJUNCT DIAGNOSTIC OR THERAPEUTIC MEASURES AND COMMENTS
Abdomen: See Peritoneum, page 33; Gallbladder, page 11; and Pelvic Inflammatory Disease, page 17				
Bone: Osteomyelitis	*General Comment:* Regardless of the type of osteomyelitis, a specific microbiologic diagnosis is essential. It is not possible to predict the microbial etiology based on epidemiology. In chronic osteomyelitis, organism(s) isolated from sinus tract drainage may not accurately reflect organisms present in bone. Ideally, empiric therapy is initiated after collection of blood and infected bone for culture. For review: *NEJM 336:999, 1997.*			
Hematogenous—Regimens refer to EMPIRIC THERAPY of acute disease				
Newborn (to 4 mo.)	S. aureus, Gm-neg. bacilli, Group B strep	(Nafcillin or oxacillin) + P Ceph 3 *(Dosage in Table 16)*	Vanco + P Ceph 3 *(Dosage in Table 16)*	Often afebrile. Localizing signs best predictor of osteo. Over ⅔ have positive blood cultures. Risk factors: Preterm and mechanical vent. *PIDJ 14:1047, 1995.* Treat for minimum of 21 days.
Children (>4 yrs) Often at or adjacent to epiphysis of long bones	S. aureus, Group A strep, coliforms rare	Nafcillin or oxacillin — Add P Ceph 3 if Gm-neg. bacteria on Gm stain. *Pediatric doses Table 16, adult below*	Vanco or clinda	With immunization, H. influenzae almost disappeared. Vanco for PRSP, pen-allergic, or high prevalence of MRSA. IV rx initially. If bacterial etiology known, then po or IV rx at home for total of 6 weeks.
Adult (>21 yrs) More often vertebral (Review: *AJM 101:550, 1996*) Vertebral osteo: *CID 20:320, 1995 & AJM 100:85, 1996)*	S. aureus most common + variety other aerobic/ anaerobic cocci & bacilli; culture before empiric rx unless blood cultures pos.	Nafcillin or oxacillin 2.0 gm q4h IV or cefazolin 2.0 gm IV q8h *See Comments*	Vanco 1.0 gm q12h IV	Rx regimens assume empiric rx and either no organism or Gm+ cocci on Gm stain. If Gram stain shows Gm-neg. bacilli, add P Ceph 3 to nafcillin or vanco or could use [CIP 750 mg bid po (400 mg IV) q12h + RIF 600 mg po qd] pending culture results. If high prevalence of MRSA, use vanco. Dx: MRI of spine. **Consider epidural abscess!**
Adult or child (special circumstances)				
Sickle cell anemia	Salmonella sp.	FQ (not in children)	P Ceph 3	Sternoclavicular joint and ribs in addition to vertebral and long bones
IV drug abuse, hemodialysis pts	―S. aureus, P. aeruginosa	PRSP* + CIP*	Vanco + CIP*	
Contiguous Osteomyelitis Without Vascular Insufficiency				
Post-reduction & internal fixation of fracture	Coliforms, S. aureus, P. aeruginosa	Natcillin 2.0 gm q4h IV + CIP 750 mg bid po	Vanco 1.0 gm q12h IV + P Ceph 3 AP	Usually necessary to remove "hardware" to achieve bone union. Revascularization if needed, e.g., pedicle muscle flaps, myocutaneous flaps.
Post-op sternotomy	S. aureus, S. epidermidis	Vanco 1.0 gm q12h IV + RIF 600-900 mg qd po		Sternal debridement establishes microbial etiology and removes necrotic bone. Use of internal mammary artery (esp. in diabetics) for CABG increases risk of sternal osteo.
Post-op prosthetic joint osteo	See *Prosthetic joint, pages 23 & 24*			
Post-nail puncture of foot through tennis shoe	P. aeruginosa	Ceftazidime 2.0 gm q8h IV or CFP 2.0 gm q12h IV	CIP 750 mg bid po (not in children)	Osteo evolves in 1–2% plantar puncture wounds in children. P. aeruginosa causes 93%. Debridement necessary to remove foreign body *(CID 21:794, 1995).* See Lung, cystic fibrosis, page 31, for CIP use in children.
Contiguous Osteomyelitis With Vascular Insufficiency				
Patients with neurologic deficit & decubiti; atherosclerotic peripheral vascular disease; diabetic with neuropathy *(see Diabetic foot, page 11)*	Polymicrobic [Gm + cocci (aerobic & anaerobic) and Gm-neg. bacilli (aerobic & anaerobic)]	Mild disease—outpatient therapy:: AM/CL 500 mg po tid. Severe—hospitalized: IMP or MER or TC/CL or PIP/TZ or AM/SB or trova or (CFP + metro) or (az-treonam + vanco + metro). *(Dosage in footnote)†*		Metal probe to bone correlates with presence of osteomyelitis *(JAMA 273:721, 1995).* **In extremity, determine extent of atherosclerotic vascular disease and revascularize if possible.** MRI helpful in documenting extent of infection. Surgical debridement for culture and removal of necrotic tissue. If neuropathy, avoid weight bearing. **Aggressive treatment** (debridement + antibiotics + revascularization) in diabetic decreases need for amputation *(CID 23:286, 1995)*

† Drug dosage: **IMP** 0.5 gm q6h IV, **MER** 1.0 gm q8h IV (not licensed indication but should be effective), **TC/CL** 3.1 gm q6h IV, **PIP/TZ** 3.375 gm q6h or 4.5 gm q8h IV, **AM/SB** 3.0 gm IV q6h, **CFP** 2.0 gm q12h IV, **metro** 1.0 gm loading dose and then 0.5 gm q6h IV or po or 1.0 gm q12h IV, **vanco** 1.0 gm q12h IV, **trova** 200 mg IV per day

NOTE: *All dosage recommendations are for adults (unless otherwise indicated) and assume normal renal function*

(Footnotes and abbreviations on page 47)

TABLE 1 (2)

ANATOMIC SITE/DIAGNOSIS/ MODIFYING CIRCUMSTANCES	ETIOLOGIES (usual)	SUGGESTED REGIMENS*		ADJUNCT DIAGNOSTIC OR THERAPEUTIC MEASURES AND COMMENTS
		PRIMARY	ALTERNATIVE§	
Bone *(continued)*				
Chronic Osteomyelitis *(AJM 101:550, 1996)* By definition, implies presence of dead bone	S. aureus, Enterobacteriaceae, P. aeruginosa	Empiric rx not indicated. Base systemic rx on results of culture, sensitivity testing. If acute exacerbation of chronic osteo, rx as acute hematogenous osteo.		Important adjuncts to be considered: removal of orthopedic hardware, surgical debridement, vascularized muscle flaps, distraction osteogenesis (Ilizarov) techniques. Antibiotic-impregnated cement & hyperbaric oxygen adjunctive. NOTE: RIF + (vanco or β-lactam) very effective in animal models + one clinical trial of S. aureus chronic osteo *(SMJ 79:947, 1986)*. Quinolone rx: *CID:25,1327, 1997.*
Breast				
Postpartum				
Mastitis	S. aureus	Dicloxacillin 500 mg q6h po or cefazolin 1.0 gm q8h IV	Clinda 300 mg q6h po	If no abscess, increased frequency of nursing may hasten response.
Abscess		Nafcillin or oxacillin 2.0 gm q4h IV or cefazolin 1.0 gm q8h IV	Vanco 1.0 gm q12h IV	With abscess, d/c nursing. I&D usually required.
Non-puerperal abscess	S. aureus, Bacteroides sp., Peptostreptococcus	Clinda 300 mg q6h po or IV or [(nafcillin/oxacillin IV as above or cefazolin IV as above) + metro 7.5 mg/kg q6h IV]	AM/CL 875/125 mg q12h po or AM/SB 1.5 gm q6h IV or (vanco + metro)	If subareolar, most likely anaerobes; if not subareolar, staph. Need pretreatment aerobic/anaerobic cultures. Surgical drainage for abscess.
Central Nervous System				
Brain abscess				
Primary or contiguous source *Reference: CID 25:763, 1997*	Streptococci (60–70%), Bacteroides (20–40%), Enterobacteriaceae (25–33%), S. aureus (10–15%). Rare: Nocardia *(Table 10A, page 76)*	P Ceph 3 (cefotaxime 2.0 gm q4h IV or ceftriaxone 2.0 gm q12h IV) + metro 7.5 mg/kg q6h or 15 mg/kg q12h IV	Pen G 20–24 mu IV qd + metro	If CT scan suggests cerebritis *(JNS 59:972, 1983)*, abscesses <2.5 cm and pt neurologically stable and conscious, start antibiotics and observe. Otherwise, surgical drainage necessary. Neurologic deterioration usually mandates surgery. Experience with Pen G (HD) + metro without P Ceph 3 or PRSP has been good. We use P Ceph 3 because of frequency of isolation of Enterobacteriaceae. S. aureus rare without positive blood culture and/or signs of endocarditis. Strep. milleri group esp. prone to produce abscess.
		Duration of rx unclear; rx until response by neuroimaging (CT/MRI)		
Post-surgical, post-traumatic	S. aureus, Enterobacteriaceae	(Nafcillin or oxacillin) 2.0 gm q4h IV + P Ceph 3	Vanco 1.0 gm q12h IV + P Ceph 3	If hospital-acquired and MRSA a consideration, substitute vanco for nafcillin or oxacillin. P Ceph 3 dose as for brain abscess, primary.
HIV-1 infected (AIDS)	Toxoplasma gondii	See *Table 12, page 91*		
Subdural empyema: In adult 60–90% are extension of sinusitis or otitis media. Rx same as primary brain abscess. Surgical emergency: must drain *(CID 20:372, 1995)*.				
Encephalitis/encephalopathy *(See Table 14, page 102)*	Herpes simplex, arboviruses, rabies; rarely: listeria, cat-scratch disease	No empiric antibiotic unless Gram stain positive. Start IV acyclovir while awaiting results of CSF PCR for H. simplex.		Newly recognized strain of bat rabies. May not require a break in the skin. Eastern equine encephalitis causes focal MRI changes in basal ganglia and thalamus *(NEJM 336:1867, 1997)*. Cat-scratch ref.: *PIDJ 14:866, 1995.*

(Footnotes and abbreviations on page 47)   NOTE: All dosage recommendations are for adults *(unless otherwise indicated) and assume normal renal function*

TABLE 1 (3)

ANATOMIC SITE/DIAGNOSIS/ MODIFYING CIRCUMSTANCES	ETIOLOGIES (usual)	SUGGESTED REGIMENS*		ADJUNCT DIAGNOSTIC OR THERAPEUTIC MEASURES AND COMMENTS
		PRIMARY	ALTERNATIVE§	
Central Nervous System *(continued)*				
Meningitis, "Aseptic": Pleocytosis of 100s of cells, CSF glucose normal, neg. culture for bacteria *(see Table 14, page 99)*	Enteroviruses, HHV-2,LCM, HIV, other viruses, drugs (NSAIDs, metronidazole, carbamazepine, TMP/SMX, IVIG), rarely leptospirosis	For all but leptospirosis, IV fluids and analgesics. D/C drugs that may be etiologic. For lepto (doxy 100 mg q12h IV or po) or (Pen G 5 mu q6h IV) or (AMP 0.5–1.0 gm q6h IV). Repeat LP if suspect partially-treated bacterial meningitis.		If readily available, culture or PCR CSF for enterovirus. Antiviral drug active vs enterovirus (Pleconaril) in clinical trial. HHV-2 unusual without concomitant genital herpes. For lepto: positive epidemiologic history and concomitant hepatitis, conjunctivitis, dermatitis, nephritis. Drug-induced: *ArIM 159:1185, 1999.*
Meningitis, Bacterial: Goal is empiric rx, then CSF Gram stain is negative—immunocompetent *(modified from NEJM 336:708, 1997)*				
Empiric Therapy—CSF Gram stain is negative; then empiric therapy, give empiric rx, do head CT, then do LP.				
Age: Preterm to <1 month	Group B strep 49%, E. coli 18%, listeria 7%, misc. Gm-negatives 10%, misc. Gm-positives 10%	AMP + cefotaxime Intraventricular rx not recommended. Repeat CSF exam/culture 24–36 hrs after start of rx. *For dosage, see Table 16*	AMP + gentamicin	Primary and alternative regimens active vs Group B strep, most coliforms, and listeria. If premature infant with long nursery stay, S. aureus, enterococci, and resistant coliforms potential pathogens. Optional empiric regimens: [nafcillin + (ceftazidime or cefotaxime)]. If high risk of MRSA, use vanco + cefotaxime. Alter regimen after culture/sensitivity data available.
Age: 1–3 months	S. pneumo, meningococci, H. influenzae now rare, rarely <1 mo. pathogens above	AMP + (cefotaxime or ceftriaxone) + dexamethasone *For dexamethasone dose, see Comment. For other dosage, see Table 16*	Vanco + (cefotaxime or ceftriaxone) + dexamethasone	Value of dexamethasone for other than H. flu uncertain, but still recommended *(PIDJ 14:490, 1995)*. Give 1st dose 15–20 min. prior to or concomitant with 1st dose of antibiotic. Dose: Either (0.4 mg/kg q12h IV x2 d.) OR (0.15 mg/kg IV q6h x4 d.) Steroid refs: *CID 20:685, 1995; NEJM 336:708, 1997; JAMA 278:925, 1997.*
Age: 3 mos.–50 yrs NOTE: *Large vanco dose—see footnote[2]*	S. pneumo (includes DRSP)[1], meningococci, H. influenzae now very rare, listeria unlikely if young and immunocompetent. Statement from Am. Acad. of Peds.: *Peds 99:289, 1997*	Adult dosage: [(Cefotaxime 2.0 gm q4–6h IV OR ceftriaxone 2 gm IV q12h) + (dexamethasone) + vanco (see footnote[2])] Dexamethasone: 0.4 mg/kg q12h IV x2 d. Give with or just before 1st dose of antibiotic to block TNF production. *See footnote regarding drug-resistant S. pneumo[1] See footnote[3] for rest of ped. dosage*	[(MER 1.0 gm q8h IV) (Peds: 40 mg/kg IV q8h)] + dexamethasone + vanco *(see footnote[3])*	In U.S., empiric Pen G not recommended; Pen G 4 mu IV q4h used in countries with low prevalence of drug-resistant S. pneumoniae (DRSP).[1] **For pts with severe pen. allergy:** chloro (for meningococcus) + TMP/SMX (for listeria if immunocompromised) *(NEJM 341:233, 1999)*. In U.S. (but not elsewhere), 60–80% of strains sensitive to clinda. If pen G MIC ≥2, cross-resistance to ceftriaxone nearly 100%, to cefotaxime/ceftriaxone 29%. The standard alternative for pts with severe pen. allergy was chloramphenicol. However, high failure rate in pts with DRSP *(Ln 339:405, 1992; Ln 342:240, 1993).* For meningococcal prophylaxis, see *Table 15, page 113.* Dexamethasone meta-analysis: *JAMA 278:925, 1997.* Meropenem ref.: *PIDJ 18:581, 1999.*

[1] **Drug-resistant S. pneumoniae (DRSP)** *(DMID 29:249, 1997; MMWR 48:649, 1999; Clin Micro Rev 11:628, 1998)*. Definition: susceptible (MIC <0.1 μg/ml), intermediate (MIC 0.1–1 μg/ml), resistant (MIC ≥2 μg/ml). Prevalence of resistance: Geographic variability ranging from 2–53%; in U.S., prevalence gradually rising. Cross-resistance to erytho, tetracycline, chloramphenicol, and TMP/SMX. So far, **no** vanco resistance, RIF resistance rare (0.5%). Also active in vitro: Levo, trova, spar, gatifloxacin, moxifloxacin; reports of ↑ FQ resistance *(NEJM 341:233, 1999)*. If pen G MIC ≥2, cross-resistance to ceftriaxone nearly 100%, to cefotaxime/ceftriaxone

[2] Low and erratic penetration of vanco into the CSF *(PIDJ 16:895, 1997)*. Consequently, the recommended dosage in children is 15 mg/kg q6h IV. Limited clinical data in adults given 15 mg/kg q6h (double the standard dose); however, in areas with high ↑ prevalence of DRSP, the empiric use of the higher vanco dose seems reasonable.

[3] Dosage of drugs used to rx children ≥1 mo. of age: Cefotaxime 200 mg/kg/d IV div. q6–8h; ceftriaxone 100 mg/kg/d IV div. q12h; vanco 15 mg/kg IV q6h.

(Footnotes and abbreviations on page 47)   NOTE: *All dosage recommendations are for adults (unless otherwise indicated) and assume normal renal function*

TABLE 1 (4)

ANATOMIC SITE/DIAGNOSIS/ MODIFYING CIRCUMSTANCES	ETIOLOGIES (usual)	SUGGESTED REGIMENS*		ADJUNCT DIAGNOSTIC OR THERAPEUTIC MEASURES AND COMMENTS
		PRIMARY	ALTERNATIVE§	
Central Nervous System (continued)				
Meningitis, Bacterial/Empiric Therapy/Negative CSF Gram Stain (continued)				
Age: >50 yrs or alcoholism or other debilitating associated disease(s)	S. pneumo, listeria, Gram-neg. bacilli. Note absence of meningo-coccus.	(AMP 2.0 gm IV q4h) + (ceftriaxone 2.0 gm IV q12h or cefotaxime 2.0 gm IV q6h) + (dexamethasone 0.4 mg/kg q12h IV x2 d.; 1st dose before or concomitant with 1st dose of antibiotic)	MER 1.0 gm q8h IV + dexamethasone. **For severe pen. allergy, see Comment**	Not sure what to do if severe pen. allergy precludes use of a penicillin, cephalosporin or MER. As in box immediately above, chloro has failed against DRSP. TMP/SMX is alternative for listeria (CID 24:1, 1997). Hence could use vanco (for S. pneumo) + TMP/SMX (for listeria and some Gm-neg. bacilli—pending culture results). MER active vs listeria in vitro [JAC 36(Suppl. A):1, 1995]; CSF levels appear adequate (JAC 34:175, 1994) but no clinical data.
Any age with impaired cellular immunity, e.g., high-dose steroids	Listeria, Gram-neg. bacilli	(AMP 2.0 gm IV q4h) + (ceftazidime 2.0 gm IV q8h)		
Post-neurosurgery or post-head trauma	S. pneumoniae most common if CSF leak. Other: S. aureus, coliforms, P. aeruginosa	Vanco (until known not MRSA) 1.0 gm q6-12h† IV + ceftazidime 2.0 gm q8h IV	MER should work, 1.0 gm q8h IV, but not an FDA-approved indication	If culture-proven coliform or pseudomonas meningitis, some add intrathecal gentamicin 4 mg q12h into lateral ventricles). MER does not have seizure potential of IMP.
Ventriculitis/meningitis due to infected ventriculo-peritoneal (atrial) shunt	S. epidermidis, S. aureus, coliforms, diphtheroids (rare), P. acnes	**Child:** [(Vanco 15 mg/kg q6h IV) + (either cefotaxime 50 mg/kg q6h IV or ceftriaxone 50 mg/kg q12h IV)]. **Adult:** Vanco 1.0 gm q6-12h† IV + RIF 600 mg qd po	(either cefotaxime 50 mg/kg q12h IV + RIF 600 mg	Early shunt removal usually necessary for cure. Refs.: Adv PID 11:29, 1996; IDCP 4:277, 1995. For adults, can use P Ceph 3 alone if positive Gram stain for Gm-neg. bacilli.
Empiric Therapy—Positive CSF Gram stain (NEJM 336:708, 1997)				
Gram-positive diplococci	S. pneumoniae	Vanco 15 mg/kg IV q6-12h† + either (ceftriaxone 2.0 gm IV q12h or cefotaxime 2.0 gm IV q6h) ± dexamethasone 0.4 mg/kg q12h IV x2 d		**For severe penicillin allergy: vanco + RIF 600 mg qd (po or IV),** Dexamethasone: (1) does not reduce penetration of vanco into CSF of **children**, so ceftriaxone + vanco OK; (2) in **adults**, probably OK based on animal model data (AAC 43:876, 1999).
Gram-negative diplococci	N. meningitidis	Pen G 4 million units IV q4h; chloro if pen. allergic		No clinical data to support use of dexamethasone (CID 20:685, 1995)
Gram-positive bacilli or coccobacilli	Listeria monocytogenes	AMP 2.0 gm IV q4h + gentamicin 2 mg/kg loading dose then 1.7 mg/kg q8h		Listeria reference: CID 24:1, 1997. If pen.-allergic, use TMP/SMX 15-20 mg/kg div. q6-8h.
Gram-negative bacilli	H. influenzae, coliforms, P. aeruginosa	Ceftazidime 2.0 gm IV q8h + gentamicin 2 mg/kg 1st dose then 1.7 mg/kg q8h		Other possible drugs: aztreonam, CIP, MER, trova. CIP rx success: CID 25:936, 1997.
Specific Therapy for S. pneumoniae—Positive culture of CSF with in vitro susceptibility results available				
S. pneumoniae	Pen G MIC <0.1 µg/ml	Aq. pen G 4 million units IV q4h		For severe pen. allergy: (Vanco + 600 mg RIF/d) or chloro.

1 Low and erratic penetration of vanco into the CSF (PIDJ 16:895, 1997). Consequently, the recommended dosage in children is 15 mg/kg q6h IV. There are limited clinical data in adults given 15 mg/kg q6h (double the standard dose). However, in areas with high or ↑ prevalence of DRSP, the empiric use of the higher vanco dose seems reasonable.

NOTE: All dosage recommendations are for adults (unless otherwise indicated) and assume normal renal function

(Footnotes and abbreviations on page 47)

TABLE 1 (5)

ANATOMIC SITE/DIAGNOSIS/ MODIFYING CIRCUMSTANCES	ETIOLOGIES (usual)	SUGGESTED REGIMENS*		ADJUNCT DIAGNOSTIC OR THERAPEUTIC MEASURES AND COMMENTS
		PRIMARY	ALTERNATIVE[1]	
Central Nervous System/Meningitis, Bacterial/Specific therapy for S. pneumoniae (continued)				
NOTE: A 2nd CSF exam after 24–48 hrs is suggested both because of difficulty treating resistant S. pneumo and because dexamethasone (if used) may impair clinical assessment	Pen G MIC >0.1 μg/ml and/or ceftriaxone MIC >0.5 μg/ml	CHILDREN: [(Ceftriaxone 100 mg/kg IV q12h or cefotaxime 50–75 mg/kg IV q6h) + vanco 15 mg/kg IV q6h] + dexamethasone 0.4 mg/kg q12h IV x2 d. ADULTS: [(Ceftriaxone 2.0 gm IV q12h) + (vanco 15 mg/kg q6–12h[1])] ± dexamethasone		In experimental S. pneumo meningitis, vanco + ceftriaxone synergistic even with high ceftriaxone MIC (AAC 37:1630, 1993). In children, dexamethasone does not ↓ vanco penetration of CSF (AAC 39:1988, 1995). MER may work but little clinical experience. Rx if severe penicillin allergy: vanco IV + [RIF 600 mg qd (po or IV)]
N. meningitidis		Treat as for Gram-stain positive: Gram-neg. diplococci	Prophylaxis, Table 15, page 113	Rare isolates chloro-resistant (NEJM 339:368, 917, 1998).
Listeria monocytogenes		Treat as for Gram-stain positive: Gram-pos. bacilli		Lab may report as diphtheroids.
Meningitis, chronic Defined as symptoms + CSF pleocytosis for ≥4 wks	M. tbc—40%, cryptococcosis—7%, neoplastic—8%, enigmatic—34% (QJM 63:283, 1987)	Treatment depends on etiology. No urgent need for empiric therapy.		Long list of possibilities: bacteria, parasites, fungi, viruses, neoplasms, vasculitis, and other miscellaneous etiologies—See IDCP 1:158, 1992
Meningitis, HIV-1 infected (AIDS)	As in adults >50 yrs, also consider cryptococci, M. tuberculosis, syphilis, HIV aseptic meningitis, Listeria monocytogenes	If etiology not identified: rx as adult >50 yrs + obtain CSF/serum cryptococcal antigen (see Comments)	For crypto rx, see Table 10A, page 74	C. neoformans most common etiology in AIDS pt. H. influenzae, pneumococci, TBc, syphilis, viral, histoplasma and coccidioides also need to be considered. Obtain blood cultures. L. monocytogenes risk >60x ↑, 3/4 present as meningitis (CID 17:224, 1993).
Ear				
External otitis				
"Swimmer's ear"	Pseudomonas sp., Enterobacteriaceae, Proteus spp., (Fungi rare) Acute infection usually 2° S. aureus	Eardrops: [(polymyxin B + neomycin + hydrocortisone) qid] or [ofloxin 0.3% soln bid] For acute disease: dicloxacillin 500 mg 4x/d		Rx should include gentle cleaning. Recurrences prevented (or decreased) by drying with alcohol drops (⅓ white vinegar, ⅔ rubbing alcohol) after swimming, then antibiotic drops or 2% acetic acid solution. Ointments should not be used in ear.
Chronic	Usually 2° to seborrhea	Eardrops: [(polymyxin B + neomycin + hydrocortisone) qid] + (selenium sulfide)]		Control seborrhea with dandruff shampoo containing selenium sulfide (Selsun) or [(ketoconazole shampoo) + (medium potency steroid solution, triamcinolone 0.1%)].
Diabetes mellitus, acute "malignant otitis externa"	Pseudomonas sp.	IMP 0.5 gm q6h IV or MER 1.0 gm q8h IV or CIP 400 mg q12h IV (or 750 mg q12h po) or ceftaz 2.0 gm q8h IV or CFP 2 gm q12h or (PIP 4–6 gm q4–6h IV + APAG [dose depends on drug]) or (TC 3.0 gm q4h IV + APAG)		CIP especially useful for outpatient rx with early disease. Surgical debridement usually required, but not radical excision. R/O osteomyelitis. CT or MRI scan more sensitive than x-ray. If bone involved, rx for 4–6 wks.

[1] Low and erratic penetration of vanco into the CSF (PIDJ 16:895, 1997). Consequently, the recommended dosage in children is 15 mg/kg q6h IV. There are limited clinical data in adults given 15 mg/kg q6h (double the standard dose). However, in areas with high of ↑ prevalence of DRSP, the empiric use of the higher vanco dose seems reasonable.

NOTE: All dosage recommendations are for adults (unless otherwise indicated) and assume normal renal function

(Footnotes and abbreviations on page 47)

TABLE 1 (6)

ANATOMIC SITE/DIAGNOSIS/ MODIFYING CIRCUMSTANCES	ETIOLOGIES (usual)	SUGGESTED REGIMENS*		ADJUNCT DIAGNOSTIC OR THERAPEUTIC MEASURES AND COMMENTS
		PRIMARY	ALTERNATIVE§	
Ear (continued)				
Otitis media—infants, children, adults				
Acute—Main ref.: *PIDJ 18:1, 1999*				>95% of earaches in children resolve without antimicrobial rx *(BMJ 260:1033, 1985).*
Initial empiric therapy	S. pneumo (40–50%) H. influenzae (20–25%) M. catarrhalis (10–15%) Viral (48%), esp. RSV & rhinoviruses *(NEJM 340:260, 312, 2001, 1999)*	Amox po: UD or HD— see *footnote¹ & Comment* Other dosages in footnote². Std rx is 10 days; 5 d. reported effective *(JAMA 279:1736, 1748, 1998; PIDJ 18854, 1999).* TMP/SMX, and clarithro/azithro are no longer considered 1st-line alternatives due to ↓ activity vs DRSP and/or poor activity vs H. influenzae.	AM/CL po: HD¹, ceftriaxone po, or ceftriaxone 50 mg/kg IM x1 (ped dose only)	Spontaneous resolution in 90% pts infected with M. catarrhalis, 50% with H. influenzae, and only 10% with S. pneumoniae. Risk of DRSP ↑ with age <2 yrs, antibiotics last 3 mos., and/or daycare attendance. Selection of drug based on (1) effectiveness against β-lactamase producing H. influenzae and M. catarrhalis and (2) effectiveness against S. pneumo, including DRSP. Of 16 FDA-approved drugs for acute otitis media, many lack data for efficacy vs DRSP. Limited data on efficacy of cefprozil and cefpodoxime vs DRSP. Cefaclor, loracarbef, cefixime, and ceftibuten less active vs DRSP than other agents listed.
Treatment if rx failure after 3 days	DRSP	AM/CL–HD, cefuroxime, or IM ceftriaxone (in children) x3 days See dosage in footnotes	Clindamycin, tympano-centesis	Definition of failure: no change in ear pain, fever, bulging TM or otorrhea after 3 days of rx. Tympanocentesis will allow culture. Newer FQs active vs DRSP, but not approved for use in children. Vanco is active vs DRSP.
After >48 hours of naso-tracheal intubation	Pseudomonas sp. Klebsiella Enterobacter	P Ceph 3 AP or CFP or IMP or MER or TC/CL or CIP. (For dosages, see Ear, malignant otitis externa)		With nasotracheal intubation >48 hrs, about ½ pts will have otitis media with effusion.
Recurrent acute Little benefit from adenoid-ectomy *(JAMA 282:945 & 987, 1999)*	Pneumococci, H. influen-zae, M. catarrhalis, Staph. aureus, Group A strep **(see Comments)**	Sulfisoxazole 50 mg/kg at bedtime or Amoxicillin 20 mg/kg qd or Azithromycin 10 mg/kg q week *(AAC 40:2752, 1996)*		Consider if ≥3 episodes in previous 6 months or ≥4/yr; or in infant, ≤6 months, 1 episode + family hx of ear infections *(CID 19:823, 1994)*. Rx daily for 6 months during winter/spring. **Use of antibiotics to prevent otitis media is a major contributor to emergence of antibiotic-resistant S. pneumo!**

¹ Amoxicillin UD or HD = amoxicillin usual dose or high dose; AM/CL HD = amoxicillin/clavulanate high dose.

² **Drugs and peds dosage (all po unless specified) for acute otitis media: Amoxicillin UD** = 40–45 mg/kg/d div q12h or q8h. **Amoxicillin HD** = 80–90 mg/kg/d div q12h or q8h. **AM/CL HD** = 80–90 mg/kg/d of amox component. Either use 875/125 AM/CL or use (500/125 + extra plain amox hd) but keep clavulanate at approx. 10 mg/kg/d. **Cefuroxime axetil** 30 mg/kg q12h. **Ceftriaxone** 50 mg/kg IM x1 initially; if treatment failure, give IM x1 for 3 days. **Clindamycin** 20–30 mg/kg/d div qid (may be effective vs DRSP but no activity vs H. influenzae).
Other drugs suitable for sensitive S. pneumo: TMP/SMX 8 mg/kg/d of TMP div q12h. **Erythro-sulfisoxazole** 50 mg/kg/d of erythro div q6–8h. **Clarithro** 15 mg/kg/d div q12h; **azithro** 10 mg/kg/d x1 and then 5 mg/kg qd on days 2–5. **Cefprozil** 30 mg/kg/d div q12h; **cefpodoxime proxetil** 10 mg/kg/d div q12h as single dose; **cefaclor** 40 mg/kg/d div q8h; **loracarbef** 30 mg/kg/d div q12h. **Cefdinir** 7 mg/kg q12h. **Cefixime** 8 mg/kg qd. **Ceftibuten** 9 mg/kg qd. (not approved for infections due to S. pneumoniae).
NOTE: *All dosage recommendations are for adults (unless otherwise indicated) and assume normal renal function*

(Footnotes and abbreviations on page 47)

TABLE 1 (7)

ANATOMIC SITE/DIAGNOSIS/ MODIFYING CIRCUMSTANCES	ETIOLOGIES (usual)	SUGGESTED REGIMENS*		ADJUNCT DIAGNOSTIC OR THERAPEUTIC MEASURES AND COMMENTS
		PRIMARY	ALTERNATIVE§	
Ear (continued)				
Mastoiditis				
Acute				
Outpatient	Strep. pneumoniae 22%, S. pyogenes 16%, Staph. aureus 7%, H. influenzae 4%, P. aeruginosa 4% Others <1%	Empirically, same as Acute otitis media, above; need nafcillin/oxacillin if culture + for S. aureus.		Has become a rare entity, presumably as result of the aggressive rx of acute otitis media.
Hospitalized		Cefotaxime 1.0 gm q4h IV or (ceftriaxone 2 gm q24h IV < age 60: 1 gm q24h IV > age 60)		
Chronic	Often polymicrobic: anaerobes, S. aureus, Enterobacteriaceae, P. aeruginosa	Treatment for acute exacerbations or perioperatively. Ideally, no treatment until surgical cultures obtained. Examples of empiric regimens: IMP 0.5 gm q6h IV, TC/CL 3.1 gm q6h IV, PIP/TZ 3.375 gm q4–6h or 4.5 gm q8h IV.		May or may not be associated with chronic otitis media with drainage via ruptured tympanic membrane. Antimicrobials given in association with surgery. Mastoidectomy indications: chronic drainage and evidence of osteomyelitis by MRI or CT, evidence of spread to CNS (epidural abscess, suppurative phlebitis, brain abscess).
Eye—General Reviews: CID 21:479, 1995; IDCP 7:447, 1998				
Eyelid				
Blepharitis	Etiol. unclear. Factors include Staph. aureus & Staph. epidermidis, seborrhea, rosacea, & dry eye	Wash off debris, then topical ointment (bacitracin or erythro) bid to qid x2 wks and then qd at bedtime		If associated rosacea, add doxy 100 mg po bid x2 wks and then qd. Clean lid margins daily with dilute baby shampoo.
Hordeolum (Stye) External	Staph. aureus	Hot packs only. Will drain spontaneously		Infection of superficial sebaceous gland.
Internal	Staph. aureus	Oral PRSP + hot packs		Also called acute meibomianitis. Rarely drain spontaneously.
Conjunctiva				
Conjunctivitis of the newborn (ophthalmia neonatorum): by day of onset post-delivery				
Onset 1st day	Chemical due to AgNO₃ prophylaxis	None		
Onset 2–4 days	N. gonorrhoeae	Aq. Pen G 100,000 u/kg/d in 4 divided doses x7 d. or ceftriaxone 25–50 mg/kg qd IV x7 d.		Treat mother and her sexual partners. Hyperpurulent.
Onset 3–10 days	Chlamydia trachomatis	Erythro syrup 50 mg/kg/d (po in 4 divided doses x14 days); 20–30% failures—see Comment		No topical therapy. Diagnosis by antigen detection. Azithro susp 20 mg/kg qd x3 d. reported efficacious (PIDJ 17:1049, 1998).
Onset 2–16 days	Herpes simplex types 1, 2	See keratitis, below		
Painless suffusion (pink eye) Usually unilateral	Adenovirus (types 3 & 7 in children, 8 & 19 in adults)	No treatment		Highly contagious. Onset of ocular pain and photophobia in an adult suggests assoc. keratitis—rare.
Inclusion conjunctivitis (adult) Usually unilateral	Chlamydia trachomatis	Doxy 100 mg bid po x1–3 weeks	Erythro 250 mg qid po x1–3 weeks	Oculogenital disease. Diagnosis by culture or antigen detection or PCR—availability varies by region and institution.

(Footnotes and abbreviations on page 47)

NOTE: All dosage recommendations are for adults (unless otherwise indicated) and assume normal renal function

TABLE 1 (8)

ANATOMIC SITE/DIAGNOSIS/ MODIFYING CIRCUMSTANCES	ETIOLOGIES (usual)	SUGGESTED REGIMENS*		ADJUNCT DIAGNOSTIC OR THERAPEUTIC MEASURES AND COMMENTS
		PRIMARY	**ALTERNATIVE§**	
Eye, Conjunctiva *(continued)*				
Trachoma	Chlamydia trachomatis	Azithro 20 mg/kg po single dose—78% effective	Doxy 100 mg bid po x14 d. or tetracycline 250 mg qid po x14 d.	Starts in childhood and can persist for years with subsequent damage to cornea. Topical therapy of marginal benefit. Avoid doxy/tetracycline in young children. Reference: CID 24:363, 1997
Suppurative				
Non-gonococcal	Staph. aureus, S. pneumoniae, H. influenzae	Ophthalmic erythro, gentamicin or bacitracin-polymyxin B	Ophthalmic tobramycin, CIP, ofloxo, poly-myxin B/trimethoprim	Often self-limited. Primary regimens are less expensive. Eye drops preferred for adults and ointments for infants or young children. Topical neomycin may cause punctate staining of cornea. Avoid chloramphenicol.
Gonococcal	N. gonorrhoeae	Ceftriaxone 125 mg IM or IV (single dose). See *Genital, page 15*		
Cornea (keratitis): Usually serious and sight-threatening. Prompt ophthalmologic consultation essential! Herpes simplex most common etiology in developed countries; bacterial and fungal infections more common in underdeveloped countries.				
Viral				
H. simplex	H. simplex, types 1 & 2	Trifluridine, one drop qh, 9x/day for up to 21 days	Vidarabine ointment	Fluorescein staining shows topical dendritic figures. 30–50% rate of recurrence within 2 years; 400 mg acyclovir po bid ↓ recurrences, p 0.005 (NEJM 339:300, 1998).
Varicella-zoster ophthalmicus	Varicella-zoster virus	Famciclovir 500 mg tid po or valacyclovir 1.0 gm tid po x10 days	Acyclovir 800 mg po 5x/day x10 days	Clinical diagnosis most common: dendritic figures with fluorescein staining in patient with varicella-zoster of ophthalmic branch of trigeminal nerve.
Bacterial		*All rx listed for bacterial, fungal, & protozoan is topical*		
Contact lens users	P. aeruginosa	Tobramycin (14 mg/ml) + piperacillin or ticarcillin eye drops (6–12 mg/ml) q15–60 min. around clock x24–72 hrs, then slow reduction	CIP or ofloxo 0.3% qtts q15–60 min qtts x24–72 hrs	Pain, photophobia, impaired vision. Recommend alginate swab for culture and sensitivity testing.
Dry cornea, diabetes, immuno-suppression	Staph. aureus, S. epidermidis, S. pneumoniae, S. pyogenes, Enterobacteriaceae, listeria	Cefazolin (50 mg/ml) + gentamicin or tobramycin (14 mg/ml) q15–60 min. around the clock for 24–72 hrs, then slow reduction	Vanco (50 mg/ml) + ceftazidime (50 mg/ml) q15–60 min. around clock x24–72 hrs, then slow reduction. See Comment	Specific therapy guided by results of alginate swab culture and sensitivity. CIP 0.3% found clinically equivalent to cefazolin + tobramycin; only concern was efficacy of CIP vs S. pneumoniae (Ophthalmology 163:1854, 1996).
Fungal	Aspergillus, fusarium, candida. No empiric therapy—see Comment	Natamycin (5%) gtts q2–3 hrs with subsequent slow reduction	Ampho B (0.05–0.15%) q2–3 hrs with subsequent slow reduction	No empiric therapy. Wait for results of Gram stain or culture in Sabouraud's medium.
Protozoan Soft contact lens users (over-night use ↑ risk 10–15 fold)	Acanthamoeba, Hartmanella	Propamidine 0.1% + neomycin/gramicidin/ polymyxin Eyedrops q waking hour x1 week and then slow taper	Polyhexamethylene biguanide 0.02% or chlorhexidine 0.02%	Uncommon. Trauma and soft contact lenses are risk factors. Corneal scrapings stained with calcofluor white shows characteristic cysts with fluorescent microscopy.

(Footnotes and abbreviations on page 47) NOTE: All dosage recommendations are for adults (unless otherwise indicated) and assume normal renal function

9

TABLE 1 (9)

ANATOMIC SITE/DIAGNOSIS/ MODIFYING CIRCUMSTANCES	ETIOLOGIES (usual)	SUGGESTED REGIMENS* PRIMARY	ALTERNATIVE§	ADJUNCT DIAGNOSTIC OR THERAPEUTIC MEASURES AND COMMENTS
Eye (continued)				
Lacrimal apparatus				
Canaliculitis	Actinomyces most common. Rarely, Arachnia.	Remove granules and irrigate with 10% sulfacetamide qtts	Irrigate with Pen G (100,000 u/ml) or clinda	Digital pressure produces exudate at punctum; Gram stain confirms diagnosis.
		Child: AM/CL or O Ceph 2	TMP/SMX	
Dacryocystitis (lacrimal sac)	S. pneumoniae, Staph. aureus, H. influenzae, S. pyogenes	Adult: O Ceph 1 or oral PRSP	Erythro	Collect exudate from lacrimal punctum for culture and sensitivity. Systemic therapy for acute disease; irrigation with antibiotic solutions for chronic disease. Adult doses in footnote.[1] Pediatric doses in Table 16, page 120.
			(See footnote for dosage)	
Endophthalmitis: Best article on etiologic agents of post-op endophthalmitis *Am J Ophthal* 122:1, 1996				
Bacterial: Haziness of vitreous key to diagnosis. Needle aspirate of both vitreous and aqueous humor for culture prior to therapy. Intravitreal administration of antimicrobials essential.				
Postocular surgery (cataracts)				All require early ophthalmologic consultation. With S. aureus or P. aeruginosa, eye may be destroyed within 24 hours. Rx must be aggressive: early vitrectomy and then intravitreal antibiotics (vanco 1 mg + amikacin 0.4 mg—each in 0.1 ml). Repeat intravitreal injection after several days. Parenteral therapy not necessary unless infection outside globe.
Early, acute onset	Staph. aureus (½) Pseudomonas sp.			
Low grade, chronic	Propionibacterium acnes, S. epidermidis, S. aureus	May require removal of lens material. Intraocular vanco.		
Post-IV filtering blebs for glaucoma	Strep. species (viridans and others), H. influenzae	Intravitreal agent and systemic AM/CL, AM/SB or P Ceph 2		
Post-penetrating trauma	Bacillus sp.	Intravitreal agent as above + systemic clinda or vanco. Do not use topical antibiotics before surgery.		
None, suspect hematogenous	S. pneumoniae, N. meningitidis, Staph. aureus	P Ceph 3 (cefotaxime 2.0 gm q4h IV or ceftriaxone 2.0 gm q24h IV) + vanco 1.0 gm q12h IV pending cultures. Intravitreal antibiotics as with early post-operative.		
IV heroin abuse	Bacillus cereus, Candida sp.	Intravitreal agent + (systemic clinda or vanco)		
Mycotic (fungal) Broad-spectrum antibiotics, often corticosteroids, indwelling venous catheters	Candida sp., Aspergillus sp.	Intravitreal ampho B 0.005-0.010 mg in 0.1 ml. *Also see Table 10, pages 71, 72 for concomitant systemic therapy. See Comment.*		With moderate/marked vitreitis, options include systemic rx + vitrectomy ± intravitreal ampho B *(CID 27:1130 & 1134, 1998).* Report of failure of ampho B lipid complex *(CID 28:1177, 1999).*
Retinitis				
Acute necrotizing retinitis	Varicella zoster, Herpes simplex	IV acyclovir 10-12 mg/kg IV q8h		Strong association of VZ virus with atypical necrotizing herpetic retinopathy *(CID 24:603, 1997).*
HIV+ (AIDS) CD4 usually <100/mm³	Cytomegalovirus	See Table 14, page 101		Occurs in 5-10% of AIDS patients

[1] **O Ceph 1** (adult doses): **Cefaclor** 250 mg q8h po; **Cefadroxil** 1.0 gm qd po; **cephalexin** 250 mg q6h po; **cephradine** 250 mg q6h po; AM/CL 875/125 mg po bid; **dicloxacillin** 125 mg q6h po; **erythro** 250 mg q6h po;
(Footnotes and abbreviations on page 47)   NOTE: *All dosage recommendations are for adults (unless otherwise indicated) and assume normal renal function*

TABLE 1 (10)

ANATOMIC SITE/DIAGNOSIS/ MODIFYING CIRCUMSTANCES	ETIOLOGIES (usual)	SUGGESTED REGIMENS*		ADJUNCT DIAGNOSTIC OR THERAPEUTIC MEASURES AND COMMENTS
		PRIMARY	ALTERNATIVE§	
Eye (continued) Orbital cellulitis (see p. 38 for erysipelas/facial)	S. pneumoniae, H. influenzae, M. catarrhalis, S. aureus, anaerobes, group A strep	P Ceph 2/3 (cefuroxime 1.5 gm q8h IV, cefotaxime 2.0 gm q8h IV, ceftizoxime 2.0 gm q12h IV), or AM/SB 1.5 gm q6h IV	TC/CL or PIP/TZ (see footnote[1] for dosages) or cefotaxime 2.0 gm q4h IV or ceftriaxone 2.0 gm q24h IV	See mucor/rhizopus, Table 10, page 75. H. influenzae becoming a rare etiology.
Foot				
"Diabetic" [G-CSF effective in small controlled study (Ln 350:855, 1997). Reviews: CID 25:1318, 1997 and NEJM 331:854, 1994]				
Previously untreated, limited in extent, no osteomyelitis	Aerobic Gm + cocci	Clinda or O Ceph 1 or oflox or AM/CL (see footnote[1] and Comment for dosage)	Clinda 300 mg qid po or cephalexin 500 mg qid x14d, 90% cure (ArIM 150:790, 1990). Oflox, AM/CL Ref.: CID 24:643, 1997.	
Chronic, recurrent, limb-threatening (See Bone, page 3, for associated osteomyelitis) **NOTE: Prognosis depends on blood supply; assess for arterial insufficiency early**	Polymicrobic: aerobic cocci, bacilli + anaerobes	If early mild: cefoxitin or [CIP + (clinda or metro)]. If septic/severe: IMP or MER or TC/CL or AM/SB or PIP/TZ or trova or [PRSP + APAG (or aztreonam) + clinda] [for dosage, see footnote[1]].	P Ceph 3 + (clinda or metro)] or trova or PIP/TZ or AM/SB or PIP/TZ + clinda] [for dosage, see Topical platelet-derived growth factor, Becaplermin, daily somewhat effective & expensive (Med Lett 40:73, 1998).	Cultures from ulcers unreliable. Prompt surgical intervention to R/O necrotizing fasciitis and for culture. X-ray to R/O gas and concomitant osteomyelitis. **Ability to insert probe to bone suggests concomitant osteomyelitis** (JAMA 273:721, 1995). MRI cannot distinguish marrow edema from osteo (Radiol 203:849, 1997). Avoidance of weight-bearing is key (NEJM 331:854, 1994).
Onychomycosis: See Table 10, page 74, fungal infections				
Gallbladder				
Cholecystitis, cholangitis, biliary sepsis, or common duct obstruction (partial: 2nd to tumor, stones, stricture)	Enterobacteriaceae (68%), Enterococci (14%), Bacteroides (10%), Clostridium sp. (7%)	[AP Pen ± metro) or (AMP + gentamicin ± metro) or TC/CL or PIP/TZ or AM/SB (for dosage, see footnote[2])]	P Ceph 3 + (metro or clinda) or Aztreonam + clinda	For severely ill pts, antibiotic rx is complementary to establishment of adequate biliary drainage (CID 19:279, 1994). 15–30% pts will require decompression; surgical, percutaneous or laparoscopic. We add metro but may not be essential. Whether empirical rx should always cover enterococci, pseudomonas and anaerobes is uncertain (CID 19:279, 1994). Enterococci of hepatobiliary origin associated with bacteremia: should be treated (IDCP 2:332, 1993). Ceftriaxone associated with biliary sludge (by ultrasound 50%, symptomatic 9%, NEJM 322:1821, 1990); clinical relevance still unclear but has led to surgery (NEJM 42:39, 1993)
Gastrointestinal				
Gastroenteritis—Empiric Therapy				
Premature infant with necrotizing enterocolitis	Associated with E. coli, Staph, epidermidis, P. aeruginosa, C. perfringens	[Ticarcillin + APAG) or P Ceph 3 for dosage, see Table 9B, pages 64, 65]	[Vanco + APAG ± clinda) or (AMP + APAG + metro)]	Pneumatosis intestinalis on x-ray confirms dx. Bacteremia-peritonitis in 30–50%. If Staph. epidermidis isolated add vanco (IV).
Infant	E. coli (enteropathogenic)	TMP/SMX (for dosage, see Table 9B, page 69)		Mild cases require hydration only.

1 **Cefoxitin** 2.0 gm q8h IV, **CIP** 750 mg bid po or 400 mg bid IV, **clinda** 300 mg po or 400 mg q8h IV, **aztreonam** 2.0 gm q8h IV, **metro** 1.0 gm IV loading dose then 0.5 gm q6h or 1.0 gm q12h IV, **amp** 2.0 gm q6h IV, **TC/CL** 3.1 gm q6h IV, **PIP/TZ** 3.375 gm q6h IV, **AM/SB** 3.0 gm q6h IV, **gati** 400 mg q24h, **oflox** 400 mg q12h, **levo** 500 mg q24h, **trova** 200 mg IV]. **APAG:** see Table 9C, page 70 for dosing of aminoglycosides.

2 **AP Pen (ticarcillin** 4.0 gm q6h IV, **PIP** 4.0 gm q6h IV), **metro** 1.0 gm IV loading dose then 0.5 gm q6h or 1.0 gm q12h IV, **amp** 2.0 gm q6h IV, **TC/CL** 3.1 gm q6h IV, **PIP/TZ** 3.375 gm q6h IV, **AM/SB** 3.0 gm q6h IV, **gent and other aminoglycosides,** see Table 9C, page 70, **IMP** 0.5 gm q6h or 1.0 gm q8h IV, **MER** 1.0 gm q24h, **aztreonam** 2.0 gm q6h IV, **see previous footnote for clinda and aztreonam dosage, P Ceph 3 dose in Table 9B, pages 64, 65.**

NOTE: All dosage recommendations are for adults (unless otherwise indicated) and assume normal renal function

(Footnotes and abbreviations on page 47)

TABLE 1 (11)

ANATOMIC SITE/DIAGNOSIS/ MODIFYING CIRCUMSTANCES	ETIOLOGIES (usual)	SUGGESTED REGIMENS*		ADJUNCT DIAGNOSTIC OR THERAPEUTIC MEASURES AND COMMENTS
		PRIMARY	ALTERNATIVE§	

Gastrointestinal *(continued)*

Gastroenteritis—Empiric Therapy (laboratory studies not performed or culture, microscopy, toxin results NOT AVAILABLE)

Mild diarrhea (≤3 uniformed stools/day, minimal associated symptomatology)	Bacterial *(see Severe, below)*, viral, parasitic. Viral usually causes mild to moderate disease. *(See AJM 106:670, 1999)*	Fluids only + lactose-free diet, avoid caffeine		For fluid replacement, see *Cholera, below.* **Antimotility:** Loperamide (Imodium) 4 mg po, then 2 mg after each loose stool to max. of 16 mg/day. Bismuth subsalicylate (PeptoBismol) 2 tablets (262 mg) po qid.
Moderate diarrhea (≥4 unformed stools/day, and/or systemic symptoms)		Antimotility agents *(see Comments)* + fluids		**Hemolytic uremic syndrome (HUS):** Risk in children infected with E. coli 0157:H7 is 8–10%. Early treatment with TMP/SMX may increase risk of HUS *(NEJM 333:364, 1995).*
Severe diarrhea (≥6 unformed stools/day, and/or temperature ≥101°F, tenesmus, blood, or fecal leucocytes) **NOTE: Severe afebrile bloody diarrhea should increase suspicion of E. coli 0157:H7 infection.**	Shigella, salmonella, C. jejuni, E. coli 0157:H7, toxin-producing C. difficile, E. histolytica. *For typhoid fever, see page 44* If recent antibiotic therapy (C. difficile toxin colitis possible), add:	FQ (CIP 500 mg q12h po, norflox 400 mg q12h po) x3–5 days Metro 500 mg tid po x10–14 days	TMP/SMX DS bid po x3–5 days. Resistance to TMP/SMX common throughout tropics. Vanco 125 mg qid po x10–14 days	**Other potential etiologies:** Cryptosporidia—no treatment in immunocompetent host *(see Table 12A and JID 170:272, 1994).* Cyclospora—usually chronic diarrhea, responds to TMP/SMX *(see Table 12A and AIM 123:409, 1995).* **Severe diarrhea** was treated with CIP 500 mg bid po or placebo; CIP ↓ duration of diarrhea and other symptoms without changing duration of fecal carriage. 4% campylobacter resistance *(CID 22:1019, 1996).*

Gastroenteritis—Specific Therapy (results of culture, microscopy, toxin assay AVAILABLE). Reference: IDCP 6:68 & 141, 1997

Amebiasis (Entamoeba histolytica, cyclospora and cryptosporidia), see Table 12A

	Campylobacter jejuni CAUTION: See Comment for quinolone reference resistance	CIP 500 mg po or norflox 400 mg po q12h x5 days or azithro 500 mg po qd x3 d.	Erythro stearate 500 mg qid po x5 days	Quinolone-resistant strains many locations: Thailand, N. Africa, Spain and Mexico; 84% of Thai isolates CIP-resistant and 7–15% azithro-resistant *(CID 26:341, 1998).* Doxy/clinda active in vitro. Risk of Guillain-Barre syndrome *(NEJM 335:208, 1996; Ln 352:635, 1998; for plasmapheresis, see AnIM 131:453, 1999).*
	C. difficile toxin positive antibiotic-associated colitis *(Recent reference: CID 26:1027, 1998)* For other causes of antibiotic-associated diarrhea, see *CID 27:702, 1998* Remember: enteric isolation indicated	Metro 500 mg tid or 250 mg qid po x10–14 days If too ill for po rx, metro 500 mg q6h IV (efficacy not established); if ileus, add vanco by infusion from above (see Comment) &/or retrograde cecal catheter &/or vanco enemas (see Comment)	(Vanco 125 mg qid po) or (bacitracin 25,000 u qid po) or (cholestyramine 4 gm po tid) x10–14 days. Teicoplanin[NUS] 400 mg po 2x/d. x 10 d. For relapses: [metro 500 mg tid po + RIF 300 mg bid po] x10 d. (see Comment)	DC antibiotic if possible; avoid antimotility agents; hydration; enteric isolation. Relapse occurs in 10–20%; retreat with metro. For refractory disease, vanco po + RIF po reported effective *(ICHE 16:459, 1995); metro + RIF should work* also but no published data. Other relapse rx regimens: metro x10 d, then [cholestyramine 4 gm po tid + lactobacillus 1 gm qid] x4 wks OR vanco 125 mg po qod x4 wks. When po rx not possible, use IV metro + vanco, 500 mg/L saline via small bowel tube and/or via pigtail catheter in cecum (severe typhlitis pts). Perfuse at 1–3 ml/min to daily max. of 2.0 gm; see *NEJM 329:583, 1993.* NOTE: IV vanco not effective. In hospital pts, exposure to P Ceph 3 may ↑ risk of C. difficile toxin diarrhea; use of BL/BLI may ↓ risk *(Aliment Pharm Ther 12:1217, 1998).* C. difficile toxin diarrhea can be community-acquired in the **absence** of antibiotic exposure *(IDCP 6:385, 1997).*
	E. coli 0157:H7 *(Ln 352:1207, 1998)* Usually afebrile	Treatment with antimicrobials controversial. In vitro, FQs induce toxin synthesis/release while killing *(Ln 353:1588, 1999).*		Natural history: 95% resolve, 5% develop HUS. TMP/SMX late in illness may not predispose to HUS *(NEJM 333:364, 1995).* General ref.: *AnIM 126:505, 1997.* Toxin terminology: *Ln 351:1003, 1998*

NOTE: All dosage recommendations are for adults (unless otherwise indicated) and assume normal renal function

(Footnotes and abbreviations on page 47)

TABLE 1 (12)

ANATOMIC SITE/DIAGNOSIS/ MODIFYING CIRCUMSTANCES	ETIOLOGIES (usual)	SUGGESTED REGIMENS* PRIMARY	ALTERNATIVE§	ADJUNCT DIAGNOSTIC OR THERAPEUTIC MEASURES AND COMMENTS
Gastroenteritis—Specific Therapy (continued)				
Listeria monocytogenes		AMP 200 mg/kg IV q6h	TMP/SMX 20 mg/kg/d IV div. q6-8h	Recently recognized cause of food poisoning, manifest as febrile gastroenteritis. Percentage with complicating bacteremia/meningitis unknown. Not detected in standard stool culture (NEJM 336:100 & 130, 1997).
Salmonella—For typhoid fever, see page 44		If patient asymptomatic or illness mild, antimicrobial therapy not indicated. If illness severe, pt septic or immunocompromised, or pt ill enough to hospitalize, antimicrobial agents indicated. (Also see typhoid fever, page 44)		
		CiP 500 mg po or norflox 400 mg po q12h x3–7 d. Resistance ↑ (Ln 353:1590, 1999)	Azithro 1.0 gm po once, then 500 mg qd x6 d (AAC 43:1441, 1999)	Other alternatives: ↑ resistance to TMP/SMX and chloro. Ceftriaxone, cefotaxime usually active (see footnote, page 17, for dosage). Primary treatment of enteritis is fluid and electrolyte replacement. No adverse effects from FQs in children with resistant organisms (Ln 348:547, 1996).
Shigella		(CiP 500 mg po) or (norflox 400 mg po) q12h x3 doses	(TMP/SMX DS bid po x3 d) or (azithro 500 mg po x1, then 250 mg qd x4 d.)	In children, peflox^{NUS} 12 mg/kg qd x3 days (CID 19:1172, 1994) and CiP suspension 10 mg/kg q12h x5 d (Ln 352:522, 1998) were effective. Cefixime was ineffective in adults (AIM 123:509, 1995). Azithro vs CiP: AnIM 126:697, 1997
Vibrio cholerae— Treatment decreases duration of disease, vol. losses, and duration of excretion		(CiP 1.0 gm po x1) or (norflox 400 mg po x3 d.) + fluids (see Comment) Single dose CiP preferred where tetra resistance is common (Ln 348:296, 1996)	Doxy 300 mg po x1 + fluids (see Comment). For children <8 yrs & in pregnancy: TMP/SMX or erythro	Primary rx is fluid. IV use (per liter): 4 gm NaCl, 1 gm KCl, 5.4 gm Na lactate, 8 gm glucose. PO use (per liter potable water): 1 level teaspoon table salt + 4 heaping teaspoons of sugar (JTMH 84:73, 1981). Volume given = fluid loss. Mild dehydration, give 5% body weight; for moderate, 7% body weight. (Reference: CID 20:1485, 1995; TRSM 89:103, 1995).
Vibrio parahemolyticus		Antimicrobial rx does not shorten course		Sensitive in vitro to FQ, doxy. Often history of seafood ingestion.
Yersinia enterocolitica— Ref.: PIDJ 14:771, 1995		CiP or norflox as for Shigella. TMP/SMX or doxy if not severe (CTID 17:405, 1993)	Ceftriaxone 2.0 gm qd IV, APAG and chloro also effective.	Mesenteric adenitis can mimic acute appendicitis. Lab diagnosis difficult: requires "cold enrichment" and/or Yersinia selective agar. Desferrioxamine rx ↑ severity, discontinue if pt on it. Iron overload states predispose to yersinia (CID 27:1362 & 1367, 1998). Tetra & TMP/SMX resistance reported (Ln 349:1825, 1997). Review: Ln 349:924, 1997).
Gastroenteritis—Specific Risk Groups—Empiric Therapy				
Anoreceptive intercourse Proctitis (distal 15 cm only)	Herpes viruses, gonococci, chlamydia, syphilis	See Genital Tract, pages 15, 16		
Colitis	Shigella, salmonella, campylobacter, E. histolytica (see Table 12A)	FQ (CiP 500 mg q12h po, norflox 400 mg q12h po) x3 days		
HIV-1 infected (AIDS) & >10 days diarrhea Acid-fast organisms:	G. lamblia	See Table 12A		For influence of highly active antiretroviral therapy, see CID 28:701, 1999
Other:	Cryptosporidium parvum, Cyclospora cayetanensis	See Table 12A		
	Isospora belli, microsporidia (Enterocytozoon bienusi, Septata intestinalis)	See Table 12A		
Neutropenic enterocolitis or "typhlitis" (CID 27:695 & 700, 1998)	Mucosal invasion by **Clostridium septicum**. Occasionally caused by Clostridium sordelli or P. aeruginosa.	As for perirectal abscess. Ensure empiric regimen includes drug active vs Clostridia species; e.g. pen G, AMP, or clinda. Empiric regimen should have predictive activity vs P. aeruginosa also.		Tender right lower quadrant. Surgical resection controversial but may be necessary.

NOTE: All dosage recommendations are for adults (unless otherwise indicated) and assume normal renal function

(Footnotes and abbreviations on page 47)

13

TABLE 1 (13)

ANATOMIC SITE/DIAGNOSIS/ MODIFYING CIRCUMSTANCES	ETIOLOGIES (usual)	SUGGESTED REGIMENS* PRIMARY	SUGGESTED REGIMENS* ALTERNATIVE§	ADJUNCT DIAGNOSTIC OR THERAPEUTIC MEASURES AND COMMENTS
Gastrointestinal—Specific Risk Groups—Empiric Therapy (continued)				
Traveler's diarrhea, self-medication. Patient usually afebrile	Toxigenic E. coli, shigella, salmonella, campylobacter, amebiasis (see Table 12), cyclospora, cryptosporidia		FQ (CIP 500 mg or norflox 400 mg or oflox 300 mg) all bid po x3 days + loperamide (Imodium) 4 mg and then 2 mg after each loose stool. Can substitute TMP/SMX-DS, bid x3 days, for FQ.	If diarrhea lasts ≥14 days (3% of travelers), pt has persistent or chronic diarrhea; for details of management of chronic diarrhea, see CID 22:124, 1996.
Prevention		Not routinely indicated. Current recommendation is to take FQ + Imodium with 1st loose stool (NEJM 328:1821, 1993).	Use in 1st 2 weeks only if activities are essential. Options: Bismuth subsalicylate (Pepto-Bismol) 2 tabs (262 mg) po qid, or FQ—cipro 500 mg po qd, norflox 400 po qd	
Gastrointestinal Infections by Anatomic Site				
Esophagitis	Candida albicans, HSV, CMV	See SANFORD GUIDE TO HIV/AIDS THERAPY		
Duodenal/Gastric Ulcer; chronic type B antral gastritis (not 2° NSAIDs) General ref: AJG 93:2336, 1998	**Helicobacter pylori** See Comment	**Rx 2x/day po for 10 days:** Omeprazole 20 mg + amox 1 gm + clarithro 500 mg. Can substitute lansoprazole 30 mg for omeprazole.	**Rx po for 2 weeks:** Bismuth (see footnote[1]) 4x/1 gm + amox 500 mg 4x/d. + metro 500 mg 4x/d. + omeprazole 20 mg 2x/d.	If active ulcer, give omeprazole 20 mg qd x18 days after 10-14 day combination rx. Many other rx regimens (AJG 93:2330, 1998). NOTE: (1) Eradication of H. pylori does not reverse symptoms of non-ulcer dyspepsia (AnIM 130:695, 1999). (2) Some question if rx of H. pylori before NSAID will ↓ ulcer risk (Ln 350:975, 1997; Ln 352:1016, 1998). Test of cure: Urea breath test if available. Stool antigen test controversial; may have false-positives (Ln 354:1209, 1999).
Whipple's disease—organism propagated in vitro (JID 176:672 & 752, 1997)		Initial IV rx: (Ceftriaxone 2.0 gm bid + streptomycin 1.0 gm qd) then po rx for 1 year with either TMP/SMX-DS bid or cefixime 400 mg daily		Rx regimen based on empiricism and retrospective analyses. TMP/SMX: CNS relapses during TMP/SMX rx reported.
Inflammatory bowel disease: Ulcerative colitis, Crohn's disease Mild to moderate Ref: AIM 100:656, 1996	Unknown	Sulfasalazine 1.0 gm po or mesalamine (5ASA) 1.0 gm q6h po. See NEJM 334:841, 1996	Coated mesalamine (Asacol) 800 mg bid or qid equally effective (AnIM 124:204, 1996). Corticosteroid enemas	Continued rx decreases relapses after initial response (AJM 93:799, 1992). Check stool for E. histolytica, (some empirically rx with metro before steroid enemas). Agranulocytosis in 0.7-10% in 1st 3 months of rx with sulfasalazine; may respond to G-CSF. Uncontrolled study suggests benefit from rifabutin + either clarithro or azithro (JAC 39:393, 1997).
Diverticulitis (NEJM 338:1521, 1998) No signs of bowel perforation (with bowel perforation, see Peritonitis, page 33)	Enterobacteriaceae, bacteroides, enterococci	(TMP/SMX-DS bid) or (CIP 500 mg bid) + [metro 500 mg q6h] po OR AM/CL 500/125 mg tid po	Parenteral regimens as for perirectal abscess or secondary peritonitis (see Comment)	First suggested regimen is designed for outpatient use; alternative is for more ill inpatients. For inpatients multiple options as for perirectal abscess (next box below) or as for peritonitis, page 33.
Perirectal abscess	Enterobacteriaceae, bacteroides (enterococci)	Multiple regimens effective. Must "cover" both Gm-neg. aerobic & Gm-neg. anaerobic bacteria. **Drugs active only vs anaerobic Gm-neg. bacilli:** clinda, metro. **Drugs active only vs aerobic Gm-neg. bacilli:** APAG, P Ceph 2/3/4, aztreonam, AP Pen, cipro TMP/SMX. **Drugs active vs both aerobic/anaerobic Gm-neg. bacteria:** cefoxitin, cefotetan, cefmetazole,[NUS] TC/CL, PIP/TZ, AM/SB, IMP, MER, gati, moxi, & trova. (Dosage: see footnotes **1 & 2,** p. 11)		**Surgical drainage is primary!** Consider underlying regional enteritis (Crohn's disease). Role of enterococci remains debatable; include drug(s) active vs enterococcus in patient with valvular heart disease. For review of antimicrobial efficacy for intra-abdominal infections, see IDCP 5(Suppl. 1):S2, 1996. Example regimens: 1. IMP 500 mg IV q6h 2. TC/CL 3.1 gm IV q6h or PIP/TZ (3.375 gm or 4.5 gm q8h IV) 3. Trova 300 mg IV qd, then 200 mg po qd (in hospital only) 4. (P Ceph 3 or 4) + metro 1.0 gm IV q12h

[1] 2 bismuth preparations: (1) In U.S., bismuth-subsalicylate (PeptoBismol) 151 mg tabs; dose is 2 tabs (302 mg) 4x/day. (2) Outside U.S., colloidal bismuth subcitrate (De-Nol) 120 mg chewable tablets; dose is 1 tablet 4x/day.

(Footnotes and abbreviations on page 47)

NOTE: All dosage recommendations are for adults (unless otherwise indicated) and assume normal renal function

TABLE 1 (14)

ANATOMIC SITE/DIAGNOSIS/ MODIFYING CIRCUMSTANCES	ETIOLOGIES (usual)	SUGGESTED REGIMENS*		ADJUNCT DIAGNOSTIC OR THERAPEUTIC MEASURES AND COMMENTS
		PRIMARY	ALTERNATIVE§	
Genital Tract: Mixture of empiric and specific treatment. Divided by sex of the patient. See Guidelines for Dx of Sexually Transmitted Diseases, MMWR 47(RR-1), 1998 & Med Lett 41:85, 1999				
Both Women & Men:				
Chancroid	H. ducreyi	Ceftriaxone 250 mg IM single dose or Azithro 1.0 gm po single dose	CIP 500 mg bid po x3 d or Erythro base 500 mg qid po x7 d	In HIV+ pts, failures reported with single dose azithro (CID 21:409, 1995; IDCP 4:407, 1995). Reference: CID 28(Suppl. 1):S14, 1999
Chlamydia, et al. non-gono-coccal or post-gonococcal urethritis, cervicitis. NOTE: Assume concomitant N. gonorrhoeae, see treatment options above	Chlamydia (50%) Myco-plasma hominis, Other known etiologies (10–15%); Ureaplasma, Trichomonas, Herpes simplex virus, Mycoplasma genitalium	[Doxy 100 mg po x7 d.) or (azithro 1.0 gm po as single dose). Evaluate and rx sex partner In pregnancy: erythro base 500 mg po qid x7 d. OR amoxicillin 500 mg po tid x7 d.	(Erythro base 500 mg qid po x7 d.) or (oflox 300 mg q12h po x7 d.) In pregnancy: erythro base 250 mg po qid x14 d. OR azithro 1.0 gm po x1	Diagnosis: PCR of voided urine (male or female) sensitive and specific; if not available culture or antigen detection. Doxy and FQ not recommended in preg-nancy. Clarithro active in vitro vs C. trachomatis, but not FDA-approved for STDs. For recurrent or persistent disease: either metro 2.0 gm po x1 + either erythro base 500 mg po qid x7 d. or erythro ethylsuccinate 800 mg po qid x7 d. Ref. on lab diagnosis: Sex Trans Dis 26(Suppl.):S8, 1999.
Gonorrhea				
Conjunctivitis (adult)	N. gonorrhoeae	Ceftriaxone 1 gm IM x1 + lavage with saline		
Disseminated gonococcal infection (DGI, dermatitis-arthritis syndrome)	N. gonorrhoeae	(Ceftriaxone 1.0 gm IV qd) or (cefotaxime 1.0 gm IV) or (ceftizoxime 1.0 gm q8h IV)—See Comment	Spectinomycin 2.0 gm q12h IM or cipro 500 mg IV q12h or oflox 400 mg IV q12h—See Comment	Continue IM or IV regimen for 24 hrs after symptoms ↓; reliable pts may be discharged 24 hrs after sx resolve to complete 7 days rx with cefixime 400 mg po bid or cipro 500 mg po bid or oflox 400 mg po bid. R/O meningitis/ endo-carditis. Treat presumptively for concomitant C. trachomatis.
Meningitis and endocarditis	N. gonorrhoeae	Ceftriaxone 1–2 gm IV q12h x10–14 d. for meningitis and 4 wks for endocarditis.		Harder to eradicate than at urogenital/anorectal sites
Pharyngitis	N. gonorrhoeae	Treat exactly as for urethritis, above		**Treat for both GC and C. trachomatis.** Screen for syphilis.
Urethritis, cervicitis, proctitis (uncomplicated)	N. gonorrhoeae (50% of pts with urethritis, cervicitis have concomitant C. tra-chomatis—**treat for both**). Dx by amplification (PCR/ LCR) of DNA in voided urine.	[(Ceftriaxone 125 mg IM x1) or (cefixime 400 mg po x1) or (cipro 500 mg po x1) or (oflox 400 mg po x1)] PLUS [(Azithro 1 gm po x1) or (doxy 100 mg po x2/d. x7 days)] Evaluate and rx sex partner.		If GC acquired in Asia or Cleveland, Ohio, do not use quinolone due to risk of resistance: MMWR 47:405, 1998. Other alternatives for **GC:** Spectinomycin 2 gm IM x1 Other single-dose cephalosporins: ceftizoxime 500 mg IM, cefotaxime 500 mg IM, cefotetan 1 gm IM, cefoxitin 2 gm IM + probenecid 1 gm po. Other single-dose quinolones: enoxacin 400 mg, lomefloxacin 400 mg, norfloxacin 800 mg, gatifloxacin 400 mg. Azithro 1 gm po x1 effective for chlamydia but need 2 gm po for GC; not recommended for GC due to GI side-effects and expense.
Granuloma inguinale (Donovanosis)	Calymmatobacterium granulomatis	Doxy 100 mg bid po x3–4 wks OR TMP/SMX-DS 2x/d. x3 wks	Erythro 500 mg qid wks OR CIP 750 mg po x3 wks	Clinical response usually seen in 1 week. Rx until all lesions healed, may take 4 weeks. Treatment failures & recurrence with doxy and TMP/SMX. Report of efficacy with FQ and chloramphenicol. Ref.: CID 25:24, 1997
Herpes simplex virus	See Table 14, page 102			

(Footnotes and abbreviations on page 47)

NOTE: All dosage recommendations are for adults (unless otherwise indicated) and assume normal renal function

15

TABLE 1 (15)

ANATOMIC SITE/DIAGNOSIS/ MODIFYING CIRCUMSTANCES	ETIOLOGIES (usual)	SUGGESTED REGIMENS*		ADJUNCT DIAGNOSTIC OR THERAPEUTIC MEASURES AND COMMENTS
		PRIMARY	ALTERNATIVE§	
Genital Tract, Both Men and Women (continued)				
Lymphogranuloma venereum	Chlamydia trachomatis, serovars. L1, L2, L3	Doxy 100 mg bid po x21 d.	Erythro 0.5 gm qid po x21 d	Dx based on serology, biopsy contraindicated because sinus tracts develop. Rectal LGV may require re-treatment.
Phthirus pubis (pubic lice, "crabs") and scabies	Phthirus pubis and Sarcoptes scabiei		[See Table 12, page 94	
Syphilis (Guidelines: [JDCP 4:407, 1995)				
Early: primary, secondary, latent: <1 year	T. pallidum	Benzathine Pen G (2.4 mu IM) x1	[[Doxy 100 mg bid po x14 d.) or (tetracycline 500 mg qid po x14 d.) or (ceftriaxone 125 mg qd IM x10 d or 250 mg every other day IM x 5 doses of 1000 mg qod IM x 4 doses)] Ref.: JID 158:881, 1988; Chemotherapy 35:140, 1989. Follow-up mandatory.	Every effort should be made to document penicillin allergy before choosing alternative (good general reference. NEJM 326:1060, 1992). All patients with early or congenital syphilis should have quantitative VDRL at 3, 6, 12 & 24 months after rx. If pt had 1° or 2°, VDRL should ↓ 2 tubes at 6 months, 3 tubes 12 months, & 4 tubes 24 months. Early latent: 2 tubes ↓ at 12 months. With 1° 50% will be RPR seronegative at 12 months, 24% negative FTA/ABS at 2–3 yrs (AnIM 114:1005, 1991). Re-treat if (1) clinical signs persist or recur. (2) a sustained 4-fold increase in titer occurs, (3) an initially high titer fails to decrease to <1:8 at 1 year. Ref. on syphilis serology: JDCP 5:351, 1996
More than 1 yrs duration (latent of indeterminate duration, cardiovascular, late benign)		Benzathine Pen G (2.4 mu IM q week x 3 = 7.2 mu total)	Doxy (100 mg bid po x28 d.) or (tetracycline 500 mg qid po x28 d.	No published data on efficacy of alternatives. The value of routine lumbar puncture in asymptomatic late syphilis is being questioned in the U.S., i.e.: No LP, rx all patients as primary recommendation. AnIM 145:465, 1985. **Indications for LP (CDC): neurologic symptoms, treatment failure, serum non-treponemal antibody titer ≥1:32, other evidence of active syphilis (aortitis, gumma, iritis), non penicillin rx, + HIV test.**
Neurosyphilis—Very difficult to treat. Includes ocular (retrobulbar neuritis) syphilis	T. pallidum	Pen G 3–4 mu q4h IV x10–14 d. OR AMP 4.0 gm IV q6h x10–14 d.	Procaine pen G 2.4 mu qd IM + probenecid 0.5 gm qid po x10 d. —See Comment	Ceftriaxone 2.0 gm qd (IV or IM) x 14 d. 23% failure rate reported (AJM 93:481, 1992). For penicillin allergy: either desensitize to penicillin or obtain infectious diseases consultation. **Serologic criteria for response to rx: 4-fold or greater ↓ in VDRL titer over 6–12 mos.** [CID 28 (Suppl. 1):S21, 1999].
HIV infection (AIDS) (See SANFORD GUIDE TO HIV/AIDS THERAPY for details)		Adding 10 d. of amoxicillin + probenecid to pen G did not change efficacy in 1° & 2° syphilis (NEJM 337:307, 1997)	For neurosyphilis, recommendations vary; some use Pen G 24 mu qd IV for 14-21 d.	Clinical presentations, serology and response to rx may be atypical (AJM 99:55, 1995). Higher doses & longer periods of rx may be required. Repeat VDRL titer (RPR) at 3, 6, 12, 24 months. Reinfection with ↑. pallidum not uncommon. Erythro should not be used as an alternative agent. Re-treat if needed (AJM 93:477, 1992); see Syphilis, early (above) for indications.
Pregnancy and syphilis		Same as for non-pregnant, some recommend 2nd dose (2.4 million units) benzathine Pen G 1 week after initial dose esp. in 3rd trimester or with 2° syphilis	Skin test for penicillin allergy. Desensitize if necessary	Monthly quantitative VDRL or equivalent. If 4-fold ↑, re-treat. Doxy, tetracycline contraindicated. Erythro not recommended because of high risk of failure to cure fetus.
Congenital syphilis		Aqueous crystalline Pen G 50,000 u/kg/dose IV q12h x7 d, then q8h x3 more days	Procaine pen G (50,000 u/kg IM for 10 d.) OR AMP 50 mg/kg q6h IV x10–14 d.	Another alternative: Ceftriaxone ≤30 days old, 75 mg/kg IV/IM qd or >30 ays old 100 mg/kg IV/IM qd. Treat 10-14 d. If symptomatic, ophthalmologic exam indicated. If more than 1 day of rx missed, restart entire course. **Need serologic follow-up!**

(Footnotes and abbreviations on page 47)

NOTE: All dosage recommendations are for adults (unless otherwise indicated) and assume normal renal function

TABLE 1 (16)

ANATOMIC SITE/DIAGNOSIS/ MODIFYING CIRCUMSTANCES	ETIOLOGIES (usual)	SUGGESTED REGIMENS*		ADJUNCT DIAGNOSTIC OR THERAPEUTIC MEASURES AND COMMENTS
		PRIMARY	ALTERNATIVE§	
Genital Tract, Both Men and Women *(continued)*				
Warts, anogenital *See Table 14*	Human papillomavirus types 6 & 11 most common; types 16, 18, 33, 35 assoc. with cervical dysplasia	Patient applied: imiquimod (Aldara) 5% cream 3X/wk x16 wks OR (podofilox 0.5% solution or gel) 2x/d. x3 d., no rx x4 d., then repeat cycle x4.	Physician applied: Cryotherapy, podophyllin, trichloroacetic acid, surgical removal, or electro-cautery	Biopsy atypical, pigmented or persistent warts. Women should have annual pap smear. HPV 16, 18, 31, 33, 35 assoc with 90% of cervical dysplasia/ Ca of cervix. Lifetime risk of HPV 16, 18 → Ca cervix is 1:30. *Ref.: AJM 102(5A):28, 1997*
		See Table 14, page 105		
Women:				
Amnionitis, septic abortion	Bacteroides, esp. Prevotella bivius; Group B,A streptococci; Enterobacteriaceae; C. trachomatis	[(Cefoxitin or TC/CL or IMP or MER or AM/SB or PIP/TZ) + doxy] OR [Clinda + (APAG or P Ceph 3)] OR Trova		D&C of uterus. In septic abortion, Clostridium perfringens may cause fulminant intravascular hemolysis. In postpartum patients with enigmatic fever and/or pulmonary emboli, **consider septic pelvic vein thrombophlebitis** *(see Vascular, septic pelvic vein thrombophlebitis, page 46).* After discharge: doxy or continue clinda. NOTE: IV clinda effective for C. trachomatis, no data on po clinda *(CID 19:720, 1994).*
		(Dosage: see footnote)[1]		
Cervicitis, mucopurulent	N. gonorrhoeae	Treat for gonorrhea, page 15		Criteria for dx: yellow or green pus on cervical swab, >10 WBC/oil field. Gram stain for GC; if negative rx for C. trachomatis. If in doubt, send swab or urine for culture, EIA or ligase chain reaction (LCR) and rx for both.
	Chlamydia trachomatis	Treat for non-gonococcal urethritis, page 15		
Endomyometritis/septic pelvic phlebitis				
Early postpartum (1st 48 hrs) (usually after C-section)	Bacteroides, esp. Prevotella bivius; Group B,A streptococci; Enterobacteriaceae; C. trachomatis	[(Cefoxitin or TC/CL or IMP or MER or AM/SB or PIP/TZ) + (doxy)] OR [(Clinda) + (APAG or P Ceph 3)] OR Trova		See *Comments under Amnionitis, septic abortion*
		(Dosage: see footnote)[1]		
Late postpartum (48 hrs to 6 wks) (usually after vaginal delivery)	Chlamydia trachomatis, M. hominis	Doxy 100 mg q12h IV or po x14 days		Tetracyclines not recommended in nursing mothers; discontinue nursing. M. hominis sensitive to tetra, clinda, not erythro *(CT/D 17:S200, 1993).*
Pelvic inflammatory disease (PID), salpingitis, tubo-ovarian abscess				
Outpatient rx: limit to pts with temp <38°C, WBC <11,000/mm³, minimal evidence of peritonitis, active bowel sounds & able to tolerate oral nourishment	N. gonorrhoeae, chlamydia, bacteroides, Enterobacteriaceae, streptococci	**Oral regimens:** (Ofloxin 400 mg bid x14 d + metro 500 mg bid x14 d) OR (ceftriaxone 250 mg IM x1 + doxy 100 mg bid x14 d)	**Parenteral regimens:** [(Cefotetan 2 gm IV q12h or cefoxitin 2 gm IV q6h) + (doxy 100 mg IV/po q12h)] [(Clinda 900 mg IV q8h) + (gentamicin 2 mg/kg loading dose, then 1.5 mg/kg q8h or single daily dosing)]	Alternative parenteral regimens: 1. Oflox 400 mg IV q12h + metro 500 mg IV q8h 2. AM/SB 3 gm IV q6h + doxy 100 mg IV/po q12h 3. Cipro 200 mg IV q12h + doxy 100 mg IV/po q12h + metro 500 mg IV q8h Remember: Evaluate and treat sex partner.

[1] **P Ceph 2** (**cefoxitin** 2.0 gm q6–8h IV, **cefotetan** 2.0 gm q12h IV, **cefuroxime** 750 mg q8h IV); **TC/CL** 3.1 gm q6h IV; **AM/SB** 3.0 gm q6h IV; **PIP/TZ** 3.375 gm q6h or 4.5 gm q8h IV; **doxy** 100 mg q12h IV or po; **clinda** 450–900 mg q8h IV; **APAG** (**gentamicin**, see Table 9C, page 70); **P Ceph 3** (**cefotaxime** 2.0 gm q8h IV, **ceftriaxone** 2.0 gm qd IV); **IMP** 0.5 gm q6h IV; **MER** 1.0 gm q8h IV; **azithro** 500 mg IV/day; **trova** 300 mg IV qd, then 200 mg po 1x/d. in hospital only.

(Footnotes and abbreviations on page 47)   NOTE: All dosage recommendations are for adults (unless otherwise indicated) and assume normal renal function

TABLE 1 (17)

ANATOMIC SITE/DIAGNOSIS/ MODIFYING CIRCUMSTANCES	ETIOLOGIES (usual)	SUGGESTED REGIMENS*		ADJUNCT DIAGNOSTIC OR THERAPEUTIC MEASURES AND COMMENTS
		PRIMARY	ALTERNATIVE§	
Genital Tract, Women (continued)				
Vaginitis—Review: IDCP 6:284, 1997				
Candidiasis Pruritus, thick cheesy discharge, pH <4.5 See Table 10	Candida albicans—80–90% C. glabrata, C. tropicalis may be increasing—they may be less susceptible to azoles	Oral azoles: Fluconazole 150 mg po x1; itraconazole 200 mg po bid x1 day	Intravaginal azoles: variety of strengths— from 1 dose to 7–14 d. Drugs available (all end in -azole): butocon, clotrim, micon, tiocon, tercon	Nystatin vag. tabs x14 d. less effective. Other rx for azole-resistant strains: gentian violet, boric acid. If recurrent candidiasis (4 or more episodes/yr): 6 mos. suppression with: fluconazole 100 mg po q week or itraconazole 100 mg po qd or clotrimazole vag. suppositories 500 mg q week.
Trichomoniasis Copious foamy discharge, pH >4.5 Treat sexual partners—see Comment	Trichomonas vaginalis	Metro (2.0 gm as single dose) or 500 mg po bid x7 d. In pregnancy, defer rx until after 1st trimester.	Options if metro-resistant: (1) metro 2–4 gm/d po/IV x10–14 d. (2) Paromomycin cream 250 mg per vagina qd x2 wks. (3) Zinc sulfate douche.	**Treat male sexual partners (2.0 gm as single dose).** Resistance to metronidazole/tinidazole rare but occurs (Ln 346:1170, 1995).
Bacterial vaginosis Malodorous vaginal discharge, pH >4.5	Polymicrobic: associated with Gardnerella vaginalis, bacteroides non-fragilis, Mobiluncus, peptococci, Mycoplasma hominis	Metro (0.5 gm po bid x7 days) or metro vaginal gel[1] (1 applicator intravaginally) 2x/d x5 d. (avoid in 1st trimester pregnancy)	Clinda (0.3 gm bid po x 7 d) or 2% clinda vaginal cream 5 gm intravaginally hs x7 d. More options in Comment	Wet prep shows cells covered with organisms "clue" cells. "Fishy" odor when discharge rx with KOH. Rx of male sex partner **not** indicated unless balanitis present. Metro: 2.0 gm po single dose not as effective as 5–7 day course (JAMA 268:92, 1992). Also, metro extended release tabs 750 mg po qd x7 d. approx. 60% effective but expensive.
Men:				
Balanitis	Candida (40%), Group B strep, Gardnerella	Oral azoles as for vaginitis		Occurs in ¼ of male sex partners of women infected with candida. Exclude circinate balanitis (Reiter's syndrome). Plasma cell balanitis (non-infectious) responds to hydrocortisone cream.
Epididymo-orchitis Age <35 years	N. gonorrhoeae, Chlamydia trachomatis	Ceftriaxone 250 mg IM x1 + doxy 100 mg po bid x10 d. or oflox 300 mg po bid po x10 d.		Also: bedrest, scrotal elevation, and analgesics.
Age >35 years or homosexual men (insertive partners in anal intercourse)	Enterobacteriaceae (coliforms)	FQ: (CiP 500 mg bid po or 400 mg po bid IV) or (oflox 200 mg bid po or IV) x10–14 d.	AM/SB, P Ceph 3, TC/CL, PIP/TZ (Dosage: see footnote 1, page 17)	Midstream pyuria and scrotal pain and edema. Also: bedrest, scrotal elevation, and analgesics.
Prostatitis—Review: AJM 106:327, 1999 Acute ≤35 years of age	N. gonorrhoeae C. trachomatis	Oflox 400 mg po x1, then 300 mg po q12h. Duration unclear, at least 7 d.		Oflox effective vs gonococci & C. trachomatis and penetrates prostate. In AIDS pts, prostate may be focus of Cryptococcus neoformans.
>35 years of age	Enterobacteriaceae (coliforms)	FQ (dosage; see Epididymo-orchitis, >35 yrs, above) or TMP/ SMX 1 DS tablet (160 mg TMP) bid po x10–14 d.		Treat as acute urinary infection, 14 days (not single dose regimen). Some authorities recommend 3–4 week rx (IDCP 4:325, 1995).

[1] 1 applicator contains 5.0 gm of gel with 37.5 mg metronidazole

NOTE: All dosage recommendations are for adults (unless otherwise indicated) and assume normal renal function

(Footnotes and abbreviations on page 47)

TABLE 1 (18)

ANATOMIC SITE/DIAGNOSIS/ MODIFYING CIRCUMSTANCES	ETIOLOGIES (usual)	SUGGESTED REGIMENS*		ADJUNCT DIAGNOSTIC OR THERAPEUTIC MEASURES AND COMMENTS
		PRIMARY	ALTERNATIVE§	
Genital Tract, Men/Prostatitis *(continued)*				
Chronic bacterial	Enterobacteriaceae (80%), enterococci (15%), P. aeruginosa	FQ (CIP 500 mg bid po x4 wks, oflox 300 mg bid po x6 wks—see *Comment*)	TMP/ SMX– DS 1 tab po bid x1–3 mos.	With rx failures consider infected prostatic calculi.
Chronic prostatitis/chronic pain syndrome (New NIH classification, *JAMA 282:236, 1999*)	The most common prostatitis syndrome. Etiology is unknown; molecular probe data suggest infectious etiology *(Clin Micro Rev 11: 604, 1998).*	Doxy 100 mg bid po x14 days	Erythro base 500 mg po qid x14 d.	Pt has sx of prostatitis, cells in prostatic secretions, but routine cultures negative. Chlamydia, ureaplasma suspected.
		α-adrenergic blocking agents		Pt has sx of prostatitis but negative cultures and no cells in prostatic secretions.
Hand *(Bites: See Skin)*				
Paronychia				
Nail biting, manicuring	Staph. aureus Anaerobes	Clinda 300 mg qid po	Erythro 500 mg po	Onset usually 2–5 days after trauma. No lymphangitis.
Contact with oral mucosa— dentists, anesthesiologists, wrestlers	Herpes simplex (Whitlow)	Acyclovir 400 mg tid po x10 days	Famciclovir or valacyclovir should work, see *Comment*	Gram stain and routine culture negative. Famciclovir/valacyclovir doses used for primary genital herpes should work; see *Table 14, page 102*
Dishwasher (prolonged water immersion)	Candida sp.	Clotrimazole (topical)		Avoid immersion of hands in water as much as possible.
Heart				
Atherosclerotic coronary artery disease *(Ln 350:430, 1997)*	Chlamydia pneumoniae— under study	Clinical trials of macrolides in progress: for commentary, see *CID 28:993, 1999; EID 4:571, 1998; AJM 106:376, 1999.*		
Infective endocarditis—Native valve—empirical rx awaiting cultures	NOTE: Diagnostic criteria include evidence of continuous bacteremia (multiple positive blood cultures), new murmur (worsening of old murmur) of valvular insufficiency, definite emboli, and echocardiographic (transthoracic or transesophageal) evidence of valvular vegetations. Von Reyn and Duke criteria compared in *CID 22:276, 1996).* Review of contemporary management issues: *Circulation 98:2936, 1998.*			
Valvular or congenital heart disease including mitral valve prolapse but no modifying circumstances *See Table 15 for prophylaxis*	Viridans strep, 30–40% "other" strep 15–25%, enterococci 5–18%, staphylococci 20–35%	[(Pen G 20 mu qd IV, continuous or div. q4h) or (AMP 12 gm qd IV, continuous or div. q4h) + (nafcillin or oxacillin 2.0 gm q4h IV) + (gentamicin 1.0 mg/kg q8h IM or IV, not once daily dosing)]	[Vanco 15 mg/kg[1] q12h IV (not to exceed 2 gm qd unless serum levels monitored) + gentamicin 1.0 mg/kg[1] q8h IM or IV	If patient not acutely ill and not in heart failure, we prefer to wait for blood culture results. If initial 3 blood cultures neg. after 24–48 hrs, obtain 2–3 more blood cultures before empiric rx started. PRSP + gentamicin coverage of enterococci may not be adequate, hence addition of penicillin G pending cultures. When blood cultures +, modify regimen from empiric to specific based on organism, in vitro susceptibilities, clinical experience.

[1] Assumes estimated creatinine clearance ≥ 80 ml/min., see *Table 17.*

(Footnotes and abbreviations on page 47)

NOTE: All dosage recommendations are for adults (unless otherwise indicated) and assume normal renal function

TABLE 1 (19)

Heart (continued)

Infective endocarditis—Native valve—culture positive (Consensus opinion on treatment by organism: JAMA 274:1706, 1995)

ANATOMIC SITE/DIAGNOSIS/ MODIFYING CIRCUMSTANCES	ETIOLOGIES (usual)	SUGGESTED REGIMENS*		ADJUNCT DIAGNOSTIC OR THERAPEUTIC MEASURES AND COMMENTS
		PRIMARY	ALTERNATIVE§	
S. viridans, S. bovis, S. bovis with penicillin G MIC ≤0.1 µg/ml	S. viridans, S. bovis	[(Pen G 12–18 mu/d IV, continuous or q4h x2 wks) PLUS (gentamicin 1 mg/kg q8h IV x2 wks)] OR (Pen G 12–18 mu/d IV, continuous or q4h x4 wks OR (ceftriaxone 2.0 gm qd IV x4 wks)	(Ceftriaxone 2.0 gm qd IV + gentamicin 1 mg/kg IV q8h both x2 wks.) If allergy pen G or ceftriaxone, use vanco 30 mg/kg/ d in 2 div. doses to 2 gm/d max. unless serum levels measured x4 wks	Also effective: (ceftriaxone 2.0 gm qd) + (netilmicin 4 mg/kg qd) x2 wks (CID 21:1406, 1995). Target gent levels: peak 3 µg/ml, trough <1 µg/ml. If very obese pt, recommend consultation for dosage adjustment. Infuse vanco over ≥1 hr to avoid "red man" syndrome. S. bovis suggests occult bowel pathology. Since relapse rate may be greater in pts ill for >3 mos. prior to start of rx, the penicillin-gentamicin synergism theoretically may be advantageous in this group.
S. viridans, S. bovis with penicillin G MIC >0.1 to <0.5 µg/ml	S. viridans, S. bovis, nutritionally variant streptococci, tolerant strep[1]	Pen G 18 mu/d IV (continuous or q4h) x4 wks PLUS gentamicin 1 mg/kg q8h IV x2 wks	Vanco 30 mg/kg/d IV in 2 divided doses to max. 2 gm/d unless serum levels documented x4 wks	Can use cefazolin for Pen G in pt with allergy that is not IgE-mediated (e.g., anaphylaxis). Alternatively can use vanco. (See comment above on gent and vanco)
For S. viridans or S. bovis with Pen G MIC ≥1.0 and enterococci susceptible to amp/Pen G, vanco, gent. NOTE: Inf. Dis. consultation suggested	"Susceptible" enterococci, S. viridans, S. bovis, nutritionally variant streptococci	[(Pen G 18–30 mu /24h IV, continuous or q4h x4–6 wks) PLUS (gentamicin 1 mg/kg q8h IV x4–6 wks)] OR (AMP 12 gm/d IV, continuous or q4h + gent as above x4–6 wks)	Vanco 30 mg/kg/d IV in 2 div. doses to max. of 2 gm/d unless serum levels measured PLUS gentamicin 1 mg/kg q8h IV x4–6 wks	4 wks of rx if symptoms <3 mos., 6 wks of rx if symptoms >3 mos. Vanco for pen-allergic pts; do not use cephalosporins. Do **not** give gent once-daily for enterococcal endocarditis. Target gent levels: peak 3 µg/ml, trough <1 µg/ml. Vanco target serum levels: peak 20–50 µg/ml; trough 5–12 µg/ml. NOTE: Because of ↑ frequency of resistance (see below), all enterococci causing endocarditis should be tested in vitro for susceptibility to penicillin, β-lactamase production, gent. susceptibility and vanco susceptibility.
Enterococci: MIC streptomycin >2000 µg/ml MIC gentamicin >500–2000 µg/ml No resistance to penicillin	Enterococci, high-level aminoglycoside resistance	Pen G or AMP IV as above x8–12 wks (approx. 50% cure)	If prolonged Pen G/amp fails, consider surgical removal of infected valve. See Comment	10–25% E. faecalis and 45–50% E. faecium resistant to high gent. levels. May be sensitive to streptomycin, check MIC. Case report of success with combination of AMP, IMP, and vanco (Scand J Inf Dis 29:628, 1997).
Enterococci: β-lactamase production test is **positive** and **no** gentamicin resistance	Enterococci, penicillin resistance	AM/SB 3.0 gm q6h PLUS gentamicin 1 mg/kg q8h IV x4–6 wks	AMP/SB 3.0 gm IV q6h PLUS vanco 30 mg/kg/d IV in 2 div. doses (check levels if >2 gm) x4–6 wks	β-lactamase **not** detected by MIC tests with standard inocula. Detection requires testing with the chromogenic cephalosporin nitrocefin. Once-daily gentamicin rx **not** efficacious in animal model of E. faecalis endocarditis (JAC 39:519, 1997).
Enterococci: β-lactamase test neg.; Pen G MIC >16 µg/ml; no gentamicin resistance	Enterococci, intrinsic Pen G/amp resistance	Vanco 30 mg/kg/d IV in 2 div. doses (check levels if >2 gm) PLUS gent. 1 mg/kg q8h (no single dose) x4–6 wks		Desired vanco serum levels: peak 20–50 µg/ml, trough 5–12 µg/ml

[1] Tolerant streptococci = MBC 32-fold greater than MIC

NOTE: All dosage recommendations are for adults (unless otherwise indicated) and assume normal renal function

(Footnotes and abbreviations on page 47)

TABLE 1 (20)

ANATOMIC SITE/DIAGNOSIS/ MODIFYING CIRCUMSTANCES	ETIOLOGIES (usual)	SUGGESTED REGIMENS* PRIMARY	ALTERNATIVE§	ADJUNCT DIAGNOSTIC OR THERAPEUTIC MEASURES AND COMMENTS
Heart; Infective endocarditis—Native valve—culture positive *(continued)*				
Enterococci: Pen/amp resistant PLUS high-level gent/strep resistant PLUS vanco resistant; usually VRE **Consultation suggested**	Enterococci, vanco-resistant, usually E. faecium	No reliable effective rx. Can try quinupristin/dalfo-pristin (Synercid) or line-zolid—see **Comment,** footnote¹, and Table 5	Teicoplanin active against a subset of vanco-resistant enterococci. Teicoplanin is no longer available in U.S.	For compassionate use of Synercid, contact Rhone-Poulenc-Rorer, 610/454-3071. Synercid activity limited to E. faecium and is usually bacteriostatic; therefore expect high relapse rate. Linezolid available for compassionate use: Pharmacia-Upjohn, 1-800-836-3535. Other regimens tried: (1) CIP + (AMP or novobiocin or RIF); (2) vanco + pen G + gent; (3) AMP + IMP, animal model (JID 173:909, 1996). See IDCP 5:528, 1996, for discussion.
Staphylococcal endocarditis— aortic and/or mitral valve infection	Staph. aureus, methicillin-sensitive	Nafcillin (oxacillin) 2 gm q4h IV x4–6 wks PLUS gentamicin 1.0 mg/kg q8h IV x3–5 d.	[(Cefazolin 2.0 gm q8h IV x4–6 wks PLUS (gentamicin 1.0 mg/kg q8h IV x3–5 d.)] OR Vanco 30 mg/kg/d IV in 2 div. doses (check levels if >2 gm/d.) x4–6 wks	Avoid cephalosporins in pts with immediate allergic reaction to penicillin; in allergic pt, vanco may not be as effective as cefazolin. No definitive data, pro or con, on once-daily gentamicin for S. aureus endo-carditis. At present, favor q8h dosing x3–5 d. ↑ recognition of IV catheter-associated S. aureus bacteremia. May need TEE to detect endocarditis. 23% of S. aureus bacteremia in association with IV catheter had endocarditis (CID 115:106 & 115, 1999).
Tricuspid valve infection (usually IVDUs)	Staph. aureus, methicillin-sensitive	Nafcillin (oxacillin) 2 gm q4h IV PLUS gentamicin 1 mg/kg q8h IV x2 wks	Nafcillin PLUS genta-micin, as in Staph. endocarditis, above	2-week regimen not recommended if metastatic infection (e.g., osteo) or left-sided endocarditis. Cloxacillin IV without gentamicin 89% successful (AnIM 125:969, 1996). 2 reports of success with **4-week oral** regimen: CIP 750 mg bid + RIF 300 mg bid. Less than 10% pts had MRSA (Ln 2:1071, 1989; AJM 101:68, 1996).
Methicillin resistance (MRSA)	Staph. aureus, methicillin-resistant	Vanco 30 mg/kg/d IV in 2 div. doses (check levels if >2 gm/day) x4–6 wks		For MRSA, no difference in duration of bacteremia or fever between pts rx with vanco or vanco + RIF (AnIM 115:674, 1991).
Slow-growing fastidious Gm-neg. bacilli	HACEK group (See Comments) (Mayo Clin Proc 72:532, 1997)	Ceftriaxone 2.0 gm qd IV x4 wks	AMP 12 gm qd (continuous or div.) x4 wks + gentamicin 1.0 mg/kg q8h IV or IM x4 wks	HACEK (acronym for Hemophilus paraInfluenzae, H. aphrophilus, Actino-bacillus, Cardiobacterium, Eikenella, Kingella). H. aphrophilus resistant to vanco, clinda, and methicillin. Penicillinase-positive HACEK organisms should be susceptible to amp-sulbactam + gentamicin. For hemophilus, see CID 24:1087, 1997.
Bartonella species AnIM 125:646, 1996	B. henselae, B. quintana	No definitive rx; aminoglycoside + surgery cured 78%; FQ or RIF or macrolide ± surgery. See Comment.		Dx: microimmunofluorescent antibody titer ≥1:1600; blood cultures only occ. positive. Surgery: without surgery, ⅓ cured; surgery + anti-infectives, 81% cure.
Infective endocarditis—culture negative				
Fever, valvular disease, and ECHO vegetations ± emboli and neg. cultures	T. whippelii, Q fever, psitta-cosis, brucellosis, barton-ella (see above), fungi	Emphasis is on diagnosis. See specific organism for treatment regimens.		For Q fever, see Clin Micro Rev 12:518, 1999. 4 pts with afebrile culture-neg. endocarditis had T. whippelii identified by PCR of resected heart valves (AnIM 131:112 & 144, 1999).

¹ Three interesting recent reports: (1) Successful rx of vanco-resistant E. faecium prosthetic valve endocarditis with Synercid without change in MIC (CID 25:163, 1997), (2) Resistance to Synercid emerged during therapy of E. faecium bacteremia (CID 24:90, 1997) and (3) super-infection with E. faecalis occurred during Synercid rx of E. faecium (CID 24:91, 1997).

NOTE: All dosage recommendations are for adults (unless otherwise indicated) and assume normal renal function

(Footnotes and abbreviations on page 47)

21

TABLE 1 (21)

ANATOMIC SITE/DIAGNOSIS/ MODIFYING CIRCUMSTANCES	ETIOLOGIES (usual)	SUGGESTED REGIMENS* PRIMARY	ALTERNATIVE§	ADJUNCT DIAGNOSTIC OR THERAPEUTIC MEASURES AND COMMENTS
Heart (continued)				
Infective endocarditis—Prosthetic valve—empiric therapy (cultures pending)				
Early (<2 months post-op)	S. epidermidis, S. aureus. Rarely, Enterobacteriaceae, diphtheroids, fungi	Vanco 15 mg/kg q12h IV + gentamicin 1.0 mg/kg q8h IV + RIF 600 mg po daily		Early surgical consultation advised. Watch for evidence of heart failure.
Late (>2 months post-op)	S. epidermidis, S. viridans, enterococci, S. aureus			
Infective endocarditis—Prosthetic valve—positive blood cultures	Staph. epidermidis	(Vanco 15 mg/kg q12h IV + RIF 300 mg q8h po) x6 wks + gentamicin 1.0 mg/kg IV x14 d.		If S. epidermidis is susceptible to methicillin in vitro (not common), then substitute natcillin (or oxacillin) for vanco.
Surgical consultation advised: retrospective analysis shows ↓ mortality of pts with S. aureus endocarditis if valve replaced during antibiotic rx (CID 26:1302 & 1310, 1998); also, retrospective study showed ↑ risk of death 2° neuro events in assoc. with coumadin rx (ArIM 159:473, 1999)	Staph. aureus	Methicillin sensitive: (Nafcillin 2.0 gm q4h IV + RIF 300 mg q8h po) x6 wks + gentamicin 1.0 mg/kg IV x14 d.		
		Methicillin resistant: (Vanco 1.0 gm q12h IV + RIF 300 mg q8h po) x6 wks + gentamicin 1.0 mg/kg IV x14 d.		
	Strep. viridans, enterococci	As for Native valve, above		
	Enterobacteriaceae or P. aeruginosa	APAG (tobramycin if P. aeruginosa) + Ceph 3 AP or P Ceph 4)	(AP Pen or P Ceph 4)	In theory, could substitute CIP for APAG, but no clinical data.
	Candida, aspergillus	Amphotericin B ± an azole, e.g., fluconazole (Table 10, page 72)		High mortality. Valve replacement plus antifungal therapy standard therapy but some success with antifungal therapy alone (CID 22:262, 1996).
Pericarditis, purulent	Staph. aureus, Strep. pneumoniae, Group A strep. Enterobacteriaceae	PRSP + APAG (Dosage, see footnote)[1]	IMP or TC/CL or PIP/TZ or AM/SB or MER or CFP (see footnote)[1]	Drainage required if signs of tamponade. If MRSA suspected use vanco 1.0 gm q12h IV.
Rheumatic fever with carditis Ref.: Ln 349:935, 1997 For acute rheumatic fever, see page 44	Post-infectious sequelae of Group A strep infection (usually pharyngitis)	Diuretics, ASA, and usually prednisone 2 mg/kg/d po		Clinical features: Carditis, polyarthritis, chorea, subcutaneous nodules, erythema marginatum. For Jones criteria: Circulation 87:302, 1993. Prophylaxis: see page 44
Joint—Also see Lyme Disease, page 42				
Septic arthritis: Treatment requires both adequate drainage of purulent joint fluid and appropriate antimicrobial therapy. There is no need to inject antimicrobials into joints. Empiric therapy after collection of blood and joint fluid for culture; review Gram stain of joint fluid. For full differential. For Ln 351:197, 1998				
Infant <3 months (neonate)	Staph. aureus, Enterobacteriaceae, Group B strep, N. gonorrhoeae	[PRSP + APAG (Dosage, see Table 16, page 120)	PRSP + APAG (If MRSA prevalent, vanco in place of PRSP)	Blood cultures frequently positive. Adjacent bone involved in ⅔ pts. Group B strep and gonococci most common community-acquired etiologies.
Children (3 months–14 years)	Staph. aureus 27%, S. pyogenes & S. pneumo 14%, H. influenzae 3%, Gm-neg. bacilli 6%, other (GC, N. meningitidis) 14%, unknown 36%	PRSP + P Ceph 3	Vanco + P Ceph 3	Marked ↓ in H. influenzae since use of conjugate vaccine. NOTE: Septic arthritis due to salmonella has no association with sickle cell disease, unlike salmonella osteomyelitis. Duration of treatment varies with specific microbial etiology.
		See Table 16 for dosage		

[1] **PRSP (nafcillin** or **oxacillin** 2.0 gm q4h IV), **APAG** (see Table 9C, page 70), **IMP** 0.5 gm q6h IV, **MER** 1.0 gm q8h IV, **TC/CL** 3.1 gm q6h or 4.5 gm q8h IV, **AM/SB** 3.0 gm q6h IV, **PIP/TZ** 3.375 gm q6h IV, **P Ceph 1 (cephalothin** 2.0 gm q4h IV or **cefazolin** 2.0 gm q8h IV), **CIP** 750 mg bid po or 400 mg bid IV, **vanco** 1.0 gm q12h IV, **RIF** 600 mg qd po, **aztreonam** 2.0 gm q8h IV, **CFP** 2.0 gm IV q12h

(Footnotes and abbreviations on page 47)

NOTE: All dosage recommendations are for adults (unless otherwise indicated) and assume normal renal function

TABLE 1 (22)

ANATOMIC SITE/DIAGNOSIS/ MODIFYING CIRCUMSTANCES	ETIOLOGIES (usual)	SUGGESTED REGIMENS*		ADJUNCT DIAGNOSTIC OR THERAPEUTIC MEASURES AND COMMENTS
		PRIMARY	ALTERNATIVE§	
Joint/Septic arthritis (continued)				
Adult (review Gram stain)				
Acute monoarticular				
Ages 15–40 (sexually active)	**N. gonorrhoeae** (see page 15), S. aureus, streptococci, rarely aerobic Gm-neg. bacilli	Gram stain negative: Ceftriaxone 1.0 gm qd IV or cefotaxime 1.0 gm q8h IV or ceftizoxime 1.0 gm q8h IV	If Gram stain shows Gm + cocci in clusters; nafcillin (or oxacillin) 2.0 gm q4h IV	For rx comments, see Disseminated GC, page 15
Age >40		All empiric choices guided by Gram stain		Differential includes gout and chondrocalcinosis (pseudogout). Look for crystals in joint fluid. Levo has appropriate in vitro spectra and should work, but no clinical data. NOTE: Substitute vanco for PRSP if MRSA suspected or proven.
No rheumatoid arthritis	**N. gonorrhoeae**, S. aureus	PRSP + P Ceph 3	PRSP + CIP	
Rheumatoid arthritis	S. aureus, streptococci, Gm-neg. bacilli	For treatment duration, see Table 3 For dosage, see footnote page 22		
Chronic monoarticular	Brucella, nocardia, mycobacteria, fungi	See Tables 2, 10, & 11		
Polyarticular, usually acute	**Gonococci**, B. burgdorferi, acute rheumatic fever, viruses: e.g., hepatitis B, rubella vaccine, parvo B19	Gram stain usually negative for GC. If sexually active, culture urethra, cervix, anal canal, throat, blood, joint fluid, and then: ceftriaxone 1.0 gm IV daily		If GC, usually associated petechiae and/or pustular skin lesions and tenosynovitis. Consider Lyme disease if exposure areas known to harbor infected ticks. See Table 9 for viral infections. Expanded differential includes gout, pseudogout, reactive arthritis (HLA-B27 pos.).
Prosthetic joint, postoperative or infection post intra-articular injection		Culture first! Isolation/ in vitro susceptibility of etiologic organisms essential.		For infections after intra-articular injections, arthroscopy for culture, joint washout, and treat specifically for 14 days. For prosthetic joints, assume adjacent bone is infected. Management of the prosthesis continues to evolve. Conservative management: remove prosthesis, obtain cultures, ± leave antibiotic-impregnated cement/beads in joint space (AAC 40:2675, 1996), and treat specifically x6 weeks (Mayo Clin Proc 74:553, 1999). (See next box for other options)
Empiric rx, no culture data	MSSE/MRSE 40%, MSSA/ MRSA 20%, Enterobacteriaceae, Pseudomonas sp.	Vanco + CIP (or aztreonam or APAG or CFP) (for dosage, see footnote page 22)	CIP 750 mg bid po + RIF 900 mg x1/d. po] or [oflox 200 mg tid po + RIF 900 mg x1/d. po]	
Culture results known; specific rx NOTE: Salvage of prosthesis unlikely after 1–2 wks of symptomatic infection (CID 29:292 & 296, 1999)	[MRSA/MRSE or MSSA/ MSSE]: **CIP/RIF susceptible**	[(CIP or oflox) + RIF] in above dosage	Oxacillin 2.0 gm q4h IV + RIF 900 mg x1/day po	Data on staph species infection of stable implants treated by debridement and prolonged oral antimicrobials: (1) po RIF + oflox x3–9 mos., 74% success (AAC 37:1214, 1993). (2) Initial IV PRSP or vanco, then po CIP + RIF x3 mos. (hip) or 6 mos. (knee). Cure in 100% (JAMA 279:1537 & 1575, 1998). (3) po TMP/SMX (20 mg/kg/d of TMP) successful in 2/3 pts with staph infection (AAC 42:3086, 1998). Most S. aureus are sensitive to RIF; most MRSA and roughly ½ of MSSE/MRSE are resistant to CIP/oflox.
	[MRSA/MRSE or MSSA/ MSSE]: **CIP and/or RIF resistant**	Vanco + RIF (if sensitive)		

(Footnotes and abbreviations on page 47)

NOTE: All dosage recommendations are for adults (unless otherwise indicated) and assume normal renal function

TABLE 1 (23)

ANATOMIC SITE/DIAGNOSIS/ MODIFYING CIRCUMSTANCES	ETIOLOGIES (usual)	SUGGESTED REGIMENS*		ADJUNCT DIAGNOSTIC OR THERAPEUTIC MEASURES AND COMMENTS
		PRIMARY	ALTERNATIVE§	
Joint/Prosthetic joint, postoperative or infection post intra-articular injection *(continued)*				
Prevention of dental-induced prosthetic joint infections		No prophylactic antibiotics recommended for dental procedures with exception of the following immunocompromised pts: (1) inflammatory arthropathies: rheumatoid arthritis, systemic lupus erythematosus, (2) disease-, drug- or radiation-induced immunosuppression, (3) insulin-dependent (type 1) diabetes, (4) 1st 2 yrs following joint placement, (5) previous prosthetic joint infections, (6) malnourishment, (7) hemophilia. **Dosing regimens** (all doses given 1 hr prior to dental procedure): **Pts not allergic to penicillin & unable to take oral medications:** Cefazolin 1 gm or ampicillin 2 gm IM or IV; **Pts allergic to penicillin & unable to take oral medications:** Clindamycin 600 mg IV. No 2nd doses are recommended for any of these dosing regimens.	**Pts not allergic to penicillin:** cephalexin, cephradine or amoxicillin 2 gm po; **Pts allergic to penicillin & unable to take oral medications:** Clindamycin 600 mg po; **Pts allergic to penicillin & unable to take oral medi-cations.** Clindamycin 600 mg IV.	For justification, see *Myths of dental-induced prosthetic-joint infection, CID 20:1420, 1995,* and multidisciplinary consensus statement, *J Am Dental Assoc 128:1004, 1997.*
Septic bursitis	Staph. aureus (>80%), M. tuberculosis (rare), M. marinum (rare)	**PRSP:** nafcillin or oxacillin IV; dicloxacillin po	P. Ceph I or vanco or (CIP + RIF 300 mg bid po)	Initially aspirate daily and treat for a minimum of 2–3 weeks. If recurrence, surgical excision of bursa—should not be necessary often if treated for 3 weeks +. Ref.: *Semin Arth & Rheum 24:391, 1995*
Kidney, Bladder and Prostate *(For excellent review, see NEJM 329:1328, 1993)*		*Other doses, see footnote page 22*		
Acute uncomplicated urinary tract infection (cystitis-urethritis) (NOTE: Routine urine culture not necessary)				
Dipstick: positive leucocyte ester-ase or hemoglobin or positive Gram stain on urine ("unspun") NOTE: Increasing resistance of E. coli to TMP/ SMX *(JAMA 281:736, 1999)*	Enterobacteriaceae (E. coli), Staph. saprophyticus, enterococci	FQ po x3 days: CIP 250 mg bid, enoxacin 200 mg bid, gati 200 or 400 mg qd, levo 250 mg qd, lomeflox 400 mg qd, moxiflox 400 mg qd, nor-flox 400 mg bid, oflox 200 mg bid	TMP/SMX DS 1 tab (160 mg TMP) bid po x3 d. Other options: O Ceph, NF, doxy, TMP, or AM/CL. Usual duration of rx is 3 d.; *for dosage, see footnote page 10.*	Single dose fostomycin 3.0 gm po x1 less effective vs E. coli than multi-dose TMP/SMX or FQ *(Med Lett 39:66, 1997).* Resistance of E. coli to TMP/SMX over 18% in 1996; hence, now suggest FQs as primary regimen. 7-day rx recommended in pregnancy [discontinue or do not use sulfon-amides (TMP/ SMX) near term (2 weeks before EDC) because of potential increase in kernicterus]. If failure on 3-day course, culture and rx 2 wks. NF not effective vs S. saprophyticus. In sexually active young women, risk of symptomatic UTI assoc. with recent intercourse, use of diaphragm/spermicide, and tx of recurrent UTIs *(NEJM 335:468, 1996).*
	C. trachomatis	Doxy 100 mg bid po x7 days	Azithro 1.0 gm single dose po	Pelvic exam for vaginitis & Herpes simplex, culture for gonococci. FDA approval of azithro is C. trachomatis urethritis, efficacy in C. trachomatis "cystitis" reported, concentration in urine exceeds MICs for C. trachomatis and many E. coli.
Risk factors for STD; Dipstick: positive leucocyte esterase or hemoglobin, negative Gram stain	Any of the above bacteria	Eradicate infection, then TMP/SMX 1 tab qd po long term	TMP/SMX 1 single-strength	In postmenopausal women, use of vaginal estrogen cream [↓ frequency of urinary tract infections *(NEJM 329:753, 1993)*]. A cost-effective alternative to continuous prophylaxis is self-administered single dose rx (TMP/SMX, 2 tabs double strength; 320/1600 mg) at symptom onset. Another alternative: 1 DS tablet TMP/SMX post-coitus.
Recurrent (3 or more episodes/year)	Coliforms	TMP/SMX (2 mg TMP/10 mg SMX)/kg po qd] or (nitrofurantoin 2 mg/kg po qd)		
Child: ≤5 yrs old and grade 3–4 reflux				

(Footnotes and abbreviations on page 47)

NOTE: All dosage recommendations are for adults (unless otherwise indicated) and assume normal renal function

TABLE 1 (24)*

ANATOMIC SITE/DIAGNOSIS/ MODIFYING CIRCUMSTANCES	ETIOLOGIES (usual)	SUGGESTED REGIMENS* PRIMARY	ALTERNATIVE§	ADJUNCT DIAGNOSTIC OR THERAPEUTIC MEASURES AND COMMENTS
Kidney, Bladder and Prostate *(continued)*				
Acute uncomplicated pyelonephritis (usually women 18–40 yrs., temperature >102°F, definite costovertebral tenderness) [NOTE: Culture of urine and blood indicated prior to therapy. Also, recent report of hemolytic uremic syndrome as result of toxin-producing E. coli UTI *(NEJM 335:635, 1996)*]				
Moderately ill (outpatient)	Enterobacteriaceae (most likely E. coli), enterococci (Gram stain of **uncentrifuged** urine may allow identification of Gm-neg. bacilli vs Gm + cocci)	An FQ po x7 d.: CIP 500 mg bid, enoxacin 400 mg bid, gati 400 mg qd, levo 500 mg qd, lome 400 mg qd, moxi 400 mg qd, oflox 400 mg bid	AM/CL,¹ O Ceph, or TMP/SMX-DS. Treat for 14 days.	In 1998 abstract, in randomized double-blind trial, bacteriologic and clinical success higher for 7 days of CIP than for 14 days o TMP/SMX; results correlated with TMP/SMX in vitro resistance. Since CIP worked with 7-d. rx, suspect other FQs effective with 7. d. of rx.
Hospitalized	E. coli most common, enterococci 2nd in frequency	FQ (IV) or (AMP + gentamicin) or P Ceph 3 or AP Pen. Treat for 14 d. *Dosages in footnote¹* Do not use P Ceph 3 for suspect or proven enterococcal infection	TC/CL or AM/SB or PIP/TZ. Treat for 14 d.	Treat IV until pt afebrile 24–48 hrs, then complete 2-wk course with oral drugs (as *Moderately ill*, above). If no clinical improvement in 3 day, we recommend imaging. On CT if single focal mass-like lesion avg. response requires 6 d, if lesions diffuse avg. response 13 d *(AJM 93:289, 1992)*. **If pt hypotensive, prompt imaging (Echo or CT) is recommended to ensure absence of obstructive uropathy.**
Complicated UTI/catheters Obstruction, reflux, azotemia, transplant, Foley catheter-related	Enterobacteriaceae, P. aeruginosa, enterococci	(AMP + gent) or PIP/TZ or TC/CL or IMP or MER ×2–3 wks	An IV FQ: CIP, gati, levo, oflox	Rule out obstruction. Often able to switch to oral quinolone or TMP/SMX in a few days. Watch out for enterococci and P. aeruginosa—not all listed drugs have predictable activity.
Asymptomatic bacteriuria				
Preschool children	Aerobic Gm-neg. bacilli and Staph. hemolyticus	Base regimen on C&S, not empirical		Diagnosis requires ≥10⁵ CFU/ml urine of same bacterial species in 2 specimens obtained 3–7 days apart.
Pregnancy	Aerobic Gm-neg. bacilli	Screen 1st trimester. If positive, rx 3 d. with amoxicillin, NF, O Ceph, TMP/SMX, or TMP alone		Screen monthly for recurrence. Some authorities treat continuously until delivery (stop TMP/SMX 2 wks before EDC); ↑ resistance of E. coli to TMP/SMX.
Before and after invasive urologic intervention, e.g., Foley catheter	Aerobic Gm-neg. bacilli	Obtain urine culture and then rx 3 d. with TMP/SMX DS, bid		In one study, single dose 2-TMP/SMX DS 80% effective *(AnIM 114:713, 1991)*.
Neurogenic bladder		No rx in asymptomatic; intermittent catheterization if possible		Reference: *IDCP 4:446, 1995*
Asymptomatic, advanced age, male or female		No treatment indicated unless in conjunction with surgery to correct obstructive uropathy		
Malacoplakia	E. coli	Bethanechol chloride + (cipro or TMP/SMX)		Chronic pyelo with abnormal inflammatory response. See *CID 29:444, 1999.*
Perinephric abscess				
Associated with staphylococcal bacteremia	Staph. aureus	PRSP or P Ceph 1 *(Dosage, see footnote p. 22)*	Vanco	Drainage, surgical or image-guided aspiration
Associated with pyelonephritis	Enterobacteriaceae	See *pyelonephritis, complicated UTI,* above		Drainage, surgical or image-guided aspiration
Prostatitis		See *prostatitis, pages 18, 19*		

¹ **AM/CL** (amoxicillin/clavulanate) 875/125 mg q12h or 500/125 mg tid po, **FQ** (IV), (**CIP** 400 mg bid, **gati** 400 mg qd, **levo** 250 mg qd, **oflox** 400 mg qd, **cefoxitin** 2.0 gm q8h IV, **P Ceph 3** (**cefotaxime** 1.0 gm q12h IV for uncomplicated infections, up to 2.0 gm q4h IV for life-threatening infections; **ceftriaxone** 2.0 gm qd IV), **AP Pen** (**PIP** 3.0 gm q6h IV, **TC/CL** 3.1 gm q6h IV, **PIP/TZ** 3.375 gm q6h or 4.5 gm q8h IV, **gentamicin** *(see Table 9C, page 70)*, **TMP/SMX** 2.0 mg/kg (TMP) q6h IV, **P Ceph 3 AP** (**ceftazidime** 2.0 gm q8h IV), **P Ceph 4** (**CFP** 2.0 gm q12h IV), **IMP** 0.5 gm q6h IV, **MER** 1.0 gm q8h IV, **PRSP: nafcillin** or **oxacillin** 2.0 gm q4h IV. For **oral cephalosporin** dosage, see *footnote page 10.* **Dicloxacillin** 500 mg po qid.

NOTE: All dosage recommendations are for adults (unless otherwise indicated) and assume normal renal function

(Footnotes and abbreviations on page 47)

TABLE 1 (25)

ANATOMIC SITE/DIAGNOSIS/ MODIFYING CIRCUMSTANCES	ETIOLOGIES (usual)	SUGGESTED REGIMENS*		ADJUNCT DIAGNOSTIC OR THERAPEUTIC MEASURES AND COMMENTS
		PRIMARY	**ALTERNATIVE§**	
Liver (for spontaneous bacterial peritonitis, see page 33)				
Cholangitis		See gallbladder, page 11		
Hepatic abscess	Enterobacteriaceae, bacteroides, enterococci, Entamoeba histolytica, Yersinia enterocolitica (rare)	AMP + APAG + metro traditional and effective but AMP-resistant Gm-neg. bacilli increasing; alternative: metro + (P Ceph 3 or cefoxitin or TC/CL or PIP/ TZ or AM/SB or FQ)	Metro (for amoeba) + either IMP or MER (Dosage, see footnote page 22)	Serological tests for amebiasis should be done on all patients; if neg., surgical drainage or percutaneous aspiration. In pyogenic abscess, ½ have identifiable GI source. If amoeba serology positive, treat with metro alone without surgery. Metro included for both E. histolytica and bacteroides. Hemochromatosis associated with Yersinia enterocolitica liver abscess (CID 18: 938, 1994); regimens listed are effective for yersinia.
Cat-scratch disease (CSD)	Bartonella henselae	Azithromycin—see page 31		Ref. on hepatosplenic CSD: CID 28:778, 1999.
Leptospirosis	Leptospirosis, see page 43			
Peliosis hepatis	Bartonella henselae and B. quintana	See page 41 and the SANFORD GUIDE TO HIV/AIDS THERAPY		
Viral hepatitis	Hepatitis A, B, C, D, E, G	See Table 14		
Lung/Bronchi				
Bronchiolitis/wheezy bronchitis (expiratory wheezing)				
Infants/children (≤ age 5)	Respiratory syncytial virus (RSV) (50%), parainfluenza (25%), other viruses (20%)	Antibiotics not useful, mainstay of rx is oxygen. Aerosolized ribavirin rx of no benefit (AJRCCM 160:829, 1999). Monoclonal antibody, palivizumab 15 mg/kg IM, efficacious for prevention (Peds 102:531, 1998). See Table 14, page 105		RSV most important. Rapid dx with antigen detection methods. Ribavirin: no data on IV ribavirin but little enthusiasm. Emphasis now on vaccine development and preventive modulation with immunoglobulins.
Bronchitis				
Infants/children (≤ age 5)	< Age 2: Adenovirus Age 2–5: Respiratory syncytial virus, parainfluenza 3 virus	Antibiotics indicated only with associated sinusitis or heavy growth on throat culture for S. pneumo., Group A strep, H. influenzae or no improvement in 1 week. Otherwise rx is symptomatic.		
Adolescents and adults with acute tracheobronchitis	Viral, Mycoplasma pneumoniae, Chlamydia pneumoniae, B. pertussis (see Persistent cough, below)	**None indicated** See Comments—antimicrobial therapy only if pneumonia present. **Take patient's temperature!** (See Comment)		Purulent sputum alone not an indication for antibiotic rx (Ln 345:665, 1995). Indications for chest x-ray: respiratory symptoms + temp >37.8°C, pulse >100/min, abnormal lung exam (rales), absence of asthma (AnIM 154:1793, 1994). If infiltrate present, see Pneumonia, below. Community outbreaks of pertussis occurring (cough ≥14 days) (JAMA 275:1672, 1996).
Persistent cough (>14 d.), afebrile: Pertussis (whooping cough) Changing epidemiology: CID 28:1230, 1999 & 28 (Suppl. 2):S112, 1999	Bordetella pertussis and occasionally Bordetella parapertussis. Also consider asthma, gastroesophageal reflux, post-nasal drip	Peds doses: Erythro estolate po 40 mg/kg/d div. q8-12h x7 d. OR Erythro base po 40 mg/kg/d div. q6h x14 d. OR TMP/SMX 5 mg/kg (TMP component) po q12h x14 d.	Adult doses: Erythro estolate 500 mg po qid x7 d. OR TMP/SMX-DS 1 tab po bid x14 d. OR clarithro 500 mg po bid x7 d.	Increasingly recognized in adults (AnIM 128:64, 1998). 3 stages of illness: catarrhal (1–2 wks), paroxysmal coughing (2–4 wks), and convalescence (1–2 wks). Erythro may abort or eliminate pertussis in catarrhal stage; erythro does not shorten paroxysmal stage; erythro will render organisms non-culturable from nasopharynx within 3–4 days (PID 15:54, 1996). **Rx aimed at ↓ spread by eradicating nasopharyngeal carriage.**
Prophylaxis of household contacts		Erythromycin—Children: 50 mg/kg/d. po div. in 4 doses. Adults: 500 mg qid po. Alternative: clarithro 7.5 mg/kg po bid x14 d.	Adults: 500 mg qid po.	Recommended by Am. Acad. Ped. red Book 1997 for all household or close contacts. Community-wide prophylaxis not recommended.

Erythromycin—Children: 50 mg/kg/d. po div. in 4 doses. Adults: 500 mg qid po.
14 days.
Alternative: clarithro 7.5 mg/kg po bid x14 d.

NOTE: All dosage recommendations are for adults (unless otherwise indicated) and assume normal renal function

(Footnotes and abbreviations on page 47)

TABLE 1 (26)

ANATOMIC SITE/DIAGNOSIS/ MODIFYING CIRCUMSTANCES	ETIOLOGIES (usual)	SUGGESTED REGIMENS*		ADJUNCT DIAGNOSTIC OR THERAPEUTIC MEASURES AND COMMENTS
		PRIMARY	ALTERNATIVE§	
Lung/Bronchitis *(continued)*				
Acute bacterial exacerbation of chronic bronchitis (ABECB), adults (almost always smokers with COPD)	Viral. S. pneumoniae. H. influenzae, Moraxella catarrhalis	**Value of antimicrobial agents** is controversial *(JAMA 273:957, 1995)*. If cost major factor in selection, TMP/SMX or doxy. If cost not a major consideration, AM/CL, O Ceph, clarithro, azithro, oflox, levo, spar, gati, moxi. *(Dosage, see footnote)*¹. Usual rx 5–10 d.		Stop smoking. Pts should receive pneumococcal and influenza vaccine. Trial of corticosteroids (methyl prednisolone) indicated if pt fails to respond *(Chest 95:563, 1989)*. CIP, lomeflox and ceftibuten have relatively poor activity vs S. pneumoniae in vitro.
Pneumonia				
Neonatal	**Viruses:** CMV, rubella, H. simplex; **Bacteria:** Group B strep, listeria, coliforms, S. aureus, P. aeruginosa; **Other:** Chlamydia trachomatis, syphilis	AMP (or nafcillin) + gentamicin (or cefotaxime). Use vanco with genta (or cefotaxime) if MRSA a concern. *For dosage, see Comment. For dosage, see Table 16, p. 120.*		Blood cultures indicated. Pneumatoceeles suggest Staph. aureus but reported with pneumococci, Group A strep, H. influenzae, & enterobacteriaceae. Drain empyemas. Consider C. trachomatis if afebrile pneumonia, staccato cough. IgM >1:8; rx with erythro or sulfisoxazole.

CONSIDER TUBERCULOSIS IN ALL PATIENTS ; ISOLATE ALL SUSPECT PATIENTS

Age 1–3 months *[Adapted from Ped. Pneumonia Guide (Can. Med. Assn. J. 156:S703, 1997)]*				
Pneumonitis syndrome. Usually afebrile	C. trachomatis, RSV, other resp. viruses, Bordetella	Erythro 10 mg/kg IV q6h x10–14 d.	Clarithro 7.5 mg/kg po bid x10–14 d (if po indicated)	Pneumonitis syndrome: cough, tachypnea, dyspnea, diffuse infiltrates, afebrile. Usually requires hospital care.
		* *For RSV, see bronchiolitis, page 26*		
Age 1–24 months *For RSV, see bronchiolitis, page 26, & Table 14*	RSV, other resp. viruses, S. pneumo, H. flu, chlamydia, mycoplasma, S. aureus (rare)	In hospital but not ICU: Cefuroxime 50 mg/kg IV q8h or q12h	In ICU: (Cefotaxime 200 mg/kg/d IV div. q8h or ceftriaxone 50–75 mg/kg IV q24h) PLUS cloxacillin 50 mg/kg IV q6h	Common "other" viruses: influenza, parainfluenza, adenovirus. S. pneumo, non-type B H. influ in 4–20%. Treat x10–14 d.
Age 3 months–5 years	Resp. viruses, S. pneumo, mycoplasma, chlamydia	Outpatient: Erythro 10 mg/kg po bid or clarithro 7.5 mg/kg po bid	In hospital (or ICU): cefuroxime 50 mg/kg IV q8h PLUS erythro 10 mg/kg IV q8h. See footnote² for rx of DRSP	If otherwise healthy and if not concomitant with or post-influenza, S. pneumoniae uncommon in this subset; suspect S. pneumo if sudden onset and large amount of purulent sputum.
Age 5 years–18 years, non-hospitalized Etiology in children: *PIDJ 17:986, 1998*	Mycoplasma and resp. viruses (influenza, parainfluenza, adeno) most common. Consider S. pneumo, Chlamydia pneumoniae *(CID 29:426, 1999)*	Clarithro 500 mg bid or azithro 500 mg po x1, then 0.25 gm/d po x4/d	Doxy 100 mg po bid (if pt over 8 yrs old) or erythro 500 mg qid. See footnote³ for rx of DRSP	Mycoplasma PCR/viral culture usually not done for outpatients. Mycoplasma/chlamydia require 2–3 wks of rx.

¹ Except for azithro & clarithro-ER, rx x10 days: **TMP/SMX** 1 double-strength tab (160 mg TMP) bid po, **doxy** 100 mg bid po, **AM/CL** 875/125 mg tid po or 500/125 mg bid po, adult dose of **O Ceph** (**cefaclor** 500 mg q8h or 500 mg CD (extended release) q12h po, **cefixime** 400 mg qd po, **cefpodoxime proxetil** 200 mg q12h po, **cefprozil** 500 mg q12h po, **loracarbef** 400 mg q12h po, **ceftibuten** 400 mg/d, **cefuroxime axetil** 250 or 500 mg q12h po, **cefdinir** 300 mg q12h or 600 mg q24h), **azithro** 500 mg po initial dose then 250 mg qd x4 (total course 5 days), **clarithro** 500 mg q12h po or **clarithro ER** 1000 mg qd x7 d, **oflox** 400 mg qd x7 d or **CIP** 750 mg q12h po), **levo** 500 mg qd po, or **spar** 400 mg qd po, **gati** 400 mg qd po, **moxi** 400 mg qd po.

² **Drug-resistant S. pneumo (DRSP) and fluoroquinolones (FQs) with enhanced activity vs S. pneumo:** Prevalence of high-level resistance of S. pneumo to pen G ↑ but geographically variable (see *DMID 29:249, 1997; MMWR 48:649, 1999)*. Ampicillin/amoxicillin intrinsically more active vs S. pneumo. If S. pneumo pen-resistance is high-level (≥2 μg/ml), **cross-resistance** as follows: **Ceftriaxone 100%, AM/CL 66%, clarithro/azithro 60%, cefuroxime 20%, levo 1%.** There are only a few documented failures of P Ceph 2/3 in rx of pen-res. S. pneumo *(NEJM 338:1861, 1998 & J Peds 132:174, 1998)*. **Major concern is reported failures of rx of meningitis due to high-level DRSP with P Ceph 2/3. FQs with enhanced activity vs S. pneumo: Levo** 500 mg IV/po qd; **spar** po 400 mg x1, then 200 mg qd; **alatrofloxa** IV 200 mg qd; **gati** 400 mg qd IV/po, **moxi** 400 mg qd po. NOTE: All dosage recommendations are for adults (unless otherwise indicated) and assume normal renal function

(Footnotes and abbreviations on page 47)

TABLE 1 (27)

ANATOMIC SITE/DIAGNOSIS/ MODIFYING CIRCUMSTANCES	ETIOLOGIES (usual)	SUGGESTED REGIMENS* PRIMARY	SUGGESTED REGIMENS* ALTERNATIVE§	ADJUNCT DIAGNOSTIC OR THERAPEUTIC MEASURES AND COMMENTS
Lung/Pneumonia (continued)				
Presumed viral pneumonia in adults: cough, no sputum, dyspnea/hypoxia, interstitial infiltrates. Also see Table 14, page 104	Influenza (Dec.-Mar. in U.S.), parainfluenza, adenovirus, RSV, hantavirus	For influenza A or B: zanamivir 10 mg inhaled bid x5 d. or oseltamivir 75 mg po bid x5 d. Start within 48 hrs of symptom onset.	For influenza A: rimantadine 100 mg po 2x/d or amantadine 100 mg po 2x/d.	Zanamivir & oseltamivir shortened course & ↓ complications of influenza A & B (Ln 352: 1877 & 1872, 1998); also efficacious in prevention (JAMA 282:31 & 75, 1999). Amantadine/rimantadine shorten course of influenza bronchitis if dose early; presumably same benefit in pneumonia; renal excretion: adjust dose for est. CrCl <90 ml/min—see Table 17.
Adults (over age 18)—Guidelines: IDSA, CID 26:811, 1998; Med Lett 40:33, 1998; Am Thor Soc: ARRD 48:1418, 1993; Brit J Hosp Med 49:346, 1993, Ln 352:1295, 1998				
Community-acquired; non-hospitalized	**Smokers:** S. pneumo, H. influenzae, Moraxella catarrhalis. **Post-viral bronchitis:** S. pneumo, rarely S. aureus. **No co-morbidity:** Mycoplasma, Chlamydia pneumoniae, viral. Rarely S. pneumo. **Alcoholic stupor:** S. pneumo, anaerobes, coliforms. **IV drug abuse:** S. aureus.	Azithro 0.5 gm po x1, then 0.25 gm/d. OR Clarithro 500 mg po bid	FQ with enhanced activity vs S. pneumo (see footnote 2, page 27) OR O Ceph 2 (dosage below)[1] OR AM/CL 875/ 125 mg po bid OR doxy 100 mg po bid	Sputum Gram stain and culture desirable. Further attempts at defining etiology depend on severity of illness, co-morbidities and local lab resources. Rx issues: None of drugs listed except FQs active vs high-level resistant S. pneumo. Neither AM/CL or O Ceph 2 active vs legionella, mycoplasma, or Chlamydia pneumoniae. ↑ resistance of S. pneumo and H. influenzae to doxy. Recent reports of FQ-resistant S. pneumo (NEJM 341:233, 1999).
		Rx duration varies: usually rx until afebrile 3-5 d. Duration of rx can range from 7-14 d.		
Community-acquired, hospitalized NOTE: Always include rx for S. pneumo in post-splenectomy, myeloma, lymphoma pts For specific rx after culture results, see below and Table 2, page 48	**Epidemic:** Legionella's. **Rabbits:** Tularemia. **Birds:** Psittacosis. **Parturient livestock or cats:** Coxiella burnetii. **Airway obstruction:** Anaerobes	**Non-ICU bed:** (P Ceph 3[2] IV + (erythro 15-20 mg/ kg/d div. q6h) OR azithro 500 mg IV once daily) OR (FQ with enhanced activity vs S. pneumo)[2] **In Intensive Care:** (P Ceph 3[2] IV + azithro 500 mg IV once daily) OR (FQ with enhanced activity vs S. pneumo; see footnote 2, page 27) Dosage in footnote[2] & in footnote 2, page 27	**Dx:** Sputum Gram stain and culture. Blood cultures. Urine legionella antigens. Pleural fluid if present. **Rx:** Major concern is ↑ prevalence of drug-resistant S. pneumo (see footnote 2, page 27). Need to know local prevalence. If local prevalence of high-level resistance >20% & pt's underlying disease ↑ likelihood that S. pneumo is etiology, start rx with enhanced activity FQ (see footnote 2, page 27) pending culture results. For Legionaire's: azithro IV requires less diluent than erythro; many prefer an FQ. Q-fever reference: CID 29:874, 1999; Clin Micro Rev 12:518, 1999
Adults—Guidelines: AJRCCM 153:1711, 1996; Med Lett 38:25, 1996				
Hospital-acquired ± mechanical ventilation. NOT neutropenic For rx of specific bacteria, see below and Table 2, page 48	**Post-CVA aspiration:** Water colonization: Legionella. **Organ failure:** Coliforms. **Mech. ventilation:** Coliforms, P. aeruginosa, S. aureus. **Airway obstruction:** Anaerobes. **Steroids:** Yeast, PCP (see AIDS)	To cover coliforms, S. pneumo & anaerobes: IMP 0.5 gm IV q6h) OR (MER 1.0 gm IV q8h) OR (P Ceph 3 AP + APAG) or (AP Pen + APAG) ± clinda) OR [(TC/CL or PIP/ TZ) + CIP] OR (P Ceph 4 ± clinda)	To include DRSP + coliforms/anaerobes: (trova 300 mg IV x1, then 200 mg IV/d. If suspect legionella: trova, levo or gati IV alone or add azithro	**Dx of ventilator-associated pneumonia:** Fever and lung infiltrates often not pneumonia (Chest 106:221, 1994). Quantitative cultures helpful: bronchoalveolar lavage (>10⁴/ml pos.) or protect. spec. brush (>10³/ml pos.). See Seminars Resp Infect 11:65, 1996; Ln 352:83, 1998. **Treatment:** Drugs active vs pen-resistant S. pneumo—vanco, levo, trova, and perhaps IMP and clinda (in U.S.). Review on use of quinolones for Legionaire's disease: AnIM 129:328, 1998. Also, if macrolide selected for Legionaire's, prefer azithro IV rather than IV erythro. **Prevention:** If possible, keep head of bed elevated 30° or more. Remove N-G, endotracheal tubes as soon as possible. If available, continuous subglottic suctioning. Limit stress ulcer prophylaxis. Ref: NEJM 340:627, 1999.
		See Comment		
		Dosages: See footnotes below & on pages 17, 25 & 27		

Dosages: See footnotes below and on pages 17, 25 & 27

NOTE: All dosage recommendations are for adults (unless otherwise indicated) and assume normal renal function

---

[1] **O Ceph 2** dosage: **Cefdinir** 300 mg po q12h; **cefpodoxime proxetil** 300 mg po q12h, **cefprozil** 250 mg po q12h, **cefuroxime axetil** 250-500 mg po q12h

[2] **P Ceph 3** (**cefotaxime** dose ranges from 2.0 gm q8h IV for severe infection to 2.0 gm q4h IV for life-threatening infection, **ceftriaxone** 2 gm qd IV < age 60; 1 gm qd IV > age 60, **ceftizoxime** not as active in vitro vs Strep pneumo) **P Ceph 3 AP** (**CFP** 2.0 gm q12h IV, **ceftazidime** 2.0 gm q8h IV), **P Ceph 4 (CFP** 2.0 gm q12h IV). **TC/CL** 3.1 gm q4h IV. If P. aeruginosa pneumonia, (**TC/CL** 3.1 gm q4h IV + **tobramycin** 5 mg/kg IV once daily) or [(**PIP/TZ** 3.375 gm q4h or 4.5 gm q8h) + **tobramycin** 5 mg/kg once daily].

(Footnotes and abbreviations on page 47)

TABLE 1 (28)

ANATOMIC SITE/DIAGNOSIS/MODIFYING CIRCUMSTANCES	ETIOLOGIES (usual)	SUGGESTED REGIMENS*		ADJUNCT DIAGNOSTIC OR THERAPEUTIC MEASURES AND COMMENTS
		PRIMARY	ALTERNATIVE§	
Lung/Pneumonia/Adults—Guidelines *(continued)*				
Hospital- or community-acquired, neutropenic pt (<500 neutrophils/mm³)	Any of organisms listed under community- & hospital-acquired: hospital-acquired + fungi (aspergillus, Candida sp.)	See *Hospital-acquired, immediately above.* Vanco not included in initial rx unless high suspicion of infected IV access or drug-resistant S. pneumo. Ampho not used unless still febrile after 3 days or high clinical likelihood. *See Comment.*		See consensus document on management of febrile neutropenic pt: *C/D 25:551, 1997.* Failures due to drug-resistant S. pneumo: *AnIM 158:868, 1998.*
Adults—Culture results (sputum, blood, pleural fluid, etc.) available to guide specific therapy. Also see *Table 2, page 48.*				
Haemophilus influenzae	β-lactamase negative	AMP IV, amox po, TMP/SMX, azithro/clarithro		25–35% strains β-lactamase positive. ↑ resistance to both TMP/SMX and doxy.
	β-lactamase positive	AM/CL, O Ceph 2/3, P Ceph 3, FQ, azithro/clarithro		
Legionella species	Hospitalized/immunocompromised	Azithro IV or levo IV or trova IV or (erythro IV ± RIF)		Active FQs: trova, spar, peflox^{NUS}, levo, moxi (not available IV), gati: Refs.: *AnIM 129:328, 1998; JAC 43:747, 1999.*
Moraxella catarrhalis	93% β-lactamase positive	AM/CL, O Ceph 2/3, P Ceph 2/3, macrolide¹, FQ, TMP/SMX. Doxy another option.		
Strep. pneumoniae	Penicillin-susceptible	AMP IV, amox po, macrolide¹, pen G IV, doxy, O Ceph 2/3		
	Penicillin-resistant, high level	FQs with enhanced activity: gati; levo, moxi, spar, trova (IV); P Ceph 3 (if susceptible); high-dose IV amp; (vanco IV ± RIF)—see *Table 5 for more data.*		
Human immunodeficiency virus infection (HIV+) + CD4 T-lymphocytes <200/mm³ or clinical AIDS Dry cough, progressive dyspnea, and diffuse infiltrate (see *Comment* reference to steroids)	Pneumocystis carinii most likely; also M. tbc, fungi, Kaposi's sarcoma, and lymphoma NOTE: AIDS pts may develop pneumonia due to DRSP or other pathogens —see next box below	*Rx listed here is for pneumocystis only; also see Table 12, page 90* TMP/SMX (IV, po if mild disease) or [(if mild) dapsone 100 mg qd po + trimethoprim 20 mg/kg/d po divided q6h]	[Clinda 900 mg q8h IV + primaquine 30 mg qd po) or (atovaquone 750 mg bid po with meals) or (pentamidine isethionate 4 mg/kg/d IV) x21d *See Comment*	Diagnostic procedure of choice is sputum induction; if negative, bronchoscopy. Pts with PCP or <200 CD4 cells/mm³ should be on anti-PCP prophylaxis for life. **Prednisone 40 mg bid po x5 d, then 20 mg qd po for 11 days is indicated with PCP (pO₂ <70 mmHg), should be given at initiation of anti-PCP rx; don't wait until pt's condition deteriorates** (*Table 12, page 90*). If PCP studies negative, consider bacterial pneumonia. TBc, cocci, histo, crypto, Kaposi's sarcoma or lymphoma. NOTE: 10–20% S. pneumoniae resistant to TMP/SMX. **Neither pentamidine nor atovaquone active vs bacterial pathogens.**
HIV-infected patients—CD4 T-lymphocytes normal Acute onset, purulent sputum and pulmonary infiltrates ± pleuritic pain. **Isolate patient until TBc excluded.**	Strep. pneumoniae, H. influenzae. Aerobic Gm-neg. bacilli (including P. aeruginosa), Legionella rare	P Ceph 3 (Dosages in footnotes on pages 17 & 25) ± erythro. Could use levo or trova IV as alternative (see Comment)		If Gram stain of sputum shows Gm-neg. bacilli, options include P Ceph 3 AP, TC/CL, PIP/TZ, IMP, or MER. FQs: Levo 500 mg po/IV qd; trova 200 mg IV qd: gati 400 mg IV/po qd; moxi 400 mg po qd
Children	Same as adult with HIV + lymphoid interstitial pneumonia (LIP)	As for HIV + adults with pneumonia. If diagnosis is LIP, rx with steroids.		In children with AIDS, LIP responsible for ⅓ of pulmonary complications, usually >1 yr of age vs PCP, which is seen at <1 yr of age. Clinically: clubbing: hepatosplenomegaly, salivary glands enlarged (take up gallium), lymphocytosis.
Chronic pneumonia with fever, night sweats and weight loss	M. tuberculosis, coccidioidomycosis, histoplasmosis	See *Tables 10, 11*		HIV+, foreign-born, alcoholism, contact with TB, travel into developing countries

¹ Macrolide = azithromycin, clarithromycin, dirithromycin, and erythromycin
(Footnotes and abbreviations on page 47)

NOTE: All dosage recommendations are for adults (unless otherwise indicated) and assume normal renal function

29

TABLE 1 (29)

ANATOMIC SITE/DIAGNOSIS/ MODIFYING CIRCUMSTANCES	ETIOLOGIES (usual)	SUGGESTED REGIMENS*		ADJUNCT DIAGNOSTIC OR THERAPEUTIC MEASURES AND COMMENTS
		PRIMARY	ALTERNATIVE¹	
Lung (continued)				
Anthrax Potential biological weapon (*JAMA* 281:1735, 1999) Review: *NEJM* 341:815, 1999	Bacillus anthracis	**Empiric:** CIP 400 mg IV q12h or levo 500 mg IV qd. Children: CIP 20–30 mg/kg/d div. 2 doses	**Specific:** Pen G 4 mU q4h IV or doxy 100 mg q12h IV. Children: <12 y/o: 50,000 U/kg pen G IV q6h; >12 y/o: pen G 4 mU q4h IV	Suspect if sudden multiple pts severe flu, fulminant course and high mortality. Dx: Chest x-ray—widened mediastinum. Peripheral blood smear: Gm-pos. bacilli visible. Pathol.: hemorrhagic mediastinitis.
		Treat for 60 days		
Post-exposure prophylaxis		Adults: CIP 500 mg po bid or doxy 100 mg po bid	Children: CIP 20–30 mg/kg/d div. q12h or, if CIP not available, doxy 5 mg/kg/d div. q12h. If anthrax confirmed, switch to amox 40 mg/kg/d div. q8h. Ref.: *MMWR* 48:69, 1999.	
Aspiration pneumonia ± lung abscess (*QJM* 88:409, 1995)	Bacteroides sp. (~15% B. fragilis), peptostreptococci, Fusobacterium sp., S. milleri group, nocardia (pts taking steroids)	Clinda 450–900 mg q8h IV (For nocardia, see Table 10, page 76)	(Cefoxitin 2.0 gm q8h IV) or (TC/CL 3.1 gm q6h IV) or (PIP/TZ 3.375 gm q6h or 4.5 gm q8h IV) [Historically Pen G (HD) has been effective]	Bronchoscopy to R/O neoplasm if pt fails to clear or recurs. Metro not as effective in putrid lung abscess as clinda. Occasionally Type 3 pneumococci, Staph. aureus, Klebsiella pneumoniae are etiologic. Spectrum of trova appropriate for aspiration; should work—no data.
Empyema. *Reference: CID 22:747, 1996 & COID 11:163, 1998*				
Neonatal	Staph. aureus	*See Pneumonia, neonatal, 5 days–1 month, page 27*		
Infants/children (1 month–5 years)	Staph. aureus, Strep. pneumoniae, H. influenzae	*See Pneumonia, age 1 month–5 years, page 27*		Drainage indicated.
Child >5 yrs to ADULT—Diagnostic thoracentesis; chest tube for empyemas				
Acute, usually parapneumonic	Strep. pneumoniae Group A strep	Cefotaxime or ceftriaxone (Dosage, see footnote² on page 28)	Vanco	Randomized trial showed benefit of intrapleural streptokinase (250,000 units in 20 ml saline with 2-hr. dwell qd x3 days) (*Thorax* 52:416, 1997). Urokinase 100,000 IU/d. x3 d. effective in double-blind study (*AJRCCM* 159:37, 1999).
	Staph. aureus	PRSP	Vanco	Gram + cocci in clusters
	H. influenzae	P Ceph 3	TMP/SMX or AM/SB	Pleomorphic Gram-negative bacilli. ↑ resistance to TMP/SMX.
Subacute/chronic	Anaerobic strep, Strep. milleri, Bacteroides sp., Enterobacteriaceae, M. tuberculosis	Clinda 450–900 mg q8h IV + P Ceph 3	(Cefoxitin) or (IMP) or (TC/CL) or (PIP/TZ) or (AM/SB) (Dosage, see footnote² on page 28)	If organisms not seen, treat as subacute. Drainage. Rule out tuberculosis or tumor. Pleural biopsy with culture for mycobacteria and histology if TBc suspected (*CID* 22:747, 1996).

(Footnotes and abbreviations on page 47)   NOTE: All dosage recommendations are for adults (unless otherwise indicated) and assume normal renal function

TABLE 1 (30)

ANATOMIC SITE/DIAGNOSIS/ MODIFYING CIRCUMSTANCES	ETIOLOGIES (usual)	SUGGESTED REGIMENS* PRIMARY	ALTERNATIVE§	ADJUNCT DIAGNOSTIC OR THERAPEUTIC MEASURES AND COMMENTS
Lung (continued)				
Cystic fibrosis: NEJM 335:179, 1996 Acute exacerbation of pulmonary symptoms Parenteral administration of 2 antibiotics x14–21 d. + intensified airway clearance of secretions *See Comment for use of inhaled tobra for chronic suppression of P. aeruginosa*	S. aureus early in disease; P. aeruginosa later in disease	**For P. aeruginosa:** [Tobra 3 mg/kg q8h IV + (ticarcillin or PIP 100 mg/ kg q6h IV)] or [tobra + ceftaz 50 mg/kg q8h IV]— see footnote†	**For S. aureus:** (1) MSSA—oxacillin/nafcillin 2.0 gm IV q4h (Peds dose, Table 16) (2) MRSA—vanco 1.0 gm q12h and check serum levels	Essential to monitor serum levels of aminoglycosides due to altered kinetics and drug accumulation in CF cells (JAC 41:215, 1998). Consensus report on FQs in pediatrics lists P. aeruginosa exacerbation in CF as an indication (PIDJ 14:1, 1995). For pts with P. aeruginosa, **inhaled tobra** led to modest ↑ in FEV₁ & ↓ bacterial density. May not work if P. aeruginosa resistant to tobra. **Dose** (age >6 yrs): 300 mg with designated inhaler bid x28 days, dc x28 d., then repeat cycle (NEJM 340:23, 1999). No major resistance so far (JID 179:1190, 1999).
	Burkholderia (Pseudomonas) cepacia	TMP/SMX 5.0 mg/kg (TMP) q6h IV	Chloramphenicol 15–20 mg/kg IV or q6h po	B. cepacia has become a major pathogen. Patients develop progressive respiratory failure, 62% mortality at 1 year. **Fail to respond to APAG, AP Pen and P Ceph 3 AP.** Patients with B. cepacia should be isolated from other CF pts.
		For other alternatives, see Table 2		

Lymph Nodes (approaches below apply to lymphadenitis without an obvious primary source)

Lymphadenitis, acute

Generalized	Etiologies: EBV, early HIV infection, syphilis, toxoplasma, tularemia, Lyme disease, sarcoid, lymphoma, systemic lupus erythematosus, and Kikuchi-Fujimoto disease. Complete history and physical examination followed by appropriate serological tests. Treat specific agent(s).			
Regional				
Cervical—see cat-scratch disease (CSD), below	CSD (B. henselae), GAS, SA, anaerobes, MTBc (scrofula), M. avium, M. scrofulaceum, M. malmoense, toxo, tularemia	History and physical exam directs evaluation. If nodes fluctuant, aspirate and base rx on Gram and acid-fast stains. Review of mycobacterial etiology: CID 20:954, 1995. Kikuchi-Fujimoto disease causes fever and benign self-limited adenopathy; the etiology is unknown (AJM 171:401, 1996).		
Inguinal				
Sexually transmitted	HSV, chancroid, syphilis, LGV	Treatment depends on specific dx		
Not sexually transmitted	GAS, SA, tularemia, CSD	Treatment depends on specific dx, geography, hx of insect bites, distal lesions may help. *See cervical adenopathy Comment.*		
Axillary	GAS, SA, CSD, tularemia, Y. pestis, sporotrichosis	*See cervical adenopathy Comment.*		
Extremity—with associated nodular lymphangitis (For full description: AnIM 118:883, 1993)	Sporotrichosis, leishmania, Nocardia brasiliensis, Mycobacterium marinum, Mycobacterium chelonae.	Treatment varies with specific etiology		A distinctive form of lymphangitis characterized by subcutaneous swellings along inflamed lymphatic channels. Primary site of skin invasion usually present; regional adenopathy variable.
Cat-scratch disease— immunocompetent patient *Also see page 41—Bartonella and SANFORD GUIDE TO HIV/AIDS THERAPY.* Axillary/epitrochlear nodes 46%, neck 26%, inguinal 17%	Bartonella henselae *See pages 36 and 41 for immunocompromised pts*	Azithro dosage—Adults (>45.5 kg): 500 mg po x1, then 250 mg/ d x4 d. Children (<45.5 kg): liquid azithro 10 mg/kg x1, then 5 mg/kg/d x4 d. Rx is controversial—see Comment	No rx; resolves in 2–6 mos. Needle aspiration relieves pain in suppurative nodes. Avoid I&D.	Clinical: Approx. 10% nodes suppurate. Atypical presentation in <5% pts, i.e. lung nodules, liver/spleen lesions, Parinaud's oculoglandular syndrome, CNS manifestations. Dx: Cat exposure. Positive IFA serology. Rarely need biopsy. Rx: Only 1 prospective randomized blinded study, used azithro (PIDJ 17:447, 1998).

† Other options: (Tobra + aztreonam 50 mg/kg q8h IV); (IMP 15–25 mg/kg q8h IV + tobra); (CIP IV/po + ceftaz IV—see comment on FQs in Cystic fibrosis and ref.: PIDJ 16:572, 1997).

NOTE: All dosage recommendations are for adults (unless otherwise indicated) and assume normal renal function

(Footnotes and abbreviations on page 47)

TABLE 1 (31)

ANATOMIC SITE/DIAGNOSIS/ MODIFYING CIRCUMSTANCES	ETIOLOGIES (usual)	SUGGESTED REGIMENS* PRIMARY	SUGGESTED REGIMENS* ALTERNATIVE§	ADJUNCT DIAGNOSTIC OR THERAPEUTIC MEASURES AND COMMENTS
Mouth				
Odontogenic infection Can result in more serious para-pharyngeal space infection (see page 35)	Oral microflora: infection polymicrobial	Clinda 300 mg q6h po	[AM/CL 875/125 mg bid or 500/125 mg tid po] or erythro 500 mg q6h po	Surgical drainage and removal of necrotic tissue essential. β-lactamase resistant organisms are ↑ in frequency. Ref.: Canad Dental Assn J 64:508, 1998
Buccal cellulitis				
Children <5 yrs	H. influenzae	Cefuroxime or P Ceph 3 Dosage: see Table 16, page 120	AM/CL or TMP/SMX	With Hib immunization, invasive H. influenzae infections have ↓ by 95%. Now occurring in infants prior to immunization.
Herpetic stomatitis	Herpes simplex virus 1 & 2	See Table 14		
Aphthous stomatitis, recurrent, HIV-neg.	Etiology unknown	Topical steroids (Kenalog in Orabase) may ↓ pain and swelling; if AIDS, see SANFORD GUIDE TO HIV/AIDS THERAPY.		
Muscle				
"Gas gangrene" Contaminated traumatic wound Can be spontaneous without trauma (CID 28:159, 1999)	Cl. perfringens, other histo-toxic Clostridium sp.	(Clinda 900 mg q8h IV) + (pen G 24 mu/d div. q4-6h IV)	Ceftriaxone 2.0 gm q12h IV or erythro 1.0 gm q6h IV (not by bolus)	Surgical debridement primary rx. Hyperbaric oxygen adjunctive: efficacy debated, consider if debridement not complete or possible (NEJM 334:1642, 1996). Clinda ↓ toxin production.
Pyomyositis	Staph. aureus, Group A strep, (rarely Gram-neg. bacilli), variety of anaerobic organisms	[PRSP (nafcillin or oxacillin 2.0 gm q4h IV)] or [P Ceph 1 (cefazolin 2.0 gm q8h IV)]	Vanco 1.0 gm q12h IV	Has been common in tropics, rare but occurs in temperate zones (IDCP 7:265, 1998). Follows exercise or muscle injury, see Necrotizing fasciitis. Now seen in HIV/AIDS (AJM 91:129, 1991). Add clinda or metro if anaerobes suspected/proven (IDCP 8:252, 1999).
Pancreas: Review—NEJM 340:1412, 1999				
Acute alcoholic (without necrosis) (idiopathic) pancreatitis	Not bacterial	None		1–9% become infected but prospective studies show no advantage to initial AMP (Ln 346:652, 1995). Observe for pancreatic abscesses or necrosis which require rx.
Pancreatic abscess, infected pseudocyst, infected necrosis	Enterobacteriaceae, entero-cocci, S. aureus, S. epider-midis, anaerobes, candida	For necrotizing pancreatitis (see Comment), start IMP (dose in footnote¹) and continue 2–4 weeks (SGO 176:480, 1993; Ar Surg 132:487, 1997).		For dx of pancreatic necrosis: contrast-enhanced CT. Accuracy >90% if >30% glandular necrosis. If infection uncertain, do CT-guided fine-needle aspiration (sens. 96%, spec. 99%)
Parotid Gland				
"Hot" tender parotitis	S. aureus, rarely aerobic Gm-neg. bacilli, mumps, rarely enteroviruses/influenza			Predisposing factors: stone(s) in Stensen's duct, dehydration. Rx depends on ID of specific etiologic organism.
"Cold" non-tender parotid swelling	Granulomatous disease (e.g., mycobacteria, fungi, sarcoidosis, Sjogren's syn-drome, drugs (Iodides, et al.), diabetes, cirrhosis, tumors			History/lab results may narrow differential; may need biopsy for dx

¹ Parenteral IV therapy for peritonitis: **TC/CL** 3.1 gm q6h, **PIP/TZ** 3.375 gm q6h or 4.5 gm q8h, **AM/SB** 3.0 gm q6h, **IMP** 0.5 gm q6h, **MER** 1.0 gm q8h, **FQ** [**CIP** 400 mg q12h, **oflox** 400 mg q12h, **levo** 500 mg qd, **trova** 300 mg qd, **gati** 400 mg qd, **moxi** 400 mg qd po (no IV)], **AMP** 1.0 gm q6h, **APAG** (see Table 9C, page 70), **cefotetan** 2 gm q12h, **cefmetazole**[NUS] 2 gm q8-12h, **P Ceph 3** [**cefotaxime** 2.0 gm q4-8h; **ceftizoxime** 2.0 gm q8h, **ceftriaxone** 2.0 gm qd, **ceftizoxime** 2 gm q4-8h), **P Ceph 4** (**CFP** 2.0 gm q12h), **clinda** 450-900 mg q8h, **metro** 1.0 gm loading then 0.5 gm q6h or 1.0 gm q12h, **AP Pen** (**ticarcillin** 4.0 gm q6h, **PIP** 4.0 gm q6h, **aztreonam** 2.0 gm q8h)

NOTE: All dosage recommendations are for adults (unless otherwise indicated) and assume normal renal function

(Footnotes and abbreviations on page 47)

TABLE 1 (32)

ANATOMIC SITE/DIAGNOSIS/ MODIFYING CIRCUMSTANCES	ETIOLOGIES (usual)	SUGGESTED REGIMENS*		ADJUNCT DIAGNOSTIC OR THERAPEUTIC MEASURES AND COMMENTS
		PRIMARY	ALTERNATIVE§	
Peritoneum/Peritonitis (Reference: CID 24:1035, 1997)				
Primary (spontaneous bacterial peritonitis, SBP) Review: CID 27:669, 1998 ESBL ref.: CID 28:683, 1999	Enterobacteriaceae 63%, S. pneumo 15%, enterococci 6–10%, anaerobes <1%. Watch out for extended-spectrum β-lactamases (ESBLs) from E. coli or Klebsiella sp.	**No ESBL:** [Cefotaxime 2.0 gm q8h IV (if life-threatening, q4h)] or [TC/CL or PIP/TZ or AM/SB] or [Ceftriaxone should be effective, 2.0 gm q24h IV] **Suspect ESBL:** (IMP or MER) or (FQ: CIP, levo, trova, gati)		One-year risk of SBP in pts with ascites and cirrhosis as high as 29% (Gastro 104:1133, 1993). 30–40% of pts have neg. cultures of blood and ascitic fluid. % positive cultures ↑ if 10 ml of ascitic fluid added to blood culture bottles. Duration of rx unclear. Suggest 2 wks if blood culture pos. One report suggests repeat paracentesis after 48 hrs of cefotaxime. If PMNs <250/mm³ and ascitic fluid sterile, success with 5 days of rx (AJM 97:169, 1994; Hepatol 5:457, 1985).
		Dosage in footnote¹		
Prevention of SBP—pts with cirrhosis and ascites		TMP/SMX-DS, 1 tab po 5 days/wk or norfloxacin 400 mg po qd	TMP/SMX ↓ peritonitis or spontaneous bacteremia from 27% to 3% (AnIM 122:595, 1995). Norfloxacin ↓ the risk from Gm-neg. bacilli but ↑ risk of staph infections and resistance to antibiotics (CID 26:1066, 1998).	
Secondary (bowel perforation, ruptured appendix, diverticula) For appendicitis and antimicrobial therapy, see IDCP 5(Suppl 1):52, 1996	Enterobacteriaceae, entero-cocci, bacteroides, P. aeru-ginosa (3–15%)	Multiple regimens effective. **Must "cover" both Gm-neg. aerobic & Gm-neg. anaerobic bacteria.** The role of enterococci remains debatable. **Drugs that have activity only vs anaerobic Gm-neg. bacilli:** clinda, metro. **Drugs active only vs aerobic Gm-neg. bacilli:** APAG, P Ceph 2/3/4, AP Pen, aztreonam, FQs. **Drugs active vs both aerobic/anaerobic Gm-neg. bacteria:** cefoxitin, cefotetan, cefmetazole,ᴺᵁˢ TC/CL, PIP/TZ, AM/SB, IMP, MER, trova (Dosage, see footnote†)		If pt has been ill for >24–48 hrs and there is absence of ongoing fecal contamination, aerobic/anaerobic culture of peritoneal exudate/abscess of help in guiding specific therapy. With large number of effective drugs, less need for aminoglycosides. When AG used, try to switch by 3 days to avoid toxic potential. In pt with severe pen allergy, can "cover" Gm-neg. aerobes with CIP or aztreonam. Remember IMP/MER are β-lactams. Useful reference: IDCP 5(Suppl):S2, 1996. In 1 study, CIP + metro was as effective as IMP alone (An Surg 223:303, 1996).
Associated with chronic ambulatory peritoneal dialysis (defined as >100 WBC/μl, >50% PMNs)	Staph. aureus (most common), Staph. epidermidis, P. aeruginosa 7%, Gm-neg. bacilli 11%, sterile 20%, M. fortuitum (rare)	If of moderate severity, can treat by adding drug to dialysis fluid—see Table 17 for dosage. Reasonable empiric combinations: vanco + P Ceph 3 AP or vanco + APAG. If severely ill, treat with same drugs IV (adjust dose for renal failure, Table 17) and via addition to dialysis fluid. Excellent reference: Perit Dialysis Int 13:14, 1993.		For diagnosis: concentrate several hundred ml of removed dialysis fluid by centrifugation. Gram stain concentrate and then inject into aerobic/anaerobic blood culture bottles. A positive Gram stain will guide initial therapy. If culture shows Staph. epidermidis, good chance of "saving" dialysis catheter; if multiple Gm-neg. bacilli cultured, consider bowel perforation and catheter removal.

¹ Parenteral IV therapy for peritonitis: **TC/CL** 3.1 gm q6h, **PIP/TZ** 3.375 gm q6h or 4.5 gm q8h, **AM/SB** 3.0 gm q6h, **IMP** 0.5 gm q6h, **MER** 1.0 gm q8h, **FQ** [**CIP** 400 mg q12h, **oflox** 400 mg q12h, **levo** 500 mg qd, **trova** 300 mg qd, gati 400 mg qd], **APAG** (see Table 9C, page 47), **cefotetan** 2 gm q12h, **cefoxitin** 2.0 gm q8h, **cefmetazole**ᴺᵁˢ 2 gm q8–12h, **P Ceph 3** [**cefotaxime** 2.0 gm q4–8h, **ceftriaxone** 2.0 gm qd, **ceftizoxime** 2.0 gm q8h, **CFP** 2.0 gm q12h], **P Ceph 4** (**cefpirome**ᴺᵁˢ 2.0 gm q12h), **clinda** 450–900 mg q8h, **metro** 1.0 gm loading then 0.5 gm q6h or 1.0 gm q12h, **AP Pen** (**ticarcillin** 4.0 gm q6h, **PIP** 4.0 gm q6h, **aztreonam** 2.0 gm q8h)

NOTE: All dosage recommendations are for adults (unless otherwise indicated) and assume normal renal function

(Footnotes and abbreviations on page 47)

TABLE 1 (33)

ANATOMIC SITE/DIAGNOSIS/ MODIFYING CIRCUMSTANCES	ETIOLOGIES (usual)	SUGGESTED REGIMENS*		ADJUNCT DIAGNOSTIC OR THERAPEUTIC MEASURES AND COMMENTS
		PRIMARY	ALTERNATIVE§	
Pharynx				
Pharyngitis—*For Practice Guideline, see CID 25:574, 1997*				
Exudative or diffuse erythema *For relationship to acute rheumatic fever, see footnote[1]* *Rheumatic fever reference: Ln 349:935, 1997*	Group A,C,G strep, "viral", infectious mononucleosis, HHV-6 *(NEJM 329:156, 1993)*, C. diphtheriae, A. haemolyticum, Mycoplasma pneumoniae	Pen V po x10 days or if compliance unlikely, benzathine pen IM x1 *See footnote[2] for adult and pediatric dosages*	Erythro x10 d. or O Ceph 2 x4–6 d or clinda or azithro x5 d. or clarithro x10 d.	Goal: Determine if Group A strep present (5–20%) rx shortens duration/severity of symptoms and ↓ risk of rheumatic fever. Rapid strep test >95% specific; sensitivity varies (60–100%). S. pyogenes Groups C & G cause pharyngitis but not risk for post-strep rheumatic fever. To prevent rheumatic fever, eradicate Group A strep. Requires 10 d. of pen V po; 4–6 d. of po P Ceph 2, 5 d. of po azithro, 10 d. of clarithro.
	Gonococci	Ceftriaxone 125 mg IM x1 + azithro or doxy *(see Comment)*	(Cipro 500 mg po x1) or (oflox 400 mg po x1) + azithro or doxy *(see Comment)*	Because of risk of concomitant genital C. trachomatis, add either (azithro 1.0 gm po x1) or (doxy 100 mg po 2x/d. x7 d.).
Asymptomatic post-rx carrier	**Group A strep**	No rx required		Routine post-rx throat culture not advised.
Multiple repeated culture-positive episodes *(CID 25:574, 1997)*	Group A strep	Clinda or AM/CL po	Parenteral benzathine pen G	Small % of pts have recurrent culture-pos. Group A strep with symptomatic pharyngitis. Hard to tell if true Group A strep infection or active viral infection in carrier of Group A strep.
		Dosages in footnote[2]		
Whitish plaques, HIV+ (thrush)	Candida albicans *(see Table 10, page 72)*			
Vesicular, ulcerative	Coxsackie A9 B1–5, ECHO (multiple types), Enterovirus 71, Herpes simplex 1,2	Antibacterial agents not indicated, but for HSV-1, 2: acyclovir 400 mg tid po x10 d.		
Membranous	C. diphtheriae	Pen G 4 mu q4h IV	Clinda 600 mg q8h IV	Diphtheria occurs in immunized individuals. Antibiotics may ↓ toxin production, ↓ spread of organisms. Penicillin superior to erythro in randomized trial *(CID 27:845, 1998)*.
	Vincent's angina (anaerobes/spirochetes)			May be complicated by F. necrophorum bacteremia, *see jugular vein phlebitis (Lemierre's), below.*

[1] Primary rationale for treatment is eradication of Group A strep (GAS) and prevention of acute rheumatic fever (ARF). Benzathine penicillin G has been shown in clinical trials to ↓ rate of ARF from 2.8 to 0.2%. This was associated with clearance of GAS on pharyngeal cultures *(CID 19:1110, 1994)*. Subsequent studies have been based on cultures, not actual prevention of ARF. Treatment ↓ duration of symptoms.

[2] Treatment of Group A strep: **PEDIATRIC DOSAGE: Benzathine penicillin** 25,000 u/kg IM to max. 1.2 mu; **Pen V** 25–50 mg/kg/d po div. q6h x10 d.; **AM/CL** 45 mg/kg/d div. q12h x10 d.; **erythro estolate** 20 mg/kg div. bid or **succinate** 40 mg/kg/d po div. bid x10 d.; **cefuroxime axetil** 20 mg/kg/d div. bid for 4–10 d. *(PIDJ 14:295, 1995)*; **cefpodoxime proxetil** 10 mg/kg div. bid x10 d.; **cefdinir** 7 mg/kg q12h x5–10 d.; **cefprozil** 15 mg/kg/d div. bid x10 d.; **clarithro** 15 mg/kg/d div. bid x10 d.; **azithro** 12 mg/kg/d x5 d., then 6 mg/kg/d x5 d. **ADULT DOSAGE: Benzathine penicillin** 1.2 mu IM x1; **Pen V** 500 mg bid or 250 mg qid x10 d.; **erythro**, dosage varies—with erythro base 500 mg qid x10 d.; **cefuroxime axetil** 250 mg bid po x4 d.; **cefpodoxime proxetil** 100 mg bid po x4 d.; **cefdinir** 300 mg q12h x5–10 d.; **cefprozil** 500 mg qd x10 d. NOTE: All O Ceph 2 drugs approved for 10 d. treatment of strep pharyngitis; increasing no. of studies show efficacy of 4–6 d.; **clarithro** 250 mg bid po x10 d.; **azithro** 500 mg po x1 and then 250 mg/d x4 d. **dirithromycin** 500 mg po qd x10 d.

(Footnotes and abbreviations on page 47)   NOTE: *All dosage recommendations are for adults (unless otherwise indicated) and assume normal renal function*

TABLE 1 (34)

ANATOMIC SITE/DIAGNOSIS/ MODIFYING CIRCUMSTANCES	ETIOLOGIES (usual)	SUGGESTED REGIMENS* PRIMARY	SUGGESTED REGIMENS* ALTERNATIVE§	ADJUNCT DIAGNOSTIC OR THERAPEUTIC MEASURES AND COMMENTS
Pharynx (continued)				
Epiglottitis (IDCP 6:500, 1997)				
Children	H. influenzae (rare), S. pyo-genes, S. pneumoniae, S. aureus	Peds dosage: Cefuroxime 50 mg/kg q8h IV or cefo-taxime 50 mg/kg q8h IV or ceftriaxone 50 mg/kg qd IV Adult dosage:See footnote†	AM/SB or TMP/SMX	Have tracheostomy set "at bedside." Chloramphenicol is effective, but poten-tially less toxic alternative agents available. Review (adults): JAMA 272:1358, 1994)
Adults	H. influenzae (rare)			
Parapharyngeal space infection [Spaces include: sublingual, submandibular (Ludwig's angina, used loosely for these), lateral pharyngeal, retropharyngeal, pretracheal]				
Poor dental hygiene, dental extractions, foreign bodies (e.g. toothpicks, fish bones)	Polymicrobic: Strep sp., anaerobes, Eikenella corrodens	(Clinda 600–900 mg IV q8h) or (pen G§ 24 mu by cont. infusion or div. q4–6h IV + metro 1.0 gm load and then 0.5 gm q6h IV)	Cefoxitin 2.0 gm IV or clinda or TC/CL or PIP/TZ or AM/SB (dosage, see footnote page 33)	Close observation of airway, ⅓ require intubation. MRI or CT to identify abscess; if present, surgical drainage. Metro may be given 1.0 gm q12h IV.
Jugular vein septic phlebitis (Lemierre's disease) (Ln 2:701, 1936; Medicine 68:85, 1989)	Fusobacterium necro-phorum in vast majority	Pen G§ 24 mu qd IV by cont. infusion or div. q4–6h IV	Clinda 600–900 mg q8h IV	Usual rx includes external drainage of lateral pharyngeal space and ligation of int. jugular vein. Emboli, pulmonary and systemic common. Erosion into carotid artery can occur.
Laryngitis (hoarseness)/tracheitis	Viral (90%)	Not indicated		
Sinuses, paranasal: Review article, CID 23:1209, 1996				
Sinusitis, acute				
Obstruction of sinus ostia, viral infection, allergens	Strep. pneumoniae 31% H. influenzae 21%, M. catar-rhalis 2%, Group A strep 2%, anaerobes 6%, viruses 15%, Staph. aureus 4%	(AM/CL 875/125 mg bid po x10 d or 500/125 mg tid) or (cefuroxime axetil 250 mg bid po x10 d) or TMP/ SMX³ or amox³. See Comment For dosage in children, see footnote 3; page 34. Also see footnote page 4 re: pen-resist. S. pneumo.	(Cefprozil 250–500 mg bid) or (cefpodoxime 200 mg bid). Rx x10 d. Severe penicillin allergy: Clarithro 500 mg po bid x10 d. (see Comment) See Comment	**If afebrile and draining, suggest symptomatic rx only, e.g., deconges-tants; consider antibacterial rx if symptoms >7–14 d.** Some experts fear rx failure with TMP/SMX and clarithro secondary to resistant H. influenzae, moraxella or DRSP. Despite ↑ prevalence of resistant organisms (DRSP, H. flu, β-lactamase + moraxella), amoxicillin (pen V) rx suggested by some. One randomized placebo-controlled trial showed no benefit of amox over placebo; criteria for sinusitis weak (Ln 349:683, 1997). A 2nd blinded randomized trial, using CT scans for dx, showed modest benefit of pen V and amox over placebo (BMJ 313:329, 1996). Regimens do not reflect rx of S. pneumo with high-level resistance to pen G; **if DRSP, would also consider an active FQ (all po): levo 500 mg qd; spar 400 mg x1, then 200 mg qd; gati 400 mg qd; or moxi 400 mg qd.** No FQs under age 18.
Diabetes mellitus, acute ketoacidosis, neutropenia, deferoxamine rx	Rhizopus sp. (Mucor) Aspergillus	See Table 10, page 75. Reference: NEJM 337:254, 1997		Usual duration 10 d.: in 1 study, results with 3 s 10 d. of TMP/SMX the same (JAMA 273:1015, 1995). CIP approved for acute sinusitis at 500 mg po bid. Not drug of 1st choice for lower respiratory tract infections due to S. pneumoniae. Should same apply to sinusitis? Cefdinir approved for sinusitis; see footnote³

---

¹ Cefuroxime 0.75–1.5 gm IV q8h; ceftriaxone 2.0 gm IV qd; cefotaxime 2.0 gm q4–8h IV.
² Penicillin may be given in divided doses q4–6h or by continuous infusion.
³ **TMP/SMX** 1 double-strength (TMP 160 mg) bid po, **cefaclor** 500 mg q6h po, **cefuroxime** 400 mg qd po, **cefdinir** 300 mg q12h po, **cefixime** 400 mg qd po. **loracarbef** 400 mg q12h po), **ceftibuten** 400 mg qd po (NOTE: poor activity vs pneumococcus), **amoxicillin** 875 mg q12h or 500 mg q8h po
(Footnotes and abbreviations on page 47)   NOTE: All dosage recommendations are for adults (unless otherwise indicated) and assume normal renal function

36

TABLE 1 (35)

ANATOMIC SITE/DIAGNOSIS/ MODIFYING CIRCUMSTANCES	ETIOLOGIES (usual)	SUGGESTED REGIMENS* PRIMARY	ALTERNATIVE§	ADJUNCT DIAGNOSTIC OR THERAPEUTIC MEASURES AND COMMENTS
Sinuses, paranasal/Sinusitis, acute *(continued)*				
Hospitalized + nasotracheal or nasogastric intubation	Gm-neg. bacilli (47%) (Pseudomonas, Acinetobacter, E. coli common), Gm + (S. aureus) 35%, yeasts 18% Polymicrobial in 80%	Remove nasotracheal tube and if fever persists, recommend sinus aspiration for C/S prior to empiric rx IMP 0.5 gm q6h IV or MER 1.0 gm q8h IV	(AP Pen) or (ceftaz + vanco) or (CFP 2.0 gm q12h IV)	After 7 d. of nasotracheal or gastric tubes, 95% have x-ray "sinusitis" (fluid in sinuses), but on transnasal puncture only 38% culture + (AJRCCM 150:776, 1994). For pts requiring mechanical ventilation for ≥1 wk, bacterial sinusitis occurs in <10% (CID 27:851, 1998). May need fluconazole if yeast on Gram stain of aspirate. Review: CID 25:1441, 1997. Epidemiology study: CID 27:463, 1998.
Sinusitis, chronic Adults	Anaerobic (Bacteroides often present (Bacteroides sp., peptostreptococci, Fusobacterium sp.). Etiologic role unclear--see Comment	Antibiotics usually not effective	Otolaryngology consultation. If acute exacerbation, rx as acute	Pathogenesis unclear and may be polyfactorial: damage to ostiomeatal complex during acute bacterial disease, allergy ± polyps, occult immunodeficiency, and/or odontogenic disease (periodontitis in maxillary teeth).
Skin				
Acne vulgaris *(NEJM 336:1156, 1997; Ln 351:1871, 1998)*				
Comedonal acne, "blackheads," "whiteheads," earliest form, no inflammation	Excessive sebum production & gland obstruction. No Propionibacterium acnes	Topical tretinoin once daily (cream 0.025 or 0.05%) or (gel 0.01 or 0.025%)	Topical adapalene 0.1% gel once daily OR azelaic acid 20% cream once daily	Goal is prevention. ↓ number of new comedones and create an environment unfavorable to P. acnes. Adapalene causes less irritation than tretinoin. Azelaic acid less potent but less irritating than retinoids.
Mild inflammatory acne: small papules or pustules	Proliferation of P. acnes + abnormal desquamation of follicular cells	Topical erythro 3% + benzoyl peroxide 5%, bid	Can substitute clinda 1% gel for erythro	Topical metro has anti-inflammatory activity but P. acnes not susceptible.
Inflammatory acne: comedones, papules & pustules. Less common: deep nodules (cysts)	Progression of above events	(Topical erythro 3% + benzoyl peroxide 5% bid) ± oral antibiotic	Oral drugs: (doxy 100 mg bid) or (minocycline 50 mg bid). Others: tetracycline, erythro, TMP/SMX, clinda	Systemic isotretinoin reserved for pts with severe widespread nodular cystic lesions that fail oral antibiotic rx; 4–5 mo. course of 0.1–1.0 mg/kg/day. Tetracyclines stain developing teeth. Doxy can cause photosensitivity. Minocycline side-effects: urticaria, vertigo, pigment deposition in skin or oral mucosa.
Acne rosacea	? Skin mite: Demodex folliculorum	Metro (topical), cream or gel	Doxy 100 mg bid po	Metro efficacious in randomized double-blind, placebo-controlled trial (Cutis 61:44, 1998).
Anthrax, cutaneous, inhalation (pulmonary, mediastinal) In biologic warfare: JAMA 281:1735, 1999; see Lung, page 30	B. anthracis Review: NEJM 341:815, 1999	Pen G 20 mu/d IV div. q6h	(CIP 750 mg po or 400 mg IV bid) or (doxy 100 mg po/IV bid)	With inhalation (pulmonary), use IV regimen. Individuals at occupational risk of exposure should be immunized. Prolonged rx (6 weeks) may be required.
Bacillary angiomatosis: See Cat-scratch disease lymphadenitis, page 31, and Bartonella, page 41				
Immunocompromised (HIV-1, bone marrow transplant) Also see SANFORD GUIDE TO HIV/AIDS THERAPY	Bartonella (Rochalimaea) henselae and quintana	Clarithro 500 mg bid po or azithro 250 mg qd po or CIP 500–750 mg bid po (see Comment)	Erythro 500 mg qid po or doxy 100 mg po bid	In immunocompromised pts with severe disease, doxy 100 mg po/IV bid + RIF 300 mg po bid reported effective (IDC No. Amer 12:37, 1998; Adv PID 11:1, 1996).

(Footnotes and abbreviations on page 47)

NOTE: All dosage recommendations are for adults (unless otherwise indicated) and assume normal renal function

TABLE 1 (36)

ANATOMIC SITE/DIAGNOSIS/ MODIFYING CIRCUMSTANCES	ETIOLOGIES (usual)	SUGGESTED REGIMENS* PRIMARY	SUGGESTED REGIMENS* ALTERNATIVE§	ADJUNCT DIAGNOSTIC OR THERAPEUTIC MEASURES AND COMMENTS
Skin *(continued)*				
Bite: Prophylaxis within 12 hrs of bite or empirical rx of established infection. *Reference: CID 14:633, 1992;* remember tetanus prophylaxis—*see Table 20.*				
Bat, raccoon, skunk	?	AM/CL 875/125 mg bid or 500/125 mg po	Doxy 100 mg bid po	In Americas, antirabies rx indicated, rabies immune globulin + vaccine. *(See Table 20C, page 128)*
Cat *(Ref.: NEJM 340:85 & 138, 1999)*	**Pasteurella multocida,** Staph. aureus	AM/CL 875/125 mg bid or 500/125 mg po	Cefuroxime axetil 0.5 gm q12h po or doxy 100 mg bid po. **Do not use cephalexin**	80% cat bites become infected. **P. multocida resistant to dicloxacillin, cephalexin, clinda; many strains resistant to erythro** (most sensitive to azithro but no clinical data). P. multocida infection develops within 24 hrs. Observe for osteomyelitis. If culture + for only P. multocida, can switch to pen G IV or Pen VK po.
Catfish sting	Toxins	*See Comments*		Present as immediate pain, erythema and edema. Resemble strep cellulitis. May become secondarily infected: AM/CL is reasonable choice for prophylaxis.
Dog Ref.: *NEJM 340:85 & 138, 1999*	**P. multocida,** S. aureus, Bacteroides, Fusobacterium sp., EF-4, Capnocytophaga	AM/CL 875/125 mg bid or 500/125 mg po	Clinda 300 mg qid po + FQ (adults) or clinda + TMP/SMX (children)	Only 5% dog bites become infected. Prophylaxis may be worthwhile (*AnEM 23:535, 1994*). Consider antirabies rx: rabies immune globulin + vaccine (*Table 20C*). May transmit blastomycosis. Capnocytophaga in splenectomized pts may cause local eschar, sepsis with DIC. **P. multocida resistant to diclox, cephalexin, clinda and erythro;** sensitive to FQs in vitro (*AAC 43:1475, 1999*)
Human	Viridans strep 100%, Staph. epidermidis 53%, corynebacterium 41%, **Staph. aureus 29%, eikenella 15%,** bacteroides 82%, peptostrep 26%	**Early** (not yet infected): AM/CL 875/125 mg bid po x5 d. **Later:** Signs of infection (usually in 3–24 hrs): (AM/SB 1.5 gm q6h IV or cefoxitin 2.0 gm q8h IV) or [TC/CL 3.1 gm q6h IV) or [PIP/TZ (3.375 gm q6h or 4.5 gm q8h) IV] Pen allergy: clinda + (either CIP or TMP/SMX)		Cleaning, irrigation and debridement most important. For clenched fist injuries, x-rays should be obtained. Bites inflicted by hospitalized patients, consider aerobic Gm-neg. bacilli. **Eikenella resistant to clinda, PRSP, metro and ± to P Ceph 1 and erythro; susceptible to FQs and TMP/SMX.** For in vitro susceptibility to FQs and macrolides: *JAC 41:391, 1998.*
Pig (swine)	Polymicrobic: Gm + cocci, Gm-neg. bacilli, anaerobes, Pasteurella sp.	AM/CL 875/125 mg bid po	P Ceph 3 or TC/CL or AM/SB or IMP	Information limited but infection is common and serious (*Ln 348:888, 1996*).
Primate, non-human	Microbiology ? Herpesvirus simiae	Acyclovir: *See Table 14B, page 107*		*CID 20:421, 1995*
Rat	Spirillum minus & Streptobacillus moniliformis	AM/CL 875/125 mg bid po	Doxy	Antirabies rx not indicated
Snake: pit viper	Pseudomonas sp., Enterobacteriaceae, Staph. epidermidis, Clostridium sp.	Primary therapy is antivenom. Penicillin generally used but would not be effective vs organisms isolated. Ceftriaxone should be more effective. Tetanus prophylaxis indicated.		
Spider				
Widow (Latrodectus)	Not infectious	None		May be confused with "acute abdomen." Diazepam or calcium gluconate helpful to control pain, muscle spasm. Tetanus prophylaxis.
Brown recluse (Loxosceles)	Not infectious	Dapsone 50 mg qd po *(see Comment)*		Most pts do well without systemic rx. Dapsone followed by excision at 6 weeks (*An Surg 202:659, 1985*) reported effective. Screen for G6PD deficiency, if positive dapsone contraindicated.
Boils, recurrent—Furunculosis				
Acute episode	Staph. aureus	Not effective: hot packs and drainage		Systemic antibiotics do not shorten course of a boil. *(See Skin, furunculosis, page 39)*

(Footnotes and abbreviations on page 47)

NOTE: *All dosage recommendations are for adults (unless otherwise indicated) and assume normal renal function*

37

TABLE 1 (37)

ANATOMIC SITE/DIAGNOSIS/ MODIFYING CIRCUMSTANCES	ETIOLOGIES (usual)	SUGGESTED REGIMENS*		ADJUNCT DIAGNOSTIC OR THERAPEUTIC MEASURES AND COMMENTS
		PRIMARY	ALTERNATIVE§	
Skin/Boils, recurrent—Furunculosis *(continued)*				
Prevention of recurrences (goal is to eliminate nasal carriage of Staph. aureus)	Staph. aureus—MSSA *For control of MRSA, see below*	Mupirocin nasal (2%, apply small amount intranasally bid x5 d.)	RiF 600 mg qd po + either [dicloxacillin 500 mg qid po x10 d. or TMP/SMX 1 double-strength tab (TMP 160 mg) bid po] x10 d.	Mupirocin intranasal effective vs S. aureus including MRSA *(JAC 19:1, 1987)*. RiF + clox/diclox also effective *(AnIM 114:101, 1991)*. Subset of pts with impaired neutrophil function responded to vitamin C, 1 gm/day *(JID 173:1502, 1997)*.
Hidradenitis suppurativa	Lesions secondarily infected: S. aureus, enterobacteriaceae, pseudomonas, anaerobes	Aspirate, base rx on culture		Caused by keratinous plugging of apocrine glands of axillary and/or inguinal areas. Many pts ultimately require surgical excision.
Methicillin-resistant S. aureus—colonization	MRSA	Mupirocin (topical 2% to nares and wounds) bid x1–2 weeks	(Novobiocin 250 mg po + RIF po) or (TMP/SMX po + RIF)	Mupirocin cleared 95% when applied to nares and wounds. But with maintenance rx 40% recurrence with acquired mupirocin resistance in 11% *(AJM 94:371, 1993; AAC 37:1334, 1993)*.
Burns				
Initial burn wound care *(NEJM 335:1581, 1996)*	Not infected	Silver sulfadiazine cream, 1%	0.5% silver nitrate solution or 11.1% mafenide acetate cream	Marrow-induced neutropenia can occur during 1st wk of sulfadiazine but resolves even if use is continued. Silver nitrate leaches electrolytes from wounds and stains everything. Mafenide inhibits carbonic anhydrase and can cause metabolic acidosis.
Burn wound sepsis	Strep pyogenes, Enterobacter sp., S. aureus, S. epidermidis, E. faecalis, E. coli, P. aeruginosa. Fungi rare. Herpesvirus rare.	(Vanco 1.0 gm q12h IV) + (amikacin 10 mg/kg loading dose then 7.5 mg/kg q12h IV) + [PIP 4.0 gm q4h IV (give ½ daily dose of AP Pen into subeschar tissues with surgical eschar removal within 12 hours)]		Monitor serum levels, 1/2 of most antibiotics ↓. Staph. aureus tend to remain localized to burn wound. If patient more toxic than expected, consider toxic shock syndrome. Candida sp. colonize but seldom invade. Pneumonia has become the major infectious complication, most often staph. Other infectious complications include septic thrombophlebitis.
Cellulitis, erysipelas				
Extremities, not associated with venous catheter *(See Comments)* *For diabetes, see below*	Group A strep, occ. Group B, C, G. Staph. aureus (uncommon but difficult to exclude)	[PRSP (nafcillin or oxacillin 2.0 gm q4h IV or if not severe, dicloxacillin 500 mg q6h po) or cefazolin 1.0 gm q8h IV]	Erythro[1] or P Ceph 1 or AM/CL or azithro or clarithro *(Dosage, see footnote, page 27)* *See Comment*	"Spontaneous" erysipelas of leg in non-diabetic is usually due to strep, Gps A, B, C and G. Hence OK to start with IV Pen G 1–2 mu q6h and observe for localized S. aureus infection. Look for tinea pedis with fissures, a common portal of entry; can often culture strep from between toes *(CID 23:1162, 1996)*. For rx of pts with lymphedema and recurrent erysipelas, see prophylaxis, Table 15. Other alternatives: clinda, gati, levo, moxi.
Facial, adult (erysipelas)	Group A strep, Staph. aureus	PRSP *(Dosage, see erysipelas of extremity, above)*	P Ceph 1 or vanco if not severe, AM/CL	**In distinction from extremity, choice of empiric therapy must have activity vs S. aureus.**
Diabetes mellitus and erysipelas	Group A strep, Staph. aureus, Enterobacteriaceae; clostridia (rare)	Early mild: P Ceph 2/3 or AM/CL. Only for severe disease: IMP or MER or trova IV *(Dosage, see page 11, Diabetic Foot)*		Prompt surgical debridement indicated to rule out necrotizing fasciitis and to obtain cultures. If septic, consider x-ray of extremity to demonstrate gas. Prognosis dependent on blood supply: assess arteries. See diabetic foot, page 11.
Erysipelas, recurrent 2° to congenital lymphedema (Milroy's disease)	S. pyogenes, Groups A, C, G	Benzathine pen G 1.2 million U IM q4wks [of minimal benefit in reducing recurrences in pts with underlying predisposing conditions *(CID 25:685, 1997)*]		Indicated only if pt is having frequent episodes of cellulitis. Pen V 250 mg po bid should be effective but not aware of clinical trials. In pen-allergic pts: erythro 500 mg po qd, azithro 250 mg po qd, or clarithro 500 mg po qd.
Dandruff (seborrheic dermatitis)	Malassezia species	Ketoconazole shampoo 2% or selenium sulfide 2.5% *(see page 6, chronic external otitis)*		

---

[1] Rapid increase of resistance of Strep. pyogenes to erythro and clinda reported from Italy *(EID 2:339, 1996)*.

(Footnotes and abbreviations on page 47)

§ NOTE: *All dosage recommendations are for adults (unless otherwise indicated) and assume normal renal function*

TABLE 1 (38)

ANATOMIC SITE/DIAGNOSIS/ MODIFYING CIRCUMSTANCES	ETIOLOGIES (usual)	SUGGESTED REGIMENS* PRIMARY	SUGGESTED REGIMENS* ALTERNATIVE§	ADJUNCT DIAGNOSTIC OR THERAPEUTIC MEASURES AND COMMENTS
Skin (continued) **Decubitus ulcers, with sepsis**	Polymicrobic: S. pyogenes (Groups A,C,G), enterococci, anaerobic strep, Enterobacteriaceae, Pseudomonas sp., Staph. aureus	IMP or MER or TC/CL or PIP/TZ *(Dosages, see footnotes, pages 11, 17, 22, 44)*	[(CIP, gati, or levo) + (clinda or metro)].	Without sepsis or extensive cellulitis local care may be adequate. Debride as needed. Topical mafenide or silver sulfadiazine adjunctive. Rule out underlying osteomyelitis. In nursing home with MRSA, vanco required for Staph. aureus.
Erythema multiforme	H. simplex type 1, mycoplasma, Strep. pyogenes, drugs (sulfonamides, phenytoin, penicillins)			Rx: Acyclovir if due to H. simplex
Erythema nodosum	Sarcoidosis, inflammatory bowel disease. M. tbc, coccidioidomycosis, yersinia, sulfonamides			Rx: NSAIDs; glucocorticoids if refractory.
Erythrasma	Corynebacterium minutissimum	Erythro 250 mg q6h po x14 d.		Coral red fluorescence with Wood's lamp. Alt: 2% aqueous clinda topically.
Furunculosis with cellulitis and/or sepsis (See Boils, recurrent, pages 37,38)	Staph. aureus	PRSP (nafcillin or oxacillin 2.0 gm q6h IV)	P Ceph 1 (cefazolin 1–2 gm q8h IV) or vanco 1.0 gm q12h IV	Surgical drainage. Hexachlorophene soap. Suppression of nasal carriage of Staph. aureus.
Hemorrhagic bullous lesions Hx of sea water-contaminated abrasion or eating raw seafood, shock	Vibrio vulnificus, V. damsela	Ceftazidime 2.0 gm q8h IV + doxy 100 mg bid (IV or po)	Either cefotaxime 2.0 gm q8h IV or CIP 750 mg bid po or 400 mg bid IV)	¾ patients have chronic liver disease. Mortality 50% (NEJM 312:343, 1985). There are no controlled studies. In Taiwan, where a number of cases are seen, the impression exists that ceftazidime is superior to tetracyclines (CID 15:271, 1992). Why not both?
No hx of saltwater exposure	Staph or strep septic shock, clostridia	See Gas gangrene, page 32		
Herpes zoster (shingles): See Table 14				
Impetigo, ecthyma—usually children "Honey-crust" lesions (non-bullous)	Group A strep impetigo	Pen VK po or O Ceph 1 or benzathine penicillin IM *(For dosages, see Table 9B)*	Mupirocin ointment tid or azithro or clarithro or erythro or O Ceph 2	24% failure with Pen VK (AJDC 144:1313, 1990). O Ceph 2 >90% cure (AAC 36:1674, 1992).
Bullous (if ruptured), thin "varnish-like" crust)	Staph. aureus impetigo	Dicloxacillin po or oxacillin po or O Ceph 1 (not cefixime) *(For dosages, see Table 9B)*	Mupirocin ointment or AM/CL or azithro or clarithro	NOTE: Cefixime not active vs Staph. aureus.
Whirlpool (Hot Tub) folliculitis	Pseudomonas aeruginosa	Usually self-limited, treatment not indicated		Decontaminate hot tub: drain and chlorinate. Also associated with exfoliative beauty aids (loofah sponges) (J Clin Micro 31:480, 1993).
Infected wound, extremity—Post-trauma (For bites, see above; for post-operative, see below) Afebrile	Polymicrobic: Staph. aureus, Group A & anaerobic strep, Enterobacteriaceae, Cl. perfringens, Cl. tetani (if water exposure, Pseudomonas sp., Aeromonas sp.)	[AM/CL 875/125 mg bid or 500/125 mg tid po) or O Ceph 1 (Dosage, page 10)	Erythro or clarithro or azithro or clinda (Dosage, page 27)	Wound cleansing and debridement. Gram stain may enable rapid diagnosis of clostridia, staph. **Antitetanus prophylaxis.** (See Table 20C, page 128) If freshwater exposure, Pseudomonas and Aeromonas species possible—FQ recommended therapy. If sea water, see hemorrhagic bullous lesions and Vibrio vulnificus, above.
Febrile, with sepsis		AM/SB or TC/CL or PiP/TZ or IMP or MER (Dosage, page 17)	PRSP (nafcillin or oxacillin 2.0 gm q4h IV) + CIP + clinda	Trova 200 mg IV qd should work for life- or limb-threatening severe infection.

(Footnotes and abbreviations on page 47)   NOTE: All dosage recommendations are for adults (unless otherwise indicated) and assume normal renal function

TABLE 1 (39)

ANATOMIC SITE/DIAGNOSIS/ MODIFYING CIRCUMSTANCES	ETIOLOGIES (usual)	SUGGESTED REGIMENS* PRIMARY	ALTERNATIVE§	ADJUNCT DIAGNOSTIC OR THERAPEUTIC MEASURES AND COMMENTS
Skin (continued)				
Necrotizing fasciitis ("flesh-eating bacteria")				
Post-surgery, trauma, streptococcal skin infections (see footnote)[1] See Gas Gangrene, p. 31, and Toxic Shock, p. 44	Streptococci, Group A, C, G; Clostridia sp.; Polymicrobic: aerobic + anaerobic; rarely, aerobic coliform alone	For treatment, see Muscle, gas gangrene. The terminology of polymicrobic wound infections is not precise. Meleney's synergistic gangrene, Fournier's gangrene, necrotizing fasciitis have a common pathophysiology. **All require prompt surgical debridement** as well as antibiotics. Dx of necrotizing fasciitis requires incision and probing. If no resistance to probing, dx = necrotizing fasciitis. If unexperienced, frozen section of biopsy (NEJM 310:1689, 1984). Need Gram stain/culture to determine if etiology is strep, clostridia or polymicrobial.		
Infected wound, post-operative				
Surgery not involving GI or female genital tract				
Without sepsis	Staph. aureus, Group A strep, Enterobacteriaceae	O Ceph 1 or AM/CL	Dicloxacillin po po	Gram stain exudate to guide treatment choice. Surgical drainage alone often adequate. Where MRSA prevalent, add vanco. In pts without sepsis after 72 hours, patient can be switched to oral therapy. Treat until pt afebrile and wound granulating.
With sepsis		TC/CL or PIP/TZ or AM/SB (Dosage, see page 17)	P Ceph 1/2/3 (Dosage, see page 17)	
Surgery involving GI tract (includes oropharynx, esophagus) or female genital tract	Above + Bacteroides sp., other anaerobes, enterococci, Group B, C strep	Cefoxitin or cefotetan or TC/CL or PIP/TZ or AM/SB or (P Ceph 2/3 + metro) or IMP or MER. Trova another option.	TC/CL or PIP/TZ or AM/SB	For all treatment options, see Peritonitis, page 33. Trova dose: 300 mg IV qd, then 200 mg po qd
Meleney's synergistic gangrene	See Necrotizing fasciitis, above			
Staphylococcal scalded skin syndrome	Toxin-producing S. aureus	Nafcillin or oxacillin 2 gm IV q4h (children: 150 mg/kg/d div. q6h) x5–7 days		Toxin causes intraepidermal split and positive Nikolsky sign. Drugs cause epiderm/dermal split, called **toxic epidermal necrolysis**—more serious (Ln 351: 1417, 1998). Biopsy differentiates.
Spleen				
Splenic abscess				
Endocarditis, bacteremia	Staph. aureus, streptococci	PRSP (nafcillin or oxacillin 2.0 gm IV)	Vanco 1.0 gm q12h IV	MRI imaging is diagnostic procedure of choice. Standard rx is splenectomy + antibiotics. Burkholderia (Pseudomonas) pseudomallei is common cause of splenic abscess in SE Asia.
Contiguous from intra-abdominal site	Polymicrobic	Treat as Peritonitis, secondary, page 33		
Immunocompromised	Candida sp.	Amphotericin B (Dosage, see Table 10, page 72)	Fluconazole	
Systemic Febrile Syndromes				
Spread by infected **TICK, FLEA, or LICE** (CID 29:888, 1999): Epidemiologic history crucial. Institute empiric therapy prior to establishing an etiologic diagnosis (JAMA 275:463, 1996).				
Babesiosis: see CID 22:611, 1996	Etiol.: B. microti et al. Vector: Usually Ixodes ticks Host: White-footed mouse & others	Do not treat if asymptomatic, young, has spleen, & immunocompetent. Clinda 1.2 gm bid IV or 600 mg tid po x7 d. + quinine 650 mg tid po x7 d. Ped. dosage: Clinda 20–40 mg/kg/d and quinine 25 mg/kg/d		Exposure endemic areas May to Sept. Can result from blood transfusion (JAMA 287:927, 1999). Usually subclinical. Illness likely in asplenic pts, pts with Lyme disease, older pts, pts with HIV. Dx: Giemsa-stained blood smear; antibody test available. PCR under study. Rx: Exchange transfusions successful adjunct, used early, in severe disease

[1] Good evidence that incidence of invasive Group A strep infection (necrotizing fasciitis and toxic shock) is increasing. Also risk of transmission in households and health care institutions (NEJM 335:547, 1996).

(Footnotes and abbreviations on page 47)

NOTE: All dosage recommendations are for adults (unless otherwise indicated) and assume normal renal function

TABLE 1 (40)

ANATOMIC SITE/DIAGNOSIS/ MODIFYING CIRCUMSTANCES	ETIOLOGIES (usual)	SUGGESTED REGIMENS*		ADJUNCT DIAGNOSTIC OR THERAPEUTIC MEASURES AND COMMENTS
		PRIMARY	ALTERNATIVE†	
Systemic Febrile Syndromes (continued)				
Bartonella				
Asymptomatic bacteremia	B. quintana	Doxy 100 mg po/IV x15 d.		Blood cultures pos. in 14% of homeless, esp. if lice/leg pain (NEJM 340:184, 1999).
Cat-scratch disease	B. henselae	See page 31 under lymphadenitis		
Bacillary angiomatosis; Peliosis hepatis—pts with AIDS	B. henselae, B. quintana	Erythro 500 mg qid po or doxy 100 mg bid po	Clarithro 500 mg bid or azithro 250 mg qd or CIP 500–750 mg bid.po	If severe, consider combination of doxy 100 mg po/IV bid + RIF 300 mg po bid (IDC No Amer 12:137, 1998; Adv PID 11:1, 1996).
Endocarditis (see page 21) (AnIM 125:646, 1996)	B. henselae, B. quintana	No definitive rx regimen: aminoglycoside + surgery. Others have used FQ or RIF or macrolide ± surgery		Hard to detect with automated blood culture systems. Need lysis-centrifugation and/or blind subculture onto chocolate agar at 7 & 14 days. Diagnosis often by antibody titer ≥1:1600.
Trench fever	B. quintana	Doxy 100 mg bid po		
Ehrlichiosis[1]				
Human monocytic ehrlichiosis (HME) (IDCP 7:252, 1998)	Ehrlichia chaffeensis (Lone Star tick is vector)	Doxy 100 mg bid po or IV x7–14 d.	Tetracycline 500 mg qid po x7–14 d. No current recommendation for children or pregnancy	30 states: mostly SE of line from NJ to Ill. to Missouri to Oklahoma to Texas. History of outdoor activity and tick exposure. April-Sept. Fever, rash (36%), leukopenia and thrombocytopenia. Blood smears no help. PCR for early dx.
Human granulocytic ehrlichiosis (HGE) (JAMA 275:199, 1996 & AnIM 125:904, 1996)	Ehrlichia equi/phagocytophilia (Ixodes tick is vector)	Doxy 100 mg bid po/IV x7–14 d.	Tetra 500 mg 4x/d. po x7–14 d. Not in children or pregnancy.	Upper Midwest, NE, West Coast & Europe. H/O tick exposure. April-Sept. Febrile flu-like illness after outdoor activity. No rash. Leukopenia/thrombocytopenia common. Dx: Up to 80% have positive blood smear. Antibody test for confirmation. Rx: Evidence for activity of erythro; RIF successful in pregnancy (CID 27:213, 1998). Chloro, new FQs active in vitro.
Human/dog granulocytic ehrlichiosis (NEJM 341:148 & 195, 1999)	Ehrlichia ewingii	Doxy 100 mg bid po/IV x7–14 d.		Previously only recognized in dogs; human cases now documented. Inclusion in granulocytes.

[1] In endemic area (New York), high % of both adult ticks and nymphs were jointly infected with both HGE and B. burgdorferi (NEJM 337:49, 1997).

(Footnotes and abbreviations on page 47)   NOTE: All dosage recommendations are for adults (unless otherwise indicated) and assume normal renal function

TABLE 1 (41)

ANATOMIC SITE/DIAGNOSIS/ MODIFYING CIRCUMSTANCES	ETIOLOGIES (usual)	SUGGESTED REGIMENS*		ADJUNCT DIAGNOSTIC OR THERAPEUTIC MEASURES AND COMMENTS
		PRIMARY	ALTERNATIVE§	
Systemic Febrile Syndromes. Spread by infected **TICK, FLEA, or LICE** (continued)				
Lyme Disease (Erythema chronicum migrans, Acrodermatitis chronica atrophicans)—Diagnosis primarily clinical: see Comment under etiology regarding serology. Review: Ln 352:557, 1998. For pediatric review: PIDJ 18:913, 1999NOTE: Think about concomitant tick-borne disease —babesiosis (JAMA 275: 1657, 1996) or ehrlichiosis.				
Tick bite; possible Ixodes acquired in endemic area	Borrelia burgdorferi	Antibiotic rx not indicated. See Comments	See NEJM 327:1769, 1992.	Transmission of B. burgdorferi occurs in ~10% of bites by infected ticks. Prompt removal of tick ↓ risk of transmission.
Early (erythema chronicum migrans) (See Comments) Treatment summary in Med Lett 39:47, 1997	**Lab tests: Lab tests support clinical dx but not basis for dx or rx.** Substantial variance in commercial antibody/ immunoblot tests (JAMA 282:62 & 79, 1999). FDA/CDC support 2-step testing: (1) antibody by ELISA/EIA/IFA; (2) If pos. Western blot. Lyme vaccine → Lyme antibody.	Doxy 100 mg bid po x14-21 d or cefuroxime axetil 500 mg bid x20 d or clarithro 500 mg bid x14-21 d or azithro 500 mg po qd x7-21 d.		Neurologic disease may develop or progress on oral regimen. Cefuroxime and doxy reported equivalent (AAC 39:661, 1995). Might prefer doxy if suspect concomitant ehrlichiosis. Azithro x7 days failed in double-blind trial vs amox (AnIM 124:785, 1996); of interest, clarithro effective in 21-day trial (AAC 40:468, 1996). Good prognosis in treated children (NEJM 335:1270, 1996).
Carditis		(Ceftriaxone 2.0 gm qd IV) or (cefotaxime 2.0 gm q4h IV) or (Pen G 24 mu qd IV) x14-21 d	Doxy (See Comments) 100 mg bid x21 d or amoxicillin 250–500 mg po tid x21 d	Doxy: Oral regimen only for mild cardiac involvement.
Facial nerve paralysis (isolated finding, early)		(Doxy 100 mg bid po) or (amoxicillin 500 mg tid po) x21-28 d	Ceftriaxone 2.0 gm qd IV x14-28 d.	LP suggested to exclude neurologic disease. If LP neg., oral regimen OK. If abnormal or not done, suggest parenteral regimen.
Meningitis For encephalopathy, see Comment		Ceftriaxone 2.0 gm qd IV x21 d.	Pen G 20 mu qd in div. dose IV or cefotaxime 2.0 gm q8h IV x21 d.	Encephalopathy: memory difficulty, depression, somnolence, or headache, CSF abnormalities. 18/18 pts improved with ceftriaxone 2 gm/d. x30 d. (JID 180:377, 1999).
Arthritis		(Doxy 100 mg bid) or (amoxicillin 500 mg qid) po, both x28 d.	(Ceftriaxone 2 gm qd IV) or (Pen G 20-24 mu/d IV) x14-28 d	
Pregnant women		None indicated	Choice should not include doxy; amoxicillin 500 mg po tid x21 d.	
Asymptomatic seropositivity		None indicated		See CID 18:112, 1994
Plague (CID 26:122, 1998)	Yersinia pestis Reservoir: rat Vector: rat flea	Gentamicin 2.0 mg/kg IV loading dose then 1.7 mg/kg q8h IV or streptomycin 1.0 gm q12h IM or IV	(Doxy 100 mg bid po or IV) or (chloramphenicol 500 mg qid po or IV)	Reference IV streptomycin: CID 19:1150, 1994. Septicemic form can occur without buboes. CDC reports 229 cases of plague in U.S. 1980-1994 (MMWR 45(RR-14), 1996). Cipro effective in vitro + animal models (JAC 41:301, 1998). Plasmid-mediated resistance to aminoglycosides reported from Madagascar.
Relapsing fever (CID 26:122, 1998) Can be tick-borne or louse-borne	Borrelia recurrentis and other borrelia sp.	Doxy 100 mg bid po	Erythro 500 mg qid po	Jarisch-Herxheimer in most patients (occurs in ~2 hrs). Not prevented by prior steroids. Dx: Examine peripheral blood smear during fever for spirochetes.
Rickettsial diseases				
Spotted fevers (NOTE: Rickettsial pox not included)				
Rocky Mountain spotted fever (RMSF) (CID 27:1353, 1998) NOTE: Can mimic Ehrlichiosis. Pattern of rash important	R. rickettsii (Dermacentor ticks)	Doxy 100 mg bid po or IV x7 d. or for 2 days after temp. normal	Chloramphenicol 500 mg qid po or IV x7 d. or for 2 days after temp. normal	Fever, rash (95%), petechiae 40-50%. Rash spreads from distal extremities to trunk. Dx: Immunohistology on skin biopsy; confirmation with antibody titers. Highest incidence in Mid-Atlantic states; also seen in Oklahoma, S. Dakota, Montana.

(Footnotes and abbreviations on page 47) NOTE: All dosage recommendations are for adults (unless otherwise indicated) and assume normal renal function

TABLE 1 (42)

ANATOMIC SITE/DIAGNOSIS/ MODIFYING CIRCUMSTANCES	ETIOLOGIES (usual)	SUGGESTED REGIMENS*		ADJUNCT DIAGNOSTIC OR THERAPEUTIC MEASURES AND COMMENTS
		PRIMARY	ALTERNATIVE§	
Systemic Febrile Syndromes, Spread by infected **TICK, FLEA,** or **LICE/Rickettsial diseases**/Spotted fevers *(continued)*				
Other spotted fevers, e.g., Boutonneuse fever	6 species: R. conorii et al. (multiple ticks)	As for RMSF	As for RMSF. Few reports of success with CIP	Death rate from Boutonneuse fever similar to RMSF (69%). Rash not prominent. Dx as for RMSF. High incidence rickettsial disease masquerading as dengue in Mexico *(AJTMH 55:157, 1996)*.
Typhus group—Consider in returning travelers with fever				
Louse-borne	R. prowazekii (body louse)	As for RMSF	As for RMSF	Brill-Zinsser disease is a relapse of remote past infection, e.g., WW II. Truncal rash spreads centrifugally—opposite of RMSF. A winter disease.
Murine typhus (cat flea typhus similar)	R. typhi (rat reservoir and flea vector)	As for RMSF	As for RMSF	Most U.S. cases south Texas and southern Calif. Flu-like illness. Rash in <50%. Dx based on suspicion; confirmed serologically.
Scrub typhus	O. tsutsugamushi [rodent reservoir; vector is larval stage of mites (chiggers)]	As for RMSF. NOTE: Reports of doxy and chloramphenicol resistance from northern Thailand *(Ln 348:86, 1996)*.		Limited to Far East (Asia, India). Cases imported into U.S. Evidence of chigger bite; flu-like illness. Rash like louse-borne typhus.
Tularemia, typhoidal type	Francisella tularensis. (Vector depends on geography; ticks, biting flies, mosquitoes identified)	Streptomycin 7.5–10 mg/ kg q12h (IM) x7–14 d. (Ped.: 30–40 mg/kg/d IM in 2 div. doses x7 d.)	Gentamicin 3–5 mg/kg/ d div. q8h IV x7–14 d. Add chloramphenicol if evidence of meningitis	Typhoidal form in 5–30% pts. No lymphadenopathy. Diarrhea, pneumonia common. Dx: blood cultures. Antibody confirmation. Rx: Jarisch-Herxheimer reaction may occur. P Ceph 3 is active in vitro but no clinical data. NOTE: CIP active in vitro.
Other Zoonotic Systemic Bacterial Febrile Illnesses: Obtain careful epidemiologic history				
Brucellosis *(Reviews: CID 21:283, 1995; EID 3:213, 1997)*				
Adult or child >8 years	Brucella sp. B. abortus—cattle B. suis—pigs B. melitensis—goats B. canis—dogs	[Doxy 100 mg bid po + gentamicin *(See Table 9C, page 70)*] or [doxy + streptomycin 1.0 gm qd IM] See Comment	[Doxy + RIF 600–900 mg gd po] or [TMP/SMX 1 double-strength tab (160 mg TMP) bid po + gentamicin]	Doxy 100 mg bid po x 6 weeks + strep 1.0 gm qd IM x 2 weeks, relapse rate 6%. With doxy + RIF relapse rate 14%. Doxy + RIF may be less effective than doxy + SM in pts with spondylitis *(AnIM 117:25, 1992)*. CIP alone initially effective but relapse in 25% *(AAC 36:150, 1992)*; however, oflox + RIF reported effective. Duration of rx unclear. For B. melitensis, gent for x7d. + doxy for 30d. *(AAC 41:80, 1997)*. Usual recommendation is 6 wks of rx.
Child <8 years		TMP/SMX 5 mg/kg TMP q12h po + gentamicin 2 mg/kg q8h IV or IM		
Leptospirosis	Leptospira—in urine of domestic livestock, dogs, small rodents	Pen G 20–24 mu qd IV div. q4–6h	Doxy 100 mg q12h IV or po or AMP 0.5–1.0 gm q6h IV	*CID 21:1, 1995.* Illness varies. Two-stage mild anicteric illness to severe icteric disease (Weil's disease) with renal failure and myocarditis. Dx: Can culture but slow and difficult. Usually a serologic diagnosis.
Salmonella bacteremia (enteric fever most often caused by S. typhi)	Salmonella enteritidis—a variety of serotypes	CIP 400 mg q12h IV x14 d. (switch to po 750 mg bid when clinically possible)	Ceftriaxone 2.0 gm qd IV x14d. (switch to po CIP when possible)	Usual exposure is contaminated poultry and eggs. Myriad of complications to consider, e.g., mycotic aneurysm, septic arthritis, osteomyelitis, septic shock. Sporadic reports of resistance to CIP.
Miscellaneous Systemic Febrile Syndromes				
Kawasaki syndrome 6 weeks to 12 yrs of age, peak at 1 yr of age *(CID 28:169, 1999)*	Unknown; syndrome of ↑ temp, rash, conjunctivitis, stomatitis, cervical adenitis, red hands/feet & coronary artery aneurysms	IVIG 2 gm/kg over 12 hrs + ASA 80–100 mg/kg/d po div. in 4 doses THEN ASA 3–5 mg/kg/d po 1x/d. x6–8 wks	If still febrile after 1st dose of IVIG, some give 2nd dose *(PIDJ 17: 1144, 1998)*.	IV gamma globulin (2.0 gm/kg over 10 hrs) in pts rx before 10th day of illness ↓ coronary artery lesions *(Ln 347:1128, 1996)*. A current hypothesis: disease due to toxin (superantigen) production by staph or strep species *(CID 29:586, 1999)*. See Table 14B, page 108 for IVIG adverse effects and expense.

(Footnotes and abbreviations on page 47)

NOTE: All dosage recommendations are for adults (unless otherwise indicated) and assume normal renal function

TABLE 1 (43)

ANATOMIC SITE/DIAGNOSIS/ MODIFYING CIRCUMSTANCES	ETIOLOGIES (usual)	SUGGESTED REGIMENS*		ADJUNCT DIAGNOSTIC OR THERAPEUTIC MEASURES AND COMMENTS
		PRIMARY	ALTERNATIVE§	
Systemic Febrile Diseases/Miscellaneous Systemic Febrile Syndromes (continued)				
Rheumatic Fever, acute Ref.: Ln 349:935, 1997	Post-Group A strep pharyn- gitis (not Group B, C, or G)	(1) Symptom relief: ASA 80–100 mg/kg/d. in children; 4–8 gm/d. in adults. (2) Eradicate Group A strep: Pen x10 d. (see Pharyngitis). (3) Start prophylaxis: see below.		
Prophylaxis				
Primary prophylaxis	Benzathine penicillin G 1.2 million U IM (see Pharyngitis)			Penicillin for 10 days, prevents rheumatic fever even when started 7–9 days after onset of illness.
Secondary prophylaxis (previous documented rheumatic fever)	Benzathine penicillin G 1.2 million U IM q3–4 wks			Alternative: Penicillin V 250 mg po bid or sulfadiazine (sulfisoxazole) 1.0 gm/d. po or erythro 250 mg po bid. Duration of 2° prophylaxis varies: with carditis continue 10 yrs or until age 25; without carditis continue 5 yrs or until age 18 (AnIM 118:401, 1993).
Typhoidal syndrome (typhoid fever, enteric fever) (JAMA 278:847, 1997)	Salmonella typhi, S. para- typhi	(CIP 500 mg bid po x10 d.) or (ceftriaxone 2.0 gm qd IV x5 d). If assoc. shock, give dexametha- sone a few minutes before antibiotic (see Comment)	Azithro 1 gm po day 1, then 500 mg po x6 d. (AAC 43:1441, 1999).	With shock or ↓ mental status, dexamethasone 3 mg/kg q6h then 1 mg/kg q6h x8 doses ↓ mortality (NEJM 310:82, 1984). Look for other complications, e.g., osteo, septic arthritis, mycotic aneurysm, meningitis. Other Rx options: Chloramphenicol 500 mg qid po or IV x14 d. or oflox 15 mg/kg qd x2–3 d. (AAC 40:958, 1996) or cefixime 10–15 mg/kg q12h po x8 d. (JTP 41:364, 1995). Sporadic reports of resistance to CIP.
Sepsis, Septic Shock, Toxic Shock [JAC 41(Suppl.A):41, 1998]				
Neonatal—early onset <1 week old	Group B strep, E. coli, klebsiella, enterobacter, Staph. aureus (uncom- mon), listeria (rare in US)	AMP 25 mg/kg q8h IV + cefotaxime 50 mg/kg q12h	(AMP + APAG 2.5 mg/kg q12h IV or IM) or (AMP + cefotaxime 50 mg/kg q24h IV or IM)	Blood cultures are key but only 5–10% +. Discontinue antibiotics after 72 hrs if cultures and course do not support diagnosis. In Spain, listeria predominates; in S. America, salmonella.
Neonatal—late onset 1–4 weeks old	As above + H. influenzae & S. epidermidis	(AMP 25 mg/kg q6h IV + cefotaxime 50 mg/kg q8h) or (AMP + ceftriaxone 75 mg/kg q24h IV)	AMP + APAG 2.5 mg/kg q8h IV or IM	If Staph. aureus is common, add PRSP or vanco (if MRSA prevalence is high). Reference: PIDJ 16:768, 1997.
Child; non-immunocompromised	H. influenzae, Strep. pneu- moniae, Meningococci, Staph. aureus	Cefotaxime 50 mg/kg q8h IV or ceftriaxone 100 mg/ kg q24h IV or cefuroxime 50 mg/kg q8h IV	PRSP + cefuroxime	AM/SB and TC/CL not currently approved for children. In children who have received recommended course of conjugate Hib vaccine, invasive Hib disease has virtually disappeared, without an increase in other organisms (PIDJ 14:978, 1995; EJCMID 14:935, 1995).
Adult; non-immunocompromised Source unclear but clinical possibilities include S. aureus bacteremia, occult intra- abdominal/pelvic pathology. **not neutropenic**	Gm + cocci, aerobic bacilli, Anaerobes	TC/CL or PIP/TZ or IMP or MER or [APAG + (P Ceph 3 or TC/CL or PIP/TZ) + (clinda or metro)]	[P Ceph 3/4 + either (clinda or metro)] or [IV FQ + (clinda or metro)]	Systemic inflammatory response syndrome (SIRS): 2 or more of the following: 1. Temperature >38°C or <36°C 2. Heart rate >90 beats/min. 3. Respiratory rate >20 breaths/min. 4. WBC >12,000/μl or >10% bands Sepsis: SIRS + a documented infection (+ culture) Severe sepsis: Sepsis + organ dysfunction/ hypotension or hypoperfusion abnormalities (lactic acidosis, oliguria, ↓ mental status) Septic shock: Sepsis-induced hypotension (systolic BP <90 mmHg) not responsive to >500 ml fluid challenge + peripheral hypoperfusion (CCM 20: 864,1992; JAMA 273:117, 1995).
Septic shock review: Ln 351: 1501, 1998		Add vanco only if MRSA a concern. Dosage in footnote[1]		High-dose steroids (methylprednisolone) not beneficial (NEJM 317:581 & 653, 1987).

[1] **P Ceph 3** (cefotaxime 2.0 gm q8h IV, use q4h if life-threatening; **ceftizoxime** 2.0 gm q4h IV; **ceftriaxone** 2.0 gm q4h IV; **AP Pen** (piperacillin 3.0 gm q4h IV, **ticarcillin** 3.0 gm q4h IV, **TC/CL** 3.1 gm q4h IV, **PIP/TZ** 3.375 gm q4h or 4.5 gm q8h IV, **APAG** (See Table 9C, page 70) **AMP** 30 mg/kg q4h IV, **clinda** 900 mg q8h IV, **IMP** 0.5 gm q6h IV, **MER** 1.0 gm q8h IV, **PRSP** (nafcillin or oxacillin 2.0 gm q4h IV, **aztreonam** 2.0 gm q8h IV, **metro** 1.0 gm loading dose then 0.5 gm q6h or 1.0 gm q12h IV, **vanco** 1.0 gm q12h IV, **P Ceph 3 AP** (ceftazidime 2.0 gm q8h IV, **P Ceph 4** [**CFP** 2.0 gm q12h (q8h if neutropenic) IV, **cefpirome**NUS 2.0 gm q12h IV], **CIP** 400 mg q12h IV, **oflox** 400 mg q12h IV, **levo** 500 mg qd

(Footnotes and abbreviations on page 47)   NOTE: All dosage recommendations are for adults (unless otherwise indicated) and assume normal renal function

TABLE 1 (44)

ANATOMIC SITE/DIAGNOSIS/ MODIFYING CIRCUMSTANCES	ETIOLOGIES (usual)	SUGGESTED REGIMENS*		ADJUNCT DIAGNOSTIC OR THERAPEUTIC MEASURES AND COMMENTS
		PRIMARY	ALTERNATIVE§	
Systemic Febrile Syndromes/Sepsis, Septic Shock, Toxic Shock/Adult: non-immunocompromised *(continued)*				
Injection drug users	Staph. aureus	PRSP + APAG	Vanco + APAG	In injection drug users, recommend HIV and hepatitis B/C antibody tests.
Splenectomized	Strep. pneumoniae, H. influenzae, meningococci	Cefotaxime or ceftriaxone as rx. (See Table 15, page 116 for prophylaxis)	Prescribe AM/CL for self-administration at home with onset of any fever. In penicillin-allergic patient, TMP/SMX. Immunization: pneumococcal, Hib, meningococcal.	
Child or adult; neutropenic (absolute neutrophile count <500/mm³) (See *Guidelines: CID 25:551, 1997*) For use of growth factors, e.g., G-CSF: *COID 11:401, 1998* For risk-based therapy, see *CID 29:515, 1999*	Of most concern: aerobic Gm-neg. bacilli to include P. aeruginosa. Other: S. aureus, fungi (candida, aspergillus), viridans streptococci & more. Virulent viridans strep infection recognized *(PIDJ 18: 280, 1999)*	Monotherapy: ceftazidime or IMP or CFP. MER should work but not an FDA-approved indication. *Dosages in footnote⁶ page 44 & Table 10 for APAG. See Comment for vanco use. Continue rx until absolute neutrophil count >500/mm³*	Duotherapy: [APAG] + [AP Pen or TC/CL or PIP/TZ] OR [APAG + ceftaz]	**Monotherapy: Drugs listed do not cover S. epi, MRSA, some entero-cocci, or DRSP.** Duotherapy. Synergistic some Gm-neg. bacilli. Minimal emergence of resistance. Lack of activity vs MRSA or DRSP. Aminoglycoside nephro/ototoxicity a concern. Vanco added when: IV cath inf., severe chemo-induced mucosal-membrane damage, after prophylaxis with FQs, known colonization with MRSA or DRSP, known pos. blood culture for Gm-pos. bacteria, hypotensive pt. Oral rx with CIP + AM/CL as effective as IV rx in **low-risk hospital pts** (*NEJM 341:305, 312 & 362, 1999*). Oral outpatient rx still investigational (*JAC 43:317, 1999*).
Septic shock Bacteremic shock, endotoxin shock Review: *Ln 351:1501, 1998*	Bacteremia with aerobic Gm-neg. bacteria or Gm + cocci	Proven therapeutic modalities: (1) Replete intra-vascular volume, (2) correct, if possible, disease that allowed bloodstream invasion, (3) appropriate empiric antimicrobial rx; see *suggestions under Sepsis, immunocompetent, above*		Clinical evidence of shock (confusion, oliguria/anuria). Lab evidence of endothelial damage (DIC with positive D-dimer). Peripheral vascular collapse with systemic vascular resistance <800. Systolic BP <90 mmHg or 40 mmHg below pt's normal pressure after fluid resuscitation. To date, high-dose steroids, anti-endotoxin, and anti-cytokine trials have failed (*JAMA 276:565, 1996*). Death due to progressive lactic acidosis
Toxic shock syndrome, staphylococcal				
Colonization by toxin-producing Staph. aureus of: vagina (tampon-assoc.), surgical/traumatic wounds, endometrium, burns	Staph. aureus (toxin-mediated)	PRSP (nafcillin or oxacillin 2.0 gm q4h IV)	P Ceph 1 (cefazolin 1-2 gm q8h IV)	PRSP or cephalothin have no effect on initial syndrome, but ↓ recurrences. Seek occult abscess. TSS may occur with "clean" colonized post-op wounds. Case fatality 5–15%. Consider eradication of carrier state *(page 38)*. IVIG reasonable (see *Streptococcal TSS*).
Toxic shock syndrome, streptococcal [Ref: *JID 179 [Suppl.2):S366–374, 1999*]				
Associated with invasive disease, i.e., erysipelas, necrotizing fasciitis; secondary infection of varicella (chickenpox) (*COID 7:423, 1994*). Secondary cases TSS reported (*NEJM 335:547 & 590, 1996; CID 27: 150, 1998*)	Group A, B, C, & G Strep. pyogenes	(Pen G 24 mu/d IV in div. doses) + (clinda 900 mg q8h IV) IVIG associated with ↑ 30-day survival in comparative observational study (*CID 28:800, 1999*). IVIG dose: 150 mg/kg/d x5 d.	Erythro 1.0 gm q6h IV or (ceftriaxone 2.0 gm q24h IV + clinda 900 mg q8h IV)	Definition: Isolation of Group A strep, hypotension and ≥2 of: renal impairment, coagulopathy, liver involvement, ARDS, generalized rash, soft tissue necrosis (*JAMA 269:390, 1993*). Associated with invasive disease. Surgery usually required. Mortality with fasciitis 30–50%, myositis 80% even with early rx (*CID 14:2, 1992*). Clinda ↓ toxin production. Use of NSAID may predispose to TSS. For discussion of possible reasons pen G may fail in fulminant S. pyogenes infections, see *JID 167:1401, 1993*.
Other Toxin-Mediated Syndromes —No fever unless complicated				
Botulism: 3 types Food; "Infant"; Wound *AnIM 129:221, 1998*	C. botulinum	Antitoxin. Antibiotics not indicated. *(See Comments)*	For "infant" and wound botulism, treat with amoxicillin	Antitoxin (polyvalent or type-specific). Ventilatory support. "Infant" botulism (germination of spores in vivo) may occur in adults—treat with po amoxicillin. Value of antibiotics for wound botulism untested.
Tetanus	C. tetani	Pen G 24 mu in div. dose or doxy 100 mg q12h IV	Metro 500 mg q6h or 1.0 gm q12h IV x7–10 d. (*See Comment*)	Primary rx is control of muscle spasms. Diazepam agent of choice. Morbidity less with metro than pen G (*BMJ 291:648, 1985*). Tetanus toxin and Pen G both GABA antagonists (*NEJM 332:812, 1995*).

NOTE: All dosage recommendations are for adults (unless otherwise indicated) and assume normal renal function

(Footnotes and abbreviations on page 47)

TABLE 1 (45)

ANATOMIC SITE/DIAGNOSIS/ MODIFYING CIRCUMSTANCES	ETIOLOGIES (usual)	SUGGESTED REGIMENS*		ADJUNCT DIAGNOSTIC OR THERAPEUTIC MEASURES AND COMMENTS
		PRIMARY	ALWERNATIVE[†]	
Vascular				
Cavernous sinus thrombosis	Staph. aureus, Group A strep, H. influenzae, Aspergillus/Mucor/ Rhizopus	[PRSP (nafcillin or oxacillin) 2.0 gm q4h IV] + P Ceph 3 [AP (ceftazidime 2.0 gm q8h IV] or IMP 1.0 gm q6h IV	Vanco for PRSP, 1.0 gm q12h IV or MER 1.0 gm q8h IV	CT or MRI scan for diagnosis. Heparin indicated (*Ln 338:597, 1991*). If patient diabetic with ketoacidosis or post-desferrioxamine rx or neutropenia, consider fungal: aspergillus, mucor, rhizopus, see *Table 10A, pages 71 & 75.* (*General reference: Med 65:82, 1986*)
IV line infection (*See NEJM 337:829, 1997; Ln 351:893, 1998*)				
Heparin lock, midline catheter, non-tunneled central venous catheter (subclavian, internal jugular), peripherally inserted central catheter (PICC)	Staph. epidermidis Staph. aureus	Vanco 1.0 gm q12h IV. Other rx and duration: (1) If S. aureus, remove catheter. Duration of rx controversial; recommendations vary from 2–6 wks. (2) If S. epidermidis, can try and ↓ save" catheter. 80% cure after 7–10 d. of rx.		In rare circumstance that MRSE or MRSA not present in hospital, PRSP for vanco. Culture removed catheter. With "roll" method >15 colonies (*NEJM 312: 1142, 1985*) suggests infection. Lines do not require "routine" changing when not infected. When infected, do not insert new catheter over a wire. New antibiotic-coated catheters may ↓ infection risk (*AnIM 127: 267, 1997; NEJM 340:1, 1999; JAMA 281:261, 1999*)
Tunnel type indwelling venous catheters and ports (Broviac, Hickman, Groshong, Quinton), dual lumen hemodialysis catheters (Perma-cath)	Staph. epidermidis Staph. aureus (Candida sp.) Rarely: leuconostoc or lactobacillus—both resistant to vanco (see *Table 2*)	Anecdotal reports of adjunctive benefit of putting high conc. of vanco into cath for 2–12 hrs (antibiotic lock technique) (*Ln 351:1738, 1998; CID 21:1286, 1995*). If candida, see *Hyperalimentation below and Table 10A, pages 71, 72.*		If S. epidermidis & catheter left in, vanco can cure 80% of infections limited to exit site but only 25% cure if infection in subcutaneous tunnel between skin and subclavian vein. If S. aureus & catheter left in, vanco cure rate 10% at exit site & 0% with tunnel infection (*AJM 89:137, 1990*). Similar statistics for infected "ports" (*CID 29:102, 1999*). Infected hemodialysis access catheters should be removed (*AnIM 127:275, 1997*).
Impaired host (burn, neutropenic)	As above + Pseudomonas sp., Enterobacteriaceae, Corynebacterium jeikeium, Aspergillus, Rhizopus	(Vanco + P Ceph 3 [AP] or (vanco + AP Pen or IMP or (P Ceph 3 + APAG) (*Dosage, see page 44*)		Usually have associated septic thrombophlebitis. Biopsy of vein to rule out fungi. If fungal, surgical excision + amphotericin B. Surgical drainage, ligation or removal often indicated.
Hyperalimentation	As with tunnel + Candida sp. common (see *Table 10*, re: resistant Candida species)	If Candida, amphotericin B 0.5–0.6 mg/kg qd IV, total dose 5.0 mg/kg or fluconazole 400 mg qd IV x7 d., then po for 14 d. after last positive blood culture		Remove venous catheter and discontinue antimicrobial agents if possible. Ophthalmologic consultation recommended. **Rx all patients with + blood cultures.** Amphotericin B [many authorities have recommended 3 mg/kg total dose but failures (endophthalmitis, hepatic abscesses) reported. Others, including us, prefer to use 7 mg/kg total dose especially if patient is neutropenic]. In a multicenter trial, fluconazole = ampho B (*NEJM 331:1325, 1994*).
Intravenous lipid emulsion	Staph. epidermidis Malassezia furfur	Vanco 1.0 gm q12h IV. Amphotericin B		Discontinue Intralipid *AJM 90:129, 1997*
Septic pelvic vein thrombophlebitis (with or without septic pulmonary emboli) Postpartum or postabortion or postpelvic surgery	Streptococci Bacteroides Enterobacteriaceae	Metro + P Ceph 3; cefoxitin; TC/CL; PIP/TZ; or AM/SB	IMP or MER or [clinda + (aztreonam or APAG)]	Use heparin during antibiotic regimen. Continued oral anticoagulation not recommended. Cefotetan less active than cefoxitin vs non-fragilis bacteroides. Cefotetan and cefmetazole[NUS] have methyltetrazole side-chain which is associated with hypoprothrombinemia (prevent with vitamin K).

(Footnotes and abbreviations on page 47)

NOTE: All dosage recommendations are for adults (unless otherwise indicated) and assume normal renal function

TABLE 1 (46): FOOTNOTES AND ABBREVIATIONS

* Dosages suggested are for adults, with clinically severe (often life-threatening) infections. Dosages also assume normal renal function, and not severe hepatic dysfunction. See Table 16, page 120 for pediatric dosages.

§ Alternative therapy includes these considerations: allergy, pharmacology/pharmacokinetics, compliance, costs, local resistance profiles.

AG = aminoglycoside
AHA = American Heart Association
AM/CL = amoxicillin/clavulanate (Augmentin)
AM/SB = ampicillin/sulbactam (Unasyn)
AMP = ampicillin
APAG = antipseudomonal aminoglycosidic antibiotics
AP Pen = antipseudomonal β-lactamase susceptible penicillins, e.g., piperacillin. See Table 4, page 52 for details.
ARDS = adult respiratory distress syndrome
ARF = acute rheumatic fever
ASO = antistreptolysin O
Azithro = azithromycin
CFP = cefepime
CIP or cipro = ciprofloxacin
Clarithro = clarithromycin; clarithro ER = clarithromycin extended release
Clinda = clindamycin
C&S = culture and sensitivities
CSD = cat-scratch disease (See page 31)
DIC = disseminated intravascular coagulation
Doxy = doxycycline
DRSP = drug-resistant Streptococcus pneumoniae
DS = double-strength
EBV = Epstein Barr virus
EDC = expected date of confinement
EES = erythromycin ethyl succinate
Erythro = erythromycin
ETB = ethambutol
FQ = fluoroquinolone
GAS = Group A streptococci

Gati = gatifloxacin
GC = gonorrhea (N. gonorrhoeae)
GNB = Gram-negative bacilli
HHV-2 = human herpesvirus 2
HIV-1 = human immunodeficiency virus type 1
HLGR = high-level gentamicin resistance
I = investigational
IMP = imipenem cilastatin (Primaxin)
INH = isoniazid
IVDU = intravenous drug users
IVIG = intravenous immune globulin
LCM = lymphocytic choriomeningitis virus
LCR = ligase chain reaction
Levo = levofloxacin
LRTI = lower respiratory tract infection
Macrolides = erythro, azithro, clarithro, dirithro
MER = meropenem
Metro = metronidazole
MOTT = mycobacteria other than M. tuberculosis
Moxi = moxifloxacin
MRI = magnetic resonance imaging
MSSA/MRSA = methicillin-sensitive/methicillin-resistant Staph. aureus
MSSE/MRSE = methicillin-sensitive/methicillin-resistant Staph. epidermidis
MTBc = Mycobacterium tuberculosis
NF = nitrofurantoin
NSAIDs = nonsteroidal anti-inflammatory drugs
NUS = not available in the United States

O Ceph 1, 2, 3 = oral cephalosporins—see Table 9B, page 65
Oflox = ofloxacin
P Ceph 1, 2, 3 = parenteral cephalosporins—see Table 9B, pages 64, 65
P Ceph 3 AP = third generation with enhanced antipseudomonal activity
P Ceph 4 = third generation with antistaph. and antipseudomonal activity
PCR = polymerase chain reaction
Peflox = pefloxacin
PIP/TZ = piperacillin-tazobactam
PRSP = penicillinase-resistant semisynthetic penicillins
PVE = prosthetic valve endocarditis
Rick = Rickettsia (spotted fever, Q fever)
RIF = Rifampin
R/O = rule out
SA = Staph. aureus
Skin/SC = skin and related skin structures
SM = streptomycin
Spar = sparfloxacin
STD = sexually transmitted diseases
TBc = tuberculosis
TC/CL = ticarcillin/clavulanate (Timentin)
TEE = transesophageal echocardiography
TMP/SMX = trimethoprim/sulfamethoxazole
Toxo = toxoplasmosis
Trova = trovafloxacin
UTI = urinary tract infection
Vanco = vancomycin

ABBREVIATIONS OF JOURNAL AND TEXT TITLES

AAC: Antimicrobial Agents & Chemotherapy
Adv PID: Advances in Pediatric Infectious Diseases
Adv Par: Advances in Parasitology
AIDS: AIDS
AJDC: American Journal of Diseases of Children
A/G: American Journal of Gastroenterology
AJM: American Journal of Medicine
AJRCCM: Am. Journal of Respiratory Critical Care Medicine
AJTMH: American Journal of Tropical Medicine & Hygiene
AnEM: Annals of Emergency Medicine
AnIM: Annals of Internal Medicine
An Surg: Annals of Surgery
ArIM: Archives of Internal Medicine
ARRD: American Review of Respiratory Disease

CCM: Critical Care Medicine
CID: Clinical Infectious Diseases
COID: Current Opinion in Infectious Disease
CTID: Clinical Topics in Infectious Disease
DMID: Diagnostic Microbiology and Infectious Disease
EID: Emerging Infectious Diseases
EJCMID: European J. of Clin. Micro. and Infectious Diseases
Gastro: Gastroenterology
ICHE: Infection Control and Hospital Epidemiology
IDC No Amer: Infectious Disease Clinics of North America
IDCP: Infectious Diseases in Clinical Practice
J Clin Micro: Journal of Clinical Microbiology
J Ped: Journal of Pediatrics
JAC: Journal of Antimicrobial Chemotherapy
JAMA: Journal of the American Medical Association

JID: Journal of Infectious Diseases
JNS: Journal of Neurosurgery
JTMH: Journal of Tropical Medicine and Hygiene
JTP: Journal of Tropical Pediatrics
Ln: Lancet
Med Lett: Medical Letter
MMWR: Morbidity & Mortality Weekly Report
NEJM: New England Journal of Medicine
Peds: Pediatrics
PIDJ: Pediatric Infectious Disease Journal
QJM: Quarterly Journal of Medicine
SGO: Surgery, Gynecology and Obstetrics
SMJ: Southern Medical Journal
TRSM: Transactions of the Royal Society of Medicine
WJM: Western Journal of Medicine

TABLE 2: RECOMMENDED ANTIMICROBIAL AGENTS AGAINST SELECTED BACTERIA

BACTERIAL SPECIES	ANTIMICROBIAL AGENT (See footnote[2] for abbreviations)		
	RECOMMENDED	ALTERNATIVE	ALSO EFFECTIVE[1] (COMMENTS)
Alcaligenes xylosoxidans (Achromobacter xylosoxidans)	IMP, MER, AP Pen	TMP/SMX. Some strains susc. to ceftaz (AAC 32:276, 1988)	Resistant to APAG; P Ceph 1, 2, 3, 4; aztreonam; FQ (AAC 40:772, 1996)
Acinetobacter calcoaceticus–baumannii complex	IMP or MER or [FQ + (amikacin or ceftaz)]	AM/SB (CID 24:932, 1997). Sulbactam[NUS] also effective (JAC 42: 793, 1998)	Up to 5% isolates resistant to IMP; resistance to FQs, amikacin increasing (see Table 5, page 55).
Actinomyces israeli	AMP or Pen G	Doxy, ceftriaxone	Clindamycin, erythromycin
Aeromonas hydrophila	FQ	TMP/SMX or (P Ceph 2, 3, 4)	APAG; IMP; MER; tetracycline (some resistant to carbapenems)
Arcanobacterium (C.) haemolyticum	Erythromycin	Benzathine Pen G	Sensitive to most drugs, resistant to TMP/SMX (AAC 38:142, 1994)
Bacillus anthracis (anthrax)	Pen G or CIP or doxy	Erythromycin or chloramphenicol	Rare β-lactamase-producing (pen.-resistant) strains reported (CID 19: 1009, 1994)
Bacillus cereus, B. subtilis	Vancomycin, clindamycin	FQ, IMP	
Bacteroides fragilis (ssp. fragilis)	Metronidazole	Clindamycin, trovafloxacin	Cefoxitin, IMP, MER, TC/CL, PIP/TZ, AM/SB, cefotetan, AM/CL
"DOT" group of bacteroides[2]			(not cefotetan)
Bartonella (Rochalimaea) henselae, quintana See Table 1, pages 31, 36, 41	Erythro or doxy (bacillary angiomatosis) or azithro (cat-scratch) (PIDJ 17:447, 1998)	Clarithro or CIP	Other drugs: TMP/SMX (IDC No. Amer 12: 137, 1998). Consider doxy + RIF for severe bacillary angiomatosis (IDC No Amer 12:137, 1998)
Bordetella pertussis	Erythromycin	TMP/SMX	An erythro-resistant strain reported in Arizona (MMWR 43:807, 1994)
Borrelia burgdorferi, B. afzelli, B. garinii	Ceftriaxone, cefuroxime axetil, doxy, amox (See Comments)	Penicillin G (HD), cefotaxime	Clarithro. Choice depends on stage of disease, Table 1, page 42
Borrelia recurrentis	Doxy	Erythromycin	Penicillin G
Brucella sp.	Doxy + either gentamicin or streptomycin	(Doxy + RIF) or (TMP/SMX + gentamicin)	FQ + RIF (AAC 41:80, 1997; Emerg ID 3:213, 1997; CID 21:283, 1995)
Burkholderia (Pseudomonas) cepacia	TMP/SMX or IMP or CIP	Minocycline or chloramphenicol	(Usually resistant to APAG) (AAC 37: 123, 1993) (Some resistant to carbapenems)
Burkholderia (Pseudomonas) pseudomallei	Ceftaz (continuous IV) (AAC 39: 2356, 1995) or AM/CL	TMP/SMX, IMP	(In Thailand, 12–80% strains resistant to TMP/SMX). FQ active in vitro
Campylobacter jejuni	FQ (↑ resistance, NEJM 340:1525,1999)	Erythromycin	Clindamycin, doxy, azithro, clarithro (see Table 5, page 55)
Campylobacter fetus	IMP	Gentamicin	AMP, chloramphenicol, erythromycin
Capnocytophaga ochracea (DF-1) and	Clindamycin	AM/CL, CIP, pen G	P Ceph 3, IMP, cefoxitin, FQ, (resistant to APAG, TMP/SMX)
canimorsus (DF-2)	AM/CL		
Chlamydia pneumoniae	Doxy	Erythromycin, FQ	Azithro, clarithro
Chlamydia trachomatis	Doxy or azithro	Erythromycin or oflox	Levofloxacin, trovafloxacin
Chryseobacterium (Flavobacterium) meningosepticum	Vancomycin ± RIF (CID 26:1169, 1998)	CIP, levofloxacin, sparfloxacin	In vitro susceptibilities may not correlate with clinical efficacy (AAC 41: 1301, 1997; CID 26:1169, 1998)
Citrobacter diversus (koseri), C. freundii	IMP or MER	FQ	APAG
Clostridium difficile	Metronidazole (po)	Vancomycin (po)	Bacitracin (po)
Clostridium perfringens	Pen G ± clindamycin	Doxy	Erythromycin, chloramphenicol, cefazolin, cefoxitin, AP Pen, IMP
Clostridium tetani	Metronidazole or pen G	Doxy	IMP
Corynebacterium jeikeium	Vancomycin	Pen G + APAG	
C. diphtheriae	Erythromycin	Clindamycin	RIF. Penicillin reported effective (CID 27:845, 1998)
Coxiella burnetii (Q fever) acute disease	Doxy	Erythromycin	In meningitis consider FQ (CID 20:489, 1995)
chronic disease	(CIP or doxy) + RIF	FQ + doxy x3 yrs (CID 20:489, 1995)]	Chloroquine + doxy (AAC 37:1773, 1993)
Ehrlichia chaffeensis, Ehrlichia phagocytophila	Doxy	Tetracycline, RIF (CID 27:213, 1998)	CIP, oflox, chloramphenicol also active in vitro. Resistant to clinda, TMP/SMX, IMP, AMP, erytho, & azithro (AAC 41: 76, 1997).
Eikenella corrodens	Penicillin G or AMP or AM/CL	TMP/SMX, FQ	Doxy, cefoxitin, cefotaxime, IMP **(Resistant to clindamycin, cephalexin, erythromycin, and metronidazole)**

TABLE 2 (2)   49

BACTERIAL SPECIES	ANTIMICROBIAL AGENT (See footnote[2] for abbreviations)		
	RECOMMENDED	**ALTERNATIVE**	**ALSO EFFECTIVE[1] (COMMENTS)**
Enterobacter spp. (aerogenes, cloacae)	IMP or MER or (AP Pen + APAG)	TC/CL or PIP/TZ or CIP	P Ceph 4. As many as 40% strains from ICUs may be ceftaz-resistant
Enterococcus faecalis	Penicillin G	Vancomycin	For UTI, nitrofurantoin effective. High-level gentamicin, vancomycin resistance increasing (see footnote, page 21). (See Table 5, page 55)
	Add gentamicin for endocarditis or meningitis		
Enterococcus faecium, β-lactamase +, high-level aminoglycoside resist., vancomycin resist.	No regimen of proven efficacy. Consultation recommended if pt has endocarditis or other life-threatening infection. (See Endocarditis, Table 1, page 21, & Table 5, page 55)		See discussion, page 21; quinupristin + dalfopristin (Synercid), page 66, and Table 5, page 55
Erysipelothrix rhusiopathiae	Penicillin G or AMP	P Ceph 3, FQ	IMP, AP Pen (vancomycin, APAG, TMP/SMX resistant)
Escherichia coli	Sensitive to BL/BLI, cephalosporins, FQ, TMP/SMX, APAG, nitrofurantoin, IMP. Selection of drug depends on site of infection, i.e., UTI multiple po agents; meningitis P Ceph 3 or MER		
Francisella tularensis (tularemia)	Streptomycin or gentamicin	Doxy	Chloramphenicol, CIP, RIF
Gardnerella vaginalis (bacterial vaginosis)	Metronidazole	Clindamycin	See page 18 for dosage
Hafnia alvei	Same as Enterobacter spp.		
Helicobacter pylori	See Table 1, page 14		Drugs effective in vitro often fail in vivo.
Hemophilus aphrophilus	[(Penicillin or AMP) ± gentamicin] or [AM/SB ± gentamicin]	P Ceph 2, 3 ± gentamicin	(Resistant to vancomycin, clindamycin, methicillin)
Hemophilus ducreyi (chancroid)	Azithro or ceftriaxone	Erythromycin, CIP	Most strains resistant to tetracycline, amox, TMP/SMX
Hemophilus influenzae Meningitis, epiglottitis & other life-threatening illness	Cefotaxime, ceftriaxone	TMP/SMX, IMP, MER, FQs (AMP if ß-lactamase negative) (U.S. 25–30% AMP resistance, Japan 35%)	Chloramphenicol (downgraded from 1st choice because of hematotoxicity). 9% of U.S. strains resistant to TMP/SMX (AAC 41:292, 1997)
non-life threatening illness	AM/CL, O Ceph 2/3, TMP/SMX, AM/SB		Azithro, clarithro
Klebsiella pneumoniae, Klebsiella oxytoca	P Ceph 3, FQ	APAG, TC/CL, AM/SB, PIP/TZ	AP Pen, IMP, MER, aztreonam. Outbreaks of ceftaz-resistance reported (AnIM 119:353, 1993) (See Table 4, page 53)
Klebsiella ozaenae/rhino-scleromatis	FQ	RIF + TMP/SMX	(Lancet 342:122, 1993)
Lactobacillus sp.	(Pen G or AMP) ± gentamicin	Clindamycin, erythromycin	**May be resistant to vancomycin**
Legionella sp. (36 species recognized) (NEJM 337:682, 1997)	FQ, or azithro, or (erythromycin ± RIF)	Clarithro	TMP/SMX, doxy. Most active FQs in vitro: trova, spar, levo. See AnIM 129:328, 1998
Leptospira interrogans	Penicillin G	Doxy	
Leuconostoc	Pen G or AMP	Clindamycin, erythromycin, minocycline	APAG **NOTE: Resistant to vancomycin**
Listeria monocytogenes	AMP	TMP/SMX	Erythromycin, penicillin G (high dose), APAG may be synergistic with β-lactams. **Cephalosporin-resistant!**
Moraxella (Branhamella) catarrhalis	AM/CL or O Ceph 2/3, TMP/SMX	Azithro, clarithro, dirithromycin	Erythromycin, doxy, FQs
Morganella sp.	IMP or MER or P Ceph 3 or 4 or FQ	Aztreonam, BL/BLI	APAG
Mycoplasma pneumoniae	Erythro, azithro, clarithro, dirithro, or FQ	Doxy	(Clindamycin and ß lactams NOT effective)
Neisseria gonorrhoeae (gonococcus)	Ceftriaxone, cefixime, cefpodoxime	Ofloxacin & other FQs (Table 1, page 15), spectinomycin	Kanamycin (used in Asia). FQ resistance in Asia; rare in U.S. (MMWR 47:405, 1998)
Neisseria meningitidis (meningococcus)	Penicillin G	Ceftriaxone, cefuroxime, cefotaxime	Sulfonamide (some strains), chloramphenicol. Chloro-resistant strains found in SE Asia (NEJM 339:868, 1998) (Prophylaxis: page 113)
Nocardia asteroides	TMP/SMX, sulfonamides (high dose),	Minocycline	Amikacin + (IMP or ceftriaxone or cefuroxime) for brain abscess
Nocardia brasiliensis	TMP/SMX, sulfonamides (high dose)	AM/CL	Amikacin + ceftriaxone
Pasteurella multocida	Pen G, AMP, amox	Doxy, AM/CL, P Ceph 2, TMP/SMX	Ceftriaxone, cefpodoxime, FQ (active in vitro), azithro (active in vitro) (DMID[3] 30:99, 1998; AAC 43:1475, 1999)
Plesiomonas shigelloides	CIP	TMP/SMX	AM/CL, P Ceph 1,2,3,4, IMP, MER, tetracycline, aztreonam
Proteus mirabilis (indole −)	AMP	TMP/SMX	Most agents except PRSP
vulgaris (indole +)	P Ceph 3 or FQ	APAG	IMP, aztreonam, BL/BLI

TABLE 2 (3)

BACTERIAL SPECIES	ANTIMICROBIAL AGENT *(See footnote[2] for abbreviations)*		
	RECOMMENDED	ALTERNATIVE	ALSO EFFECTIVE[1] (COMMENTS)
Providencia sp.	Amikacin or P Ceph 3 or FQ	TMP/SMX	AP Pen + amikacin, IMP
Pseudomonas aeruginosa	AP Pen, AP Ceph 3, IMP, MER, tobramycin, CIP, aztreonam. For serious inf., use AP β-lactam + APAG or CIP	For UTI, single drugs usually effective: AP Pen, AP Ceph 3, cefepime, IMP, MER, APAG, CIP, aztreonam	Resistance to ß-lactams (IMP, ceftaz) may emerge during rx. β-lactam inhibitor adds nothing to activity of TC or PIP against P. aeruginosa. Clavulanic acid has been shown to antagonize TC in vitro *(AAC 43:882, 1999)*. *(See also Table 5)*
Rhodococcus (C. equi)	[Erythromycin or IMP] + RIF	CIP (variable). Resistant strains SE Asia *(CID 27:370, 1998)*	Vancomycin active in vitro but intracellular location of R. equi may impair efficacy *(Sem Resp Inf 12:57, 1997)*
Rickettsiae species	Doxy	Chloramphenicol	FQ
Salmonella typhi	FQ, ceftriaxone	Chloramphenicol, amox, TMP/SMX, azithro (for uncomplicated disease: *AAC 43: 1441, 1999)*	Multi drug resistant strains (chloramphenicol, AMP, TMP/SMX) common in many developing countries, seen in immigrants
Serratia marcescens	P Ceph 3, IMP, MER, FQ	Aztreonam, gentamicin	TC/CL, PIP/TZ
Shigella sp.	FQ or azithro	TMP/SMX and AMP (resistance common in Middle East, Latin America). Azithro ref.: *AnIM 126:697, 1997*	
Staph. aureus, methicillin-susceptible	PRSP	P Ceph 1, vancomycin, clindamycin	IMP, BL/BLI, FQ, erythromycin, clarithro, dirithromycin, azithro
Staph. aureus, methicillin-resistant	Vancomycin	Teicoplanin[NUS], TMP/SMX (some strains resistant). Invest. drugs: *see Table 5, page 55*	Fusidic acid[NUS]. >60% CIP-resistant in U.S. (Fosfomycin + RIF), novobiocin. Partially vancomycin-resistant strains isolated *(MMWR 27:624, 1997).*
Staph. epidermidis	Vancomycin *(see page 22)*	Vancomycin + RIF	Cephalothin or PRSP if sensitive to PRSP but 75% are resistant. FQs. *(See Table 5)*
Stenotrophomonas (Xanthomonas, Pseudomonas) maltophilia	TMP/SMX	TC/CL or (aztreonam + TC/CL) *(AAC 41:2612, 1997)*	Minocycline, doxy, ceftaz. [In vitro synergy (TC/CL + TMP/SMX) and (TC/CL + CIP), AAC 39:2220, 1995; CMR 11:57, 1998]
Streptobacillus moniliformis	Penicillin G or doxy	Erythro, clindamycin	
Streptococcus, anaerobic (Peptostreptococcus)	Penicillin G	Clindamycin	Erythro, doxy, vancomycin
Streptococcus pneumoniae penicillin-susceptible	Penicillin G	Multiple agents effective, e.g., amox	See footnote, page 4
penicillin-resistant (MIC ≥2.0)	(Vancomycin ± RIF) or (levo, spar, or trova) See footnote page 4 and Table 5, page 55)		For non-meningeal infections: P Ceph 3/4, IMP, MER
Streptococcus pyogenes, Groups A, B, C, G, F, Strep. milleri (constellatus, intermedius, anginosus)	Penicillin G or V (some add gentamicin for serious Group B strep infections)	All ß lactams, erythromycin, azithro, dirithromycin, clarithro	In France, Finland & Japan, resistance to macrolides was over 50%, but ↓ in Japan to <1% *(Arch Ped 148:67, 1994).*
Vibrio cholerae	Doxy, FQ	TMP/SMX	Strain 0139 is resistant to TMP/SMX
Vibrio parahemolyticus	Antibiotic rx does not ↓ course		Sensitive in vitro to FQ, doxy
Vibrio vulnificus, alginolyticus, damsela	Doxy + ceftaz	Cefotaxime, FQ	APAG often used in combination with ceftaz
Yersinia enterocolitica	TMP/SMX or FQ	P Ceph 3 or APAG	*CID 19:655, 1994*
Yersinia pestis (plague)	Streptomycin, gentamicin	Chloramphenicol or doxy	Susceptible to FQ in vitro

[1] These agents are more variable in effectiveness than the "Recommended" or "Alternative". Selection of "Alternative" or "Also Effective" agents is based on in vitro susceptibility testing, pharmacokinetics, host factors such as auditory, renal, hepatic function, and cost.

[2] **AM/CL:** amoxicillin clavulanate; **Amox:** amoxicillin; **AMP:** ampicillin; **AM/SB:** ampicillin sulbactam; **APAG:** antipseudomonal aminoglycosides; **AP Pen:** antipseudomonal penicillin *(see page 47)*; **Azithro:** azithromycin; **BL/BLI:** β-lactam/β-lactamase inhibitor (AM/CL, TC/CL, AM/SB, or PIP/TZ); **Ceftaz:** ceftazidime; **CIP:** ciprofloxacin; **Clarithro:** clarithromycin; **DOT group:** B. distasonis, B. ovatus, B. thetaiotaomicron; **Doxy:** doxycycline **FQ:** fluoroquinolones [ciprofloxacin, ofloxacin, lomefloxacin, enoxacin, pefloxacin, levofloxacin, (not norfloxacin or sparfloxacin unless specifically indicated)]; **IMP:** imipenem + cilastatin; **MER:** meropenem; **NUS:** not available in the U.S.; **P Ceph:** parenteral cephalosporins; **PIP/TZ:** piperacillin-tazobactam; **PRSP:** penicillinase- resistant synthetic penicillins; **RIF:** rifampin; **TC/CL:** ticarcillin clavulanate; **TMP/SMX:** trimethoprim/sulfamethoxazole

TABLE 3: SUGGESTED DURATION OF ANTIBIOTIC THERAPY IN IMMUNOCOMPETENT PATIENTS[1,2]

SITE	CLINICAL SITUATION / CLINICAL DIAGNOSIS	DURATION OF THERAPY (Days)
Bacteremia	Bacteremia with removable focus (no endocarditis)	10–14 (Clin Inf Dis 14:75, 1992) (See Table 1)
Bone	Osteomyelitis, adult; acute	42
	adult; chronic	Until ESR[6] normal (often > 3 months)
	child; acute; staph. and enterobacteriaceae[3]	21
	child; acute; strep., meningococci, hemophilus[3]	14
Ear	Otitis media with effusion	10 (or 1 dose ceftriaxone).
	Recent metanalysis suggests 5 days of "short-acting" antibiotics effective for uncomplicated otitis media (JAMA 279:1736, 1998).	
Endocardium	Infective endocarditis, native valve	
	Viridans strep	14 or 28 (See Table 1, p. 20)
	Enterococci	28 or 42 (See Table 1, pp. 20,21)
	Staph. aureus	14 (R-sided only) or 28 (See Table 1, p. 21)
Gastrointestinal *Also see Table 1*	Bacillary dysentery (shigellosis)/traveller's diarrhea	3
	Typhoid fever (S. typhi): Ceftriaxone	5
	FQ[6] (ofloxacin, fleroxacin[NUS])	3–5
	Chloramphenicol	14
	Helicobacter pylori	10–14
	Pseudomembranous enterocolitis (C. difficile)	10
Genital	Non-gonococcal urethritis or mucopurulent cervicitis	7 days doxy[6] or single dose azithro[6]
	Pelvic inflammatory disease	14
Heart	Pericarditis (purulent)	28
Joint	Septic arthritis (non-gonococcal) Adult	14–28 (Ln 351:197, 1998)
	Infant/child	Rx as osteomyelitis above
	Gonococcal arthritis/disseminated GC infection	7 (See Table 1, page 15)
Kidney	Cystitis (bladder bacteriuria)	3
	Pyelonephritis	14 (7 days if cipro used)
	Recurrent (failure after 14 days rx)	42
Lung	Pneumonia, pneumococcal	Until afebrile 3–5 days (minimum 5 days)
	Pneumonia, enterobacteriaceae or pseudomonal	21, often up to 42
	Pneumonia, staphylococcal	21–28
	Pneumocystis carinii, in AIDS	21
	other immunocompromised	14
	Legionella, mycoplasma, chlamydia	14–21
	Lung abscess	Usually 28–42[4]
Meninges[5]	N. meningitidis	5–7 (IDCP 7:370, 1998)
	H. influenzae	7
	S. pneumoniae	10–14
	Listeria meningoencephalitis, gp B strep, coliforms	14–21 (longer in immunocompromised)
Multiple systems	Brucellosis (See Table 1, page 43)	42 (add SM[6] or GM[6] for 1st 7–14 days)
	Tularemia (See Table 1, pages 31, 43)	7–14
Muscle	Gas gangrene (clostridial)	10
Pharynx *Also see Pharyngitis, Table 1, page 34*	Group A strep pharyngitis	10 (O Ceph 2/3, azithromycin effective at 5 d.
	Diphtheria (membranous)	7–14
	Carrier	7
Prostate	Chronic prostatitis (TMP/SMX)[6]	30–90
	(FQ)	28–42
Sinuses	Acute sinusitis	10–14[7]
Skin	Cellulitis	Until 3 d. after acute inflammation disappears
Systemic	Lyme disease	See Table 1, page 42
	Rocky Mountain spotted fever (See Table 1, p. 42)	Until afebrile 2 days

[1] It has been shown that early change from parenteral to oral regimens (about 72 hours) is cost-effective with many infections, i.e., intra-abdominal (AJM 91:462, 1991)
[2] The recommended duration is a minimum or average time and should not be construed as absolute
[3] These times are with proviso: sx & signs resolve within 7 days and ESR[6] is normalized (J.D. Nelson, APID 6:59, 1991)
[4] After patient afebrile 4-5 days, change to oral therapy
[5] In children relapses seldom occur until 3 days or more after termination of rx. Practice of observing in hospital for 1 or 2 days after rx is expensive and non-productive. For meningitis in children, see Table 1, page 4.
[6] **Azithro** = azithromycin; **Cipro** = ciprofloxacin; **Doxy** = doxycycline; **ESR** = erythrocyte sedimentation rate; **FQ** = fluoroquinolones; **GM** = gentamicin; **rx** = treatment; **SM** = streptomycin; **TMP/SMX** = trimethoprim/sulfamethoxazole
[7] If pt not sx-free at 10 d., sinus puncture and/or rx for 7 more days (NEJM 326:319, 1992). One study reports 3 days of TMP/SMX effective (JAMA 273:1015, 1995).

52

TABLE 4
COMPARISON OF ANTIMICROBIAL SPECTRA*

(These are generalizations; there are major differences between countries, areas and hospitals depending upon antibiotic usage patterns—verify for individual location. See Table 5 for resistant bacteria)

PENICILLINS, IMIPENEM, AZTREONAM, METRONIDAZOLE, FLUOROQUINOLONES

Organisms	Penicillin V	Penicillin G	Methicillin	Nafcillin/Oxacillin	Cloxacillin/Dicloxacillin	Amp/Amox	Amox/Clav	Amp/Sulb	Ticarcillin	Ticar/Clav	Pip/Tazo	Mezlocillin	Piperacillin	Imipenem	Meropenem	Aztreonam	Metronidazole	Ciprofloxacin	Ofloxacin	Lomefloxacin	Pefloxacin	Levofloxacin	Sparfloxacin	Trovafloxacin	Gatifloxacin	Moxifloxacin
GRAM-POSITIVE:																										
Strep, Group A,B,C,G	+	+	+	+	+	+	+	+	+	+	+	+	+	+	+	0	0	±	±	0	0	+	+	+	+	+
Strep. pneumoniae	+	+	+	+	+	+	+	+	+	+	+	+	+	+	+	0	0	±	±	0	0	+	+	+	+	+
Viridans strep, milleri	+	+	+	+	+	+	+	+	+	+	+	+	+	+	+	0	0	0	0			+	+	+	+	+
Enterococcus faecalis	+	+	0	0	0	+	+	+	±	±	±	±	+	±	0	0	0	**	**		0	+	+	+	+	+
Enterococcus faecium	±	±	0	0	0	+	+	+	±	±	±	±	±	±	0	0	0	0	0			0	0	±	±	±
Staph.aureus(MSSA)	0	0	+	+	+	0	+	+	0	+	+	0	0	+	+	0	0	+	+	+	+	+	+	+	+	+
Staph.aureus(MRSA)	0	0	0	0	0	0	0	0	0	0	0	0	0	0	0	0	0	0	0	0	0	±	±	±	±	±
Staph. epidermidis	0	0	±	±	±	±	+	+	±	+	+	0	0	+	+	0	0	+	+	+	+	+	+	+	+	+
C. jeikeium	0	0	0	0	0	0	0	0	0	0	0	0	0	0	0	0		0	0						0	0
L. monocytogenes	+	0	0	0	0	+	+	+	+	+			+	+	+	0	0	+				±	+			
GRAM-NEGATIVE:																										
N. gonorrhoeae	0	0	0	0	0	0	+	+	+	+	+	+	+	+	+	+	0	+	+	+	+	+	+	+	+	+
N. meningitidis	+	0	0	0	0	+	+	+	+	+	+	+	+	+	+	+	0	+	+			+	+	+	+	+
M. catarrhalis	0	0	0	0	0	0	+	+	0	+	+	0	±	+	+	+	0	+	+	+	+	+	+	+	+	+
H. influenzae	0	0	0	0	0	0	0	0	±	+	+	±	±	+	+	+	0	+	+	+	+	+	+	+	+	+
E. coli	0	0	0	0	0	±	+	+	±	+	+	+	+	+	+	+	0	+	+	+	+	+	+	+	+	+
Klebsiella sp.	0	0	0	0	0	0	+	+	0	+	+	+	+	+	+	+	0	+	+	+	+	+	+	+	+	+
Enterobacter sp.	0	0	0	0	0	0	0	0	+	+	+	+	+	+	+	+	0	+	+	+	+	+	+	+	+	+
Serratia sp.	0	0	0	0	0	0	0	0	0	0	0	+	+	+	+	+	0	+	+	+	+	+	+	+	+	+
Salmonella sp.	0	0	0	0	0	±	+	+				+	+	+	+	+	0	+	+	+	+	+	+	+	+	+
Shigella sp.	0	0	0	0	0	±	+	+				+	+	+	+	+	0	+	+	+	+	+	+	+	+	+
Proteus mirabilis	0	0	0	0	0	±	+	+	+	+	+	+	+	+	+	+	0	+	+	+	+	+	+	+	+	+
Proteus vulgaris	0	0	0	0	0	0	+	+	0	+	+	+	+	+	+	+	0	+	+	+	+	+	+	+	+	+
Providencia sp.	0	0	0	0	0	0	+	+	+	+	+	+	+	+	+	+	0	+	+	+	+	+	+	+	+	+
Morganella sp.	0	0	0	0	0	0	±	+	0	±	+	+	+	+	+	+	0	+	+	+	+	+	+	+	+	+
Citrobacter sp.	0	0	0	0	0	0	0	0	+	+	+	+	+	+	+	+	0	+	+	+	+	+	+	+	+	+
Aeromonas sp.	0	0	0	0	0	0	0	0	+	+	+	+	+	+	+	+	0	+	+		+	+	+	+	+	+
Acinetobacter sp.	0	0	0	0	0	0	0	0	0	+	+	0	0	+	+	0	0	+	±			+	+	+	+	+
Ps. aeruginosa	0	0	0	0	0	0	0	0	+	+	+	+	+	+	+	+	0	+	±	±		+	0	±	±	±
B. (Ps.) cepacia§	0	0	0	0	0	0	0	0	0	0	0			+	+	0	0	0	0	0			±			0
S. (X.) maltophilia§	0	0	0	0	0	0	0	0	0	+	0	±	+	0	0	0	0	0	0	0	0	±	+	0		
Y. enterocolitica	0	0	0	0	0	0	±	±	±	+		+	+	+	+		0	+	+	+	+	+	+	+	+	+
Legionella sp.	0	0	0	0	0	0	0	0	0	0	0	0	0	0	0		0	+	+			+	+	+	+	+
P. multocida	+	+	0	0	0	+	+	+	+	+		+	+	+	+		0	+	+			+	+	+	+	+
H. ducreyi	+					0	+	+																		
MISC.:																										
Chlamydia sp.	0	0	0	0	0	0	0	0	0	0	0	0	0	0			0	0	+	+	+	+	+	+	+	+
M. pneumoniae	0	0	0	0	0	0	0	0	0	0	0	0	0					+	+		0	+	+	+	+	+
ANAEROBES:																										
Actinomyces	+	±	0	0	0	+	+	+					+	+	0	0		0	±							+
Bacteroides fragilis	0	±	0	0	0	0	+	+	0	+	+	0	0	+	+	0	+	0	0	0	0	0	0	+	+	+
P. melaninogenica§	+	0	0	0	0	+	+	+	+	+	+	+	+	+	+	0	+	0	±	0		+	+	+	+	+
Clostridium difficile	+[1]									±[1]				+[1]	+[1]	0	0	0	0		0	0		±[1]		±[1]
Clostridium (not difficile)	+	+				+	+	+	+	+	+	+	+	+	+	0	+	±	±	0		+	0	+		+
Peptostreptococcus sp.	+	+	+	+	+	+	+	+	+	+	+	+	+	+	+	0	+	±	±	0		+	+	+		+

+ = usually effective clinically or >60% susceptible; ± = clinical trials lacking or 30–60% susceptible; 0 = not effective clinically or <30% susceptible.

§ B. melaninogenicus → Prevotella melaninogenica, Pseudomonas cepacia → Burkholderia cepacia, Xanthomonas → Stenotrophomonas

** Most strains ±, can be used in UTI, not in systemic infection

Ticar/Clav = ticarcillin clavulanate; **Amp/Sulb** = ampicillin sulbactam; **Amox/Clav** = amoxicillin clavulanate; **MSSA** = methicillin-sensitive Staph. aureus; **MRSA** = methicillin-resistant Staph. aureus; **Pip/Tazo** = piperacillin tazobactam

[1] No clinical evidence that penicillins or fluoroquinolones are effective for C. difficile enterocolitis (but they may cover this organism in mixed intra-abdominal and pelvic infections)

TABLE 4 (2)

CEPHALOSPORINS

Generation groupings: **1st Generation** — Cefazolin; **2nd Generation** — Cefotetan, Cefoxitin, Cefuroxime; **3rd/4th Generation** — Cefotaxime, Ceftizoxime, Ceftriaxone, Cefoperazone, Ceftazidime, Cefepime; **Oral Agents / 1st Generation** — Cefadroxil, Cephalexin; **Oral Agents / 2nd Generation** — Cefaclor/Loracarbef*, Cefprozil, Cefurox. axetil; **Oral Agents / 3rd Generation** — Cefixime, Ceftibuten, Cefetamet-Piv., Cefpodox/Cefdinir[3]

Organisms	Cefazolin	Cefotetan	Cefoxitin	Cefuroxime	Cefotaxime	Ceftizoxime	Ceftriaxone	Cefoperazone	Ceftazidime	Cefepime	Cefadroxil	Cephalexin	Cefaclor/Loracarbef*	Cefprozil	Cefurox. axetil	Cefixime	Ceftibuten	Cefetamet-Piv.	Cefpodox/Cefdinir[3]
GRAM-POSITIVE:																			
Strep, Group A,B,C,G	+	+	+	+	+	+	+	+	+	+	+	+	+	+	+	+	+	+	+
Strep. pneumoniae[1]	+	+	+	+	+	+	+	+	+[1]	+	+	+	+	+	+	+	±	+	+
Viridans strep	±	+	+	+	+	+	+	+	+[1]	+	+	+	+	0	+	+	0	±	+
Enterococcus faecalis	0	0	0	0	0	0	0	0	0	0	0	0	0	0	0	0	0	0	0
Staph. aureus (MSSA)	+	+	+	+	+	+	+	+	±	+	+	+	+	+	+	0	0	0	+
Staph. aureus (MRSA)	0	0	0	0	0	0	0	0	0	0	0	0	0	0	0	0	0	0	0
Staph. epidermidis	±	±	±	±	±	±	±	±	±	±	±	±	±	±	±	0	0		±
C. jeikeium	0	0	0	0	0	0	0	0	0		0	0	0	0	0	0	0		
L. monocytogenes	0	0	0	0	0	0	0	0	0	0	0	0	0	0	0	0	0	0	0
GRAM-NEGATIVE																			
N. gonorrhoeae	+	±	±	±	±	±	+	±	±	+	0	0	±	±	±	+	±	±	+
N. meningitidis	0	±	±	+	+	±	+	±	±	+	0	0	±	±	±	±	±		
M. catarrhalis	+	+	+	+	+	+	+	+	+	+	+	0	+	+	+	+	+	+	+
H. influenzae	+	+	+	+	+	+	+	+	+	+	0		+	+	+	+	+	+	+
E. coli	+	+	+	+	+	+	+	+	+	+	+	+	+	+	+	+	+	+	+
Klebsiella sp.	+	+	+	+	+	+	+	+	+	+	+	+	+	+	+	+	+		
Enterobacter sp.	0	±	0	±	+	+	+	+	+	+	0	0	0	0	0	0	±	0	0
Serratia sp.	0	+	0	0	+	+	+	+	+	+	0	0	0	0	0	±	±	0	0
Salmonella sp.					+		+	+			0								
Shigella sp.											0								
Proteus mirabilis	+	+	+	+	+	+	+	+	+	+	+	+	+	+	+	+	+	+	+
Proteus vulgaris	0	+	+	+	+	+	+	+	+	+	0	0	0	0	0	+	+	+	±
Providencia sp.	0	+	+	+	+	+	+	+	+	+	0	0	0	0	±	+	+	+	
Morganella sp.	0	+	+	±	+	+	+	+	+	+	0	0	0	0	±	0	0	0	0
C. freundii	0	0	0	0	0	0	0	0	0	+	0	0	0	0	0	0	0	0	0
C. diversus	0	±	±	±	+	+	+	+	+	+	0	0	0	0	0		+		
Citrobacter sp.	0	±	±	±	+	+	+	+	+	+		0	±	0	±	+	+	±	+
Aeromonas sp.	0	+	±	+	+	+	+	+	+	+						+	+	+	
Acinetobacter sp.	0	0	0	0	+	+	+	0	+	±	0	0	0	0	0	0	0		
Ps. aeruginosa	0	0	0	0	±	±	±	+	+	+	0	0	0	0	0	0	0		0
B. (Ps.) cepacia[§]	0	0	0	0	+	+	+	+	+	±	0	0	0	0	0	0	+		
S. (X.) maltophilia[§]	0	0	0	0	0	0	±	±	0		0	0	0	0	0	0	0		
Y. enterocolitica	0	±	±	±	+	+	+	±	±	+						+	+	+	
Legionella sp.	0	0	0	0	0	0	0	0	0	0	0	0	0	0	0	0	0	0	0
P. multocida					+	+	+				0					+			
H. ducreyi				+	+	+	+		+										
ANAEROBES:																			
Actinomyces					+	+													
Bacteroides fragilis	0	+[2]	+	0	0	±	0	0	0	0		0	0	0	0	0	0	0	
P. melaninogenica[§]		+	+	+	+	+	±	+	+	0			+	+	+	+		+	
Clostridium difficile			0		0	0		0		0									
Clostridium (not difficile)		+	+	+	+	+	+	+	+					+	+	0			
Peptostreptococcus sp.		+	+	+	+	+	+	+	+	+		+	+	+	+	+			

+ = usually effective clinically or >60% susceptible; ± = clinical trials lacking or 30–60% susceptible; 0 = not effective clinically or <30% susceptible; blank = data not available.

§ B. melaninogenicus → Prevotella melaninogenica, P. cepacia → Burkholderia cepacia, Xanthomonas → Stentrophomonas

* A 1-carbacephem best classified as a cephalosporin

1 Ceftaz 8–16x less active than cefotax/ceftriax, effective only vs Pen-sens strains (AAC 39:2193, 1995). Oral cefuroxime, cefprozil, cefpodoxime most active in vitro vs resistant S. pneumo (PIDJ 14:1037, 1995).

2 Cefotetan is less active against B. ovatus, B. distasonis, B. thetaiotamicron

3 Cefpodox = Cefpodoxime proxetil

MSSA = methicillin-sensitive Staph. aureus; **MRSA** = methicillin-resistant Staph. aureus

TABLE 4 (3)

Column groups: **AMINOGLYCOSIDES** (Gentamicin, Tobramycin, Amikacin, Netilmicin) · Chloramphenicol · Clindamycin · **MACROLIDES** (Erythro/Dirithro, Azithromycin, Clarithromycin) · **TETRACYCLINES** (Doxycycline, Minocycline) · **GLYCOPEPTIDES** (Vancomycin, Teicoplanin) · Fusidic Acid · Trimethoprim · TMP/SMX · **URINARY TRACT AGENTS** (Nitrofurantoin, Norfloxacin, Enoxacin) · Rifampin · Metronidazole · Quinupristin/dalfopristin · Linezolid

Organisms	Gen	Tob	Ami	Net	Chlor	Clin	Ery/Dir	Azi	Clar	Doxy	Mino	Vanc	Teic	Fus	Trim	TMP/SMX	Nitro	Norf	Enox	Rif	Metro	Q/D	Lin
GRAM-POSITIVE:																							
Strep Group A,B,C,G	0	0	0	0	+	+	+	+	+	±	+	+	+	±	+	+[2]	+	0	0	+	0	+	+
Strep. pneumoniae	0	0	0	0	+	+	+	+	+	+	+	+	+	±	±	±	+	0	±	+	0	+	+
Enterococcus faecalis	S	S	S	S	±	0	0	0	0	0	0	+	+		+	+[2]	±	0	0	±	0	0	+
Enterococcus faecium	S	0	0	0	±	0	0	0	0	0	0	±	±		0	0	0	0	0	0	0	0	+
Staph.aureus(MSSA)	+	+	+	+	±	+	±	+	+	±	+	+	+	+	+	+	+	±	+	+	0	+	+
Staph.aureus(MRSA)	0	0	0	0	0	0	0	0	0	0	0	+	+	+	+		0	0		+	0	+	+
Staph. epidermidis	±	±	±	±	0	0	±		±	0	0	+	±	+	+	±		±	+	+	0	+	+
C. jeikeium	0	0	0	0	0	0	0	0	0	0	0	+	±	+	+	0	0	0	0	+	0	+	+
L. monocytogenes	S	S	S	S		+	+	+	+	+	+	+	+		+	+				+	0	+	+
GRAM-NEGATIVE:																							
N. gonorrhoeae	0	0	0	0	+	0	±	±	±	±	±	0		+	0	±	+	+	+	+	0	+	
N. meningitidis	0	0	0	0	+	0	+		+	+	+	0	0	+	±	+				+	0	0	0
M. catarrhalis§	+	+	+	+	+	0	+	+	+	+	+					+	+			+	0	+	±
H. influenzae	+	+	+	+	+	0	±	+	+	+	+	±	±		+	+		+	+	+	0	±	±
Aeromonas	0				+					+	+	0			+					0	0		
E. coli	+	+	+	+	+	0	0	0	0	+		0	0	0	+	+	+	+	+	0	0	0	0
Klebsiella sp.	+	+	+	+	±	0	0	0	0	±	±	0	0	0	+	+	±	+	+	0	0	0	0
Enterobacter sp.	+	+	+	+	0	0	0	0	0	0	0	0	0	0	±		±	+	+	0	0	0	0
Salmonella sp.	+	+	+	+	+	0	0	±	0	±	±	0	0	0	±	±	+	+	+	0	0	0	0
Shigella sp.	+	+	+	+	+	0	0	±	0	±	±	0	0	0	±	±	+	+	+	0	0	0	0
Serratia marcescens	+	+	+	+	0	0	0	0	0	0	0	0	0	0	0	±	0	+		0	0		0
Proteus vulgaris	+	+	+	+	±	0	0	0	0	0	0	0	0	0	0	0	0	+	+	0	0	0	0
Acinetobacter sp.	0	+	0			0	0	0	0	0	0	0	0	0	0	0	0	±		0	0		0
Ps. aeruginosa	+	+	+	+	0	0	0	0	0	0	±	0	0	0	0	0	0	+	+	0	0	0	0
B. (Ps.) cepacia§	0	0	0	0	+	0				0	0	0	0	0	+	+	0	0	0	0			0
S. (X.) maltophilia§	0	0	0	0	+	0	0	0	0	0	0			0	0	+	0	0	0				0
Y. enterocolitica	+	+	+		+	0	0	0	0	0	0			0		+				0	0		0
F. tularensis	+				+					+					+					+	0	0	
Brucella sp.	+				+	0	0	0	0	+	+	0	0		+	+				+	0	0	
Legionella sp.							+	+	+	+	+			±	+	+						+	±
H. ducreyi					+	+	+	+				0			±		+			0			
V. vulnificus	0	0	0		+					0	0				0								
MISC.:																							
Chlamydia trachomatis	0	0	0	0	+	±	+	+	+	+	+			0	0		0	0		+	0		
M. pneumoniae	0	0	0	0	+	0	+	+	+	+	+			0						0	+		
Rickettsia sp.	0	0	0	0	+			±		+	+	0	0	0						0			
Mycobacterium avium		+						+	+											0	0		+
ANAEROBES:																							
Actinomyces	0	0	0	0	+	+	+	+	+	+	+	+		+						0			
Bacteroides fragilis	0	0	0	0	+	+	0	0	0	±	±	0		+	0			0	0		+		0
P. melaninogenica§	0	0	0	0	+	+		+	+	±	±	0		+				0	0		+	+	
Clostridium difficile	0	0	0	0	±							+	+							0	+	±	±
Clostridium (not difficile)**						+	±	+	+	+	+	+	+	+						+	+	+	
Peptostreptococcus sp	0	0	0	0	+	+	±	+	±	+	+	0	0	+							+		+

+ = usually effective clinically or >60% susceptible; ± = clinical trials lacking or 30–60% susceptible; 0 = not effective clinically or <30% susceptible; S = synergistic with penicillins (ampicillin); blank = data not available. Antimicrobials such as azithromycin have high tissue penetration and some such as clarithromycin are metabolized to more active compounds, hence in vivo activity may exceed in vitro activity.

[1] In vitro results discrepant, + in one study, 0 in another *[JAC 31(Suppl. C):39, 1993]*

[2] Although active in vitro, TMP/SMX is not clinically effective for Group A strep pharyngitis or for infections due to E. faecalis.

§ B. melaninogenicus → Prevotella melaninogenica, P. cepacia → Burkholderia cepacia, Xanthomonas → Stentrophomonas

** Vancomycin, metronidazole given po active vs C. difficile; IV vancomycin not effective

Dirithro = dirithromycin; **Erythro** = erythromycin; **TMP/SMX** = trimethoprim/sulfamethoxazole; **MSSA** = methicillin-sensitive Staph. aureus; **MRSA** = methicillin-resistant Staph. aureus; **S** = potential synergy in combination with penicillin, ampicillin, vancomycin, or teicoplanin

TABLE 5: TREATMENT OPTIONS FOR SELECTED HIGHLY RESISTANT BACTERIA (NEJM 335:1445, 1996)*

ORGANISM/RESISTANCE	THERAPEUTIC OPTIONS		COMMENT[1]
E. faecalis. Resistant to:			
Vanco + strep/gentamicin (MIC >500 µg/ml); β-lactamase neg. (JAC 40:161, 1997).	Penicillin G or AMP (systemic infections); Nitrofurantoin, fosfomycin (UTI only). Usually resistant to Synercid		Non BLA+ strains of E. faecalis resistant to penicillin and AMP recently described in Spain, but unknown (except BLA+ strains) so far in U.S. and elsewhere (AAC 40:2420, 1996).
Penicillin (β-lactamase producers)	Vanco, AM/SB		Appear susceptible to AMP and penicillin by standard in vitro methods. Most use direct test for β-lactamase to identify in lab (JCM 31:1965, 1993).
E. faecium Resistant to:			
Vanco and high levels (MIC >500 µg/ml) of streptomycin and gentamicin	Penicillin G or AMP (systemic infections); fosfomycin, nitrofurantoin (UTI only).		For strains with pen/AMP MICs of >8 ≤64 µg/ml there is anecdotal evidence that high-dose (300 mg/kg/day) AMP rx may be effective.
Penicillin, AMP, vanco, & high-level resist. to streptomycin and gentamicin	Quinupristin/dalfopristin (Synercid) is bacteriostatic against most strains of E. faecium (7.5 mg/ kg IV q8h) Can try combinations of cell-active antibiotics with other agents as well as chloramphenicol, RIF, or doxy. Nitrofurantoin or fosfomycin may work for UTI.		For strains with Van B phenotype (vanco R, teico S), teicoplanin[NUS], preferably in combination with streptomycin or gentamicin if not highly AG resistant, may be effective. Synercid roughly 70% effective in clinical trials to date. Linezolid available on compassionate use protocol (800-836-3535). **Infectious disease consultation imperative!**
S. aureus. Resistant to:			
Methicillin (Ln 349:1901, 1997; Clin Micro Rev 10:781, 1997)	Vanco	Other alternatives include teicoplanin[NUS], TMP/SMX (test susceptibility first), doxy, minocycline (some strains), or quinupristin/dalfopristin. Fusidic acid[NUS] fosfomycin, RIF, novobiocin, FQ may be active but must be used in combination regimens to prevent in vivo emergence of resistance. **Investigational drugs with activity against MRSA include linezolid (800-836-3535), daptomycin (215-370-6266), L4333328, evernomicin.**	
Vanco, methicillin (VRMRSA) NEJM 339:520, 1998	Unknown, but high-dose vanco with or without a 2nd agent (see Comments for MRSA) likely effective		So far, clinical isolates of VRMRSA have had only low levels (MIC ≤8 µg/ml) of vanco resistance (MMWR 27:624, 1997; JAC 40:135, 1997). Some call these strains VISA or GISA. Quinupristin/dalfopristin and linezolid (I) (see Comment on E. faecium above) active in vitro against VRMRSA.
S. epidermidis. Resistant to:			
Methicillin	Vanco (+ RIF and gentamicin for prosthetic valve endocarditis)		
Methicillin, glycopeptides	Quinupristin/dalfopristin (see comments on E. faecium)		Vanco more active than teicoplanin[NUS] (Clin Microbial Rev 8:585, 1995). New FQs (levofloxacin, gatifloxacin, moxifloxacin) active in vitro, but development of resistance is a potential problem.
S. pneumoniae Resistant to:			
Penicillin G (MIC >0.1 ≤1.0)	Ceftriaxone or cefotaxime. High-dose penicillin (≥10 million units/day) or AMP (amox) likely effective for nonmeningeal sites of infection (e.g., pneumonia)		IMP, cefepime, cefpodoxime, cefuroxime also active (IDCP 3:75, 1994). MER less active than IMP (AAC 38:898, 1994). Levo, spar, gati, moxi, trova also have good activity (AAC 38:898, 1994).
Penicillin G (MIC ≥2.0)	(Vanco ± RIF) or an active FQ: levo, spar, gati, moxi. Alternatives if non-meningeal infection: ceftriax/cefotax, IMP, MER, high-dose AMP		High-dose cefotaxime (300 mg/kg/day, max. 24 gm/day) effective in meningitis due to strains with cefotaxime MICs as high as 2 µg/ml (AAC 40:218, 1996). Review: IDCP 6(Suppl 2):S21, 1997.
Penicillin, erythro, tetracycline, chloramphenicol, TMP/SMX	Vanco ± RIF		60–80% of strains susceptible to clindamycin (Diag Microbial Inf Dis 25:201, 1996). Levofloxacin, gatifloxacin, moxifloxacin, sparfloxacin active in vitro (AAC 40:2431, 1996).
Acinetobacter baumannii. Resistant to:			
IMP, AP Ceph 3, AP Pen, APAG, FQ	AM/SB (subbactam alone is active against some A. baumannii, JAC 42:793, 1998)		6/8 patients with A. baumannii meningitis (7 organisms resistant to IMP) cured with AM/SB (CID 24:932, 1997). Various combinations of FQs and AGs, IMP and AGs, or AP Pens or AP Ceph 3s with AGs may show activity against **some** multiresistant strains (AAC 41:881, 1997; AAC 41:1073, 1997). IV colistin also effective (CID 26:1008, 1999).
Campylobacter jejuni. Resistant to: FQs	Erythro, azithro, clarithro, doxy, clindamycin		Strains resistant to **both** FQs and macrolides have been reported from Thailand (IJAA 8:37, 1997) and
Klebsiella pneumoniae (producing ESBL)			
Resistant to: Ceftazidime, P Ceph 3, aztreonam	IMP, MER, FQ	P Ceph 4, TC/CL, PIP/TZ	P Ceph 4, TC/CL, PIP/TZ show in vitro activity, but have not been proven entirely effective in animal models (IJAA 8:37, 1997) and some strains which hyperproduce ESBLs are primarily resistant to TC/CL and PIP/TZ (JCM 34:358, 1996)

* Footnotes at top of next page

TABLE 5 (2)

ORGANISM/RESISTANCE	THERAPEUTIC OPTIONS	COMMENT[1]
Pseudomonas aeruginosa. Resistant to: IMP, MER	CIP (check susceptibility), APAG (check susceptibility)	Many strains remain susceptible to aztreonam & ceftazidime or AP Pens (*JAC 36:1037, 1995*). Combinations of (AP Pen & APAG) or (AP Ceph 3 + APAG) may show in vitro activity (*AAC 39:2411, 1995*). IV colistin may have some utility (*CID 28:1008, 1999*)

[1] Guideline on prevention of resistance: *CID 25:584, 1997.* **Abbreviations: AGs** = aminoglycosides; **AP Pen** = antipseudomonal β-lactamase susceptible penicillins; **AM/SB** = ampicillin/sulbactam, **AP Ceph 3** = third generation parenteral cephalosporin with enhanced antipseudomonal activity, **APAG** = antipseudomonal aminoglycosidic antibiotics. **Azithro** = azithromycin. **BL** = beta-lactamase. **CIP** = ciprofloxacin, **Clarithro** = clarithromycin, **Doxy** = doxycycline. **Erythro** = erythromycin; **ESBLs** = extended spectrum β-lactamases, **FQ** = fluoroquinolone, **Gati** = gatifloxacin, **IMP** = imipenem cilastatin, **Levo** = levofloxacin, **MER** = meropenem, **Moxi** = moxifloxacin, **PIP/TZ** = piperacillin-tazobactam, **R** = resistant, **RIF** = rifampin, **S** = sensitive, **Spar** = sparfloxacin, **TC/CL** = ticarcillin/clavulanate, **Vanco** = vancomycin, **VISA** = vancomycin intermediately-resistant Staph. aureus, **VRMRSA** = vancomycin-resistant, methicillin-resistant Staph. aureus.

TABLE 6: RISK CATEGORIES OF ANTIMICROBICS IN PREGNANCY

DRUG	FDA PREGNANCY RISK CATEGORIES*
Antibacterial Agents	
Aminoglycosides:	
Amikacin, gentamicin, isepamicin, netilmicin, streptomycin & tobramycin	D
Beta Lactams (*CPh 27;49, 1994*)	
Penicillins; pens + BLI; cephalosporins	B
Aztreonam	B
Imipenem/cilastatin	C
Meropenem	B
Chloramphenicol, clindamycin	C
Ciprofloxacin, oflox, levoflox, sparflox, gatiflox, moxiflox	C
Fosfomycin	B
Macrolides:	
Erythromycins/azithromycin	B
Clarithromycin	C
Metronidazole	B
Nitrofurantoin	B
Sulfonamides/trimethoprim	C
Tetracyclines	D
Vancomycin	C

DRUG	FDA PREGNANCY RISK CATEGORIES*
Antifungal Agents: (*CID 27:1151, 1998*)	
Amphotericin B preparations	B
Fluconazole, itraconazole, ketoconazole	C
flucytosine	C
Terbinafine	B
Antiparasitic Agents:	
Albendazole/mebendazole	C
Chloroquine, eflornithine	C
Ivermectin	C
Mefloquine	C
Pentamidine	C
Praziquantel	B
Pyrimethamine/pyrisulfadoxine	C
Quinidine	C
Quinine	X
Antimycobacterial Agents:	
Capreomycin	C
Clofazimine/cycloserine	C
Dapsone	"avoid"[1]
Ethambutol	"safe"[1]
Thalidomide	X

DRUG	FDA PREGNANCY RISK CATEGORIES*
Antimycobacterial Agents *(continued)*	
Ethionamide	"do not use"[1]
INH, pyrazinamide, rifampin	C
Rifabutin	B
Antiviral Agents:	
Abacavir	C
Acyclovir, famciclovir, valacyclovir	B
Amantadine, rimantadine	C
Amprenavir, indinavir	C
Cidofovir	C
Delavirdine, efavirenz, nevirapine	C
Didanosine (ddI)	B
Foscarnet	C
Ganciclovir	C
Interferons	C
Lamivudine/stavudine	C
Nelfinavir, ritonavir, saquinavir	B
Oseltamivir	C
Ribavirin	X
Zalcitabine/zidovudine	C
Zanamivir	B

* **FDA Pregnancy Categories: A**—studies in pregnant women, no risk; **B**—animal studies no risk, but human not adequate or animal toxicity but human risk; **C**—animal studies show toxicity, human studies inadequate but benefit of use may exceed risk; **D**—evidence of human risk, but benefits may outweigh; **X**—fetal abnormalities in humans, risk > benefit.
Abbreviations: BLI = β-lactamase inhibitor; **FQ** = fluoroquinolones
[1] From CDC: TB Core Curriculum, 3rd Ed., 1994

TABLE 7: ANTIMICROBIAL AGENTS ASSOCIATED WITH PHOTOSENSITIVITY

The following drugs are known to cause photosensitivity in some individuals. There is no intent to indicate relative frequency or severity of reactions.
Source: 1998 Drug Topics Red Book, Medical Economics, Montvale, NJ. Listed in alphabetical order:

Amantadine, azithromycin, benznidazole, ciprofloxacin, clofazimine, dapsone, doxycycline, enoxacin, flucytosine, griseofulvin, interferons, levofloxacin, lomefloxacin, norfloxacin, ofloxacin, pefloxacin, pyrazinamide, saquinavir, sparfloxacin, sulfonamides, tetracyclines, tretinoins, trimethoprim.

The approximate phototoxic potential among fluoroquinolones (from *CID 28:352, 1999*) is: lomefloxacin, fleroxacin > sparfloxacin > enoxacin > pefloxacin > ciprofloxacin, [levofloxacin, norfloxacin, moxifloxacin, ofloxacin, trovafloxacin].

8A: PHARMACOKINETICS: Route, Half-life, Protein-binding (See Table 8B for serum levels)

DRUG	ROUTES OF ADMIN.	ORAL WC	ORAL % AB	SERUM t/2 hrs[1]	PROTEIN BOUND %
PENICILLINS					
Natural					
Penicillin G	IV,IM,PO	N	15	0.5	65
Pen'ase Resist.					
Clox;Dicloxacillin	PO	N	35	0.5	95–98
Nafcillin	IV,IM			0.5	90
Oxacillin	IV,IM,PO	N	30	0.5	94
Aminopenicillins					
Amoxicillin	PO	Y	75	1.2	17
AM/CL	PO	Y	75	1.2	20/30
Ampicillin	IV,IM,PO	N	40	1.2	18–22
AM/SB	IV,IM			1.2	28/38
Antipseudomonal					
Indanyl carb.	PO	N	35	1.0	50
Mezlo;Piperacillin	IV			1.1	16–42
PIP/TZ	IV			1.0	16–48
Ticarcillin;TC/CL	IV			1.2	45/30
CEPHALOSPORINS					
1st Generation					
Cefadroxil	PO	Y	90	1.5	20
Cefazolin	IV,IM			1.9	73–87
Cephalexin	PO	Y	90	1.0	5–15
Cephradine	PO	N	90	1.3	6–20
2nd Generation					
Cefaclor	PO	N	93	0.8	22–25
Cefaclor-CD	PO	Y		0.8	22–25
Cefamandole	IV,IM			1.0	56–78
Cefonicid	IV,IM			4.0	98
Cefotetan	IV,IM			4.2	78–91
Cefoxitin	IV,IM			0.8	65–79
Cefprozil	PO	Y	95	1.3–1.8	65
Cefuroxime	IV,IM			1.5	33–50
Cefurox.-axetil	PO	Y	52	1.5	50
Loracarbef[2]	PO	N	~90	1.2	25
3rd Generation					
Cefdinir	PO	N	25	1.7	60–70
Cefixime	PO	Y	50	3.1	65
Cefoperazone	IV,IM			1.9	82–93
Cefotaxime	IV,IM			1.5	30–51
Cefpodoxime proxetil	PO	Y	46	~2.3	40
Ceftazidime	IV,IM			1.8	< 10
Ceftibuten	PO	N	–	2.4	65
Ceftizoxime	IV,IM			1.7	30
Ceftriaxone	IV,IM			8	85–95
4th Generation					
Cefipime	IV			2.0	20
CARBAPENEMS					
Imipenem	IV,IM			1.0	15–25
Meropenem	IV			1.0	
MONOBACTAMS					
Aztreonam	IV,IM			2.0	56
AMINOGLYCOSIDES					
Parenteral: amikacin, gentamicin, isepamicin[NUS], kanamycin, netilmicin, sisomicin[NUS], tobramycin have similar pharmacokinetics:	IV,IM			2.5	0–10
Neomycin	PO		<3		0–10

DRUG	ROUTES OF ADMIN.	ORAL WC	ORAL % AB	SERUM t/2 hrs[1]	PROTEIN BOUND %
MACROLIDES					
Azithromycin	PO	Y	37	12/68	12–50
	IV			12/68	7–51
Clarithromycin	PO	Y	50	5–7	65–70
Dirithromycin	PO	Y	10	8	15–30
Erythromycins	PO	N	18–45	2–4	70–74
MISCELLANEOUS					
Chloramphenicol	PO,IV,IM	N	80	1.5–3.5	60–80
Clindamycin	PO,IV,IM	Y	90	2.4	85–94
Doxycycline	PO,IV	Y	93	18	93
Fosfomycin	PO	N	30–37	5.7	<10
Metronidazole	PO,IV		90	6–14	20
Minocycline	PO	Y	95	16	76
Rifabutin	PO	Y	≥20	45	85
Rifampin	PO	N	100	2–5	80
Quinu/dalfo (Synercid)	IV			1.5	
TMP/SMX	PO,IV		90–100	11/9	40–70
Vancomycin	IV			4–6	<10–55
FLUOROQUINOLONES					
Ciprofloxacin	PO,IV	Y	70	4	20–40
Gatifloxacin	PO,IV	N	96	7–8	20
Levo;Ofloxacin	PO,IV	N	98	7	24–38
Lomefloxacin	PO	Y	>95	8	10
Moxifloxacin	PO	N	89	10–14	50
Norfloxacin	PO	N	30–40	4	10–15
Sparfloxacin	PO	N	92	20	–
Trovafloxacin	PO,IV	Y	88	11	76
ANTIVIRALS					
Abacavir	PO	Y	83	1.5	50
Acyclovir	PO,IV	Y	15–30	2.5	9–33
Amantadine	PO	Y	90	15	67
Amprenavir	PO	Y	—	—	90
Cidofovir	IV			2.5	<6
Delavirdine	PO		85	5.8	98
Didanosine(ddI)	PO	N	33	1.6	<5
Efavirenz	PO	N		40–55	99
Famciclovir	PO	Y	77	1.6–2.9	<25
Foscarnet	IV			3	17
Ganciclovir	PO/IV	Y	6–9	3.6	1–2
Indinavir	PO		65	2	60
Lamivudine(3TC)	PO	N	86	5–7	36
Nelfinavir	PO	Y	20–80	3.5–5.0	Unknown
Nevirapine	PO	N	>90	25–30	60
Oseltamivir	PO	Y	75	1–3/ 6–10[3]	
Ribavirin	PO	Y	52	30–60	0
Rimantadine	PO	Y	>90	27–36	
Ritonavir	PO		Good	3–5	98–99
Saquinavir–soft gel	PO		>4	–	98
Stavudine (d4T)	PO	Y	86–99	1.0	<1
Valacyclovir	PO	Y	75–90	2.5	9–33
Zalcitabine(ddC)	PO	N	>80	1.2	<4
Zidovudine(ZDV)	PO,IV	N	65	1.1	10–30

Abbreviations: **WC** = with meals, **Y** = yes, **N** = no, **AB** = absorption (oral) (bioavailability), **AM/CL** = amoxicillin clavulanate, **AM/SB** = ampicillin sulbactam, **NUS** = not licensed in the U.S., **I** = investigational, **TC/CL** = ticarcillin clavulanate, **TMP/SMX** = trimethoprim/sulfamethoxazole, **PIP/TZ** = piperacillin tazobactam, **Quinu/dalfo** = quinupristin/dalfopristin

[1] Assumes creatinine clearance >80 ml/min.
[2] A 1-carbacephem but classified as a cephalosporin
[3] Oseltamivir/oselt. carboxylate

TABLE 8B: PHARMACOKINETICS: Peak Serum Levels[1] and Biliary Excretion

DRUG	DOSE/ ROUTE	PEAK SERUM LEVEL (μg/ml)	BILIARY EXCRE- TION[2] %
PENICILLINS			
Natural			
Benzathine Pen G	1.2 million U IM	0.15	
Penicillin G	12 million U qd IV	20	500
Penicillin V	500 mg PO	5–6	
Pen'ase Resistant			
Clox;Dicloxacillin	500 mg PO	7–18	6
Nafcillin/Oxacillin	500 mg IV	40–57	>100/20–30
Aminopenicillins			
Amoxicillin	250 mg PO	4–5	100–3000
AM/CL (875/125)	875 mg PO	11.6/2.2	100–3000
Ampicillin	500 mg PO	3–6	100–3000
	2 gm IV	47	
AM/SB (2 gm/1gm)	3 gm IV	109–150	
Antipseudomonal			
Indanyl carb (382 mg)	1 tab (382mg)PO	6.5	
Mezlocillin	3 gm IV	263	1000–6000
Piperacillin	4 gm IV	400	100–6000
PIP/TZ (3/0.375 gm)	3.375 gm IV	209	>100
4/0.5 gm	4.5 gm IV	209	>100
Ticarcillin	3 gm IV	260	
TC/CL (3/0.1 gm)	3.1 gm IV	324	
CEPHALOSPORINS			
1st Generation			
Cefadroxil	500 mg PO	16	22
Cefazolin	1 gm IV	188	29–300
Cephalexin	500 mg PO	18–38	216
Cephradine	1 gm IV	86	10–400
	500 mg PO	16	
2nd Generation			
Cefaclor	500 mg PO	9.3	≥60
Cefaclor-CD	500 mg PO	8.4	
Cefamandole	2 gm IV	165	300–400
Cefonicid	1 gm IV	220	<10
Cefprozil	500 mg PO	10.5	
Cefuroxime	1.5 gm IV	100	35–80
Cefuroxime axetil	250 mg PO	4.1	
Loracarbef[4]	200 mg PO	8	
Cephamycins			
Cefotetan	1 gm IV	124	2–21
Cefoxitin	1 gm IV	110	280
3rd Generation			
Cefdinir	300 mg PO	1.6	
Cefixime	400 mg PO	3–5	800
Cefoperazone	1 gm IV	153	800–1200
Cefotaxime	1 gm IV	100	15–75
Cefpodoxime proxetil	200 mg PO	2.9	115
Ceftazidime	1 gm IV	60	13–54
Ceftibuten	400 mg PO	15	
Ceftizoxime	1 gm IV	132	34–82
Ceftriaxone	1 gm IV	150	200–500
4th Generation			
Cefepime	2 gm IV	193	∝5

DRUG	DOSE/ ROUTE	PEAK SERUM LEVEL (μg/ml)	BILIARY EXCRE- TION[2] %
CARBAPENEMS			
Imipenem	500 mg IV	40	Minimal
Meropenem	500 mg IV	26	3–300
MONOBACTAMS			
Aztreonam	1 gm IV	125	115–405
AMINOGLYCOSIDES			
Amikacin	7.5 mg/kg IV	38	30
Genta;Tobra- mycin	1.25 mg/kg IV	4–8	10–60
Kanamycin	500 mg IM	14–29	1
Netilmicin	2.0 mg/kg IV	7	
FLUOROQUINOLONES			
Ciprofloxacin	750 mg PO	1.8–2.8	2800–4500
	400 mg IV	4.6	
Gatifloxacin	400 mg PO/IV	4.2–4.6	
Levofloxacin	500 mg PO/IV	5.7/6.2	See oflox
Lomefloxacin	400 mg PO	1.4	700
Moxifloxacin	400 mg PO	4.5	
Norfloxacin	400 mg PO	1.4–1.8	1000
Ofloxacin	400 mg PO/IV	4.6/5.2– 7.2	210–1886
Sparfloxacin	400 mg PO	1.3	
Trovafloxacin	200 mg PO/IV	3.1/3.1	1500
MACROLIDES			
Azithromycin	500 mg PO	0.4	High
	500 mg IV	3.6	
Clarithromycin	500 mg PO	2–3	7000
Dirithromycin	500 mg PO	0.4	
Erythromycin			
oral[3]	500 mg PO	0.1–2	
estolate	500 mg PO	2	
lacto/glucep	500 mg IV	3–4	
MISCELLANEOUS			
Antibacterial			
Chloramphenicol	1.0 gm PO	11–18	
Clindamycin	150 mg PO	2.5	250–300
	600 mg IV	10	250–300
Doxycycline	100 mg PO	1.5–2.1	200–3200
Fosfomycin	3.0 gm PO	26	
	20 mg/kg IV	130	
Metronidazole	500 mg PO	20–25	100
	500 mg IV	20–25	100
Minocycline	200 mg PO	2.0–3.5	200–3200
Polymyxin B	30,000 u/kg IV	1–8	
Quinu/dalfo (Synercid)	7.5 mg/kg IV	Approx. 5.0	
Rifampin	600 mg po	7.0	10,000
Sulfisoxazole	2–4 gm PO	11–25	40–70
	2–4 gm IV	11–25	40–70
Tetracycline	250 mg PO	1.5–2.2	200–3200
TMP/SMX–DS (160 mg TMP/ 800 mg SMX)	1 tab po	TMP 1–2 SMX 40–60	100–200
(160 mg TMP/ 800 mg SMX)	2 ampuls IV	TMP: 9 SMX: 105	40–70
Vancomycin	1 gm IV	20–50[5]	50

[1] Traditionally, peak serum levels are determined on serum obtained 1 hr after the start of the infusion of the 3rd dose. However, if dosing is qd and the pt is critically ill, it is reasonable to measure the peak level after the 1st or 2nd dose.

[2] Peak concentration in bile divided by peak concentration in serum x 100. If blank = no data

[3] Erythromycin oral includes base, stearate, ethyl succinate, lactobionate, and gluceptate

[4] A 1-carbacephem but classified as a cephalosporin

[5] In renal failure pts, assay method (fluorescent polarization immunoassay) may overestimate serum level; use enzyme mult. immunoassay *(JAC 36:411, 1995).*

TABLE 8B (2)

DRUG	DOSE/ROUTE	PEAK SERUM LEVEL (μg/ml)	DRUG	DOSE/ROUTE	PEAK SERUM LEVEL (μg/ml)
ANTIFUNGAL			**ANTIVIRAL**		
Ampho B—standard	0.4–0.7 mg/kg IV	0.5–3.5	Abacavir	300 mg po	0.9–1.7
ABLC[1]	5 mg/kg IV	1.7 ± 0.8	Acyclovir	5 mg/kg IV	9.8
AB chole. complex[1]	4 mg/kg IV	2–9	Aman/Rimantadine	100 mg po	0.1–0.4
Liposom. AB[1]	2.5 mg/kg IV	31 ± 18	Amprenavir	1200 mg po	5.4
Fluconazole	400 mg po	6.7	Delavirdine	400 mg po	19 ± 11
Flucytosine	2.5 gm po	30–45	Didanosine (ddl)	300 mg po	1.6
Itraconazole,oral soln	200 mg po	2 (fasting)	Efavirenz	600 mg po	13 μM
ANTIMYCOBACTERIAL			Famciclovir	500 mg po	3–4
Ethambutol	25 mg/kg po	2–6	Foscarnet	57 mg/kg IV	155 (517 μM)
Ethionamide	1 gm po	20	Ganciclovir	5 mg/kg IV	8.3
Isoniazid	300 mg po	3–5	Indinavir	800 mg po	Data unclear
Pyrazinamide	20–25 mg/kg po	30–50	Lamivudine (3TC)	2 mg/kg po	1.5
Rifampin	600 mg po	8–24	Nelfinavir	750 mg po	3–4
Streptomycin	1 gm IV	25–50	Nevirapine	200 mg po	2
ANTIPARASITIC			Oseltamivir	75 mg po	0.65/3.5[2]
Albendazole	400 mg po	1.3	Ribavirin	400 mg po	0.6
Dapsone	100 mg po	1.8	Ritonavir	300 mg po	7.8
Ivermectin	12 mg po	46	Saquinavir (gel)	1200 mg po	Not clear
Mefloquine	1.0 gm po	0.5–1.2	Stavudine (d4T)	70 mg po	1.4
Pentamidine	4.0 mg/kg IV	0.5–3.4	Valacyclovir	1000 mg po	5.6
Pyrimethamine	25 mg po	0.1–0.3	Zalcitabine (ddC)	0.5 mg po	7.6 ng/ml
Praziquantel	20 mg/kg po	0.2–2.0	Zidovudine (ZDV)	200 mg po	1.2
Quinine	650 mg po	3–10			

[1] **Abbreviations: ABLC** = ampho B lipid complex; **AB chole** = ampho B cholesterol complex; **Liposom. AB** = liposomal ampho B   [2] Oseltamivir/oselt. carboxylate

TABLE 8C: CEREBROSPINAL FLUID CONCENTRATIONS OF ANTIMICROBIALS (see footnote)[1]

DRUG	CSF/BLOOD (%)	CSF LEVEL POTENTIALLY THERAPEUTIC[1]	DRUG	CSF/BLOOD (%)	CSF LEVEL POTENTIALLY THERAPEUTIC[1]
Antibacterial Drugs			Erythro/Clarithro/ Azithromycin	2–13 for erythro	0
Penicillins			Metronidazole	30–100	+
Ampicillin	13–14	+	Sulfisoxazole	$\propto$80	+[6]
Nafcillin	9–20	+	TMP/SMX	<41	+[6]
Penicillin G, high dose	5–10	+[2]	Vancomycin, HD[7]	7–14	+[7]
Piperacillin	30	±[3]	**Antifungal Drugs**		
Ticarcillin	40	±[3]	Ampho B, Itraconazole	0	0
Cephalosporins (no activity vs listeria)			Fluconazole	50–94	+
Cefazolin	1–4	0	Flucytosine	60–100	+
Cefepime	10	No data	**Antimycobacterial Drugs**		
Cefotaxime	10	+	Cycloserine	80–100	+
Cefoxitin	3	±[3]	Ethambutol	25–50	0
Ceftazidime	20–40	+	Isoniazid	20–90	+
Ceftriaxone	8–16	+	Pyrazinamide	85–100	+
Cefuroxime	17–88	+	Rifampin	7–56	+
Other beta-lactams			**Antiviral Drugs**[8]		
Aztreonam	3–52	±	Abacavir	18	No data
Imipenem	8.5	+[4]	Acyclovir	50	+
Meropenem	21	+	Didanosine	12–85	+
Aminoglycosides	0–30	0[3]	Foscarnet	13–103	+
Chloramphenicol, IV	45–89	+	Ganciclovir	41	+
Clindamycin	<1	0	Lamivudine	6–11	No data
Fluoroquinolones			Saquinavir	Negligible	0
Ciprofloxacin	26	+[5]	Stavudine	16–97	+
Gatifloxacin	36	Under study	Zalcitabine	9–37	+
Sparfloxacin	No data	No data	Zidovudine	60	+
Levofloxacin	30–50	+	No data for delavirdine, indinavir, nelfinavir, nevirapine, or ritonavir		
Trovafloxacin	23	Under study			

[1] CSF concentrations are those reported with inflammation unless indicated. "Therapeutic CSF level" is a judgment based on drug dose and organism susceptibility. As a general rule, CSF concentration should be ≥10x above MBC for bactericidal effect. [2] Does not apply to penicillin-resistant S. pneumoniae. [3] Does not apply to P. aeruginosa meningitis; levels borderline for coliforms; in individual pts, may need to add intrathecal gentamicin 5–10 mg. [4] Avoid for meningitis rx due to seizure potential. [5] Concentration inadequate for streptococci. [6] Most neisseria resistant. Not cidal vs coliforms. [7] Need high doses for resistant pneumococci (PJID 16:895, 1997). [8] Data do not imply inflamed meninges. Reference: CID 27:1117, 1998

TABLE 9A
SELECTED ANTIBACTERIAL AGENTS—ADVERSE REACTIONS—OVERVIEW

Adverse reactions in individual patients represent all-or-none occurrences, even if rare. After selection of an agent, the physician should read the manufacturer's package insert [statements in the product labeling (package insert) must be approved by the FDA].

Numbers = frequency of occurrence (%); + = occurs, incidence not available; ++ = significant adverse reaction; 0 = not reported; R = rare, defined as <1%. NOTE: Important reactions in bold print.

| ADVERSE REACTIONS | PENICILLINS, CARBAPENEMS, MONOBACTAMS, AMINOGLYCOSIDES | | | | | | | | | | | | | | | | | | | | |
| | PRSP | | | | | AMINO-PENICILLINS | | | | AP PENS | | | | | | | AMINO-GLYCOSIDES | | | | |
	Penicillin G,V	Cloxacillin	Dicloxacillin	Nafcillin	Oxacillin	Amoxicillin	Amox/Clav	Ampicillin	Amp/Sulb	Piperacillin	Pip/Taz	Ticarcillin	Ticar/Clav	Imipenem	Meropenem	Aztreonam	Amikacin	Gentamicin	Kanamycin	Netilmicin	Tobramycin
Local, phlebitis	+			++	+				3	4	1	3		3	1	4					
Hypersensitivity	+													3	3						
Fever	+	+	+	+	+	+	+	+	+	+	2	+	+	+		2	+				+
Rash	3	4	4	4	4	5	3	5	2	1	4	3	2	+	+	2	+				1
Photosensitivity	0	0	0	0	0	0	0	0	0	0	0	0	0	0		0					
Anaphylaxis	R	0	0	R	R	0	R	R	+	0	0	+	+	+		+					
Serum sickness	4									+	+	+	+	+		+					
Hematologic																					
+ Coombs	3	0	0	R	R	+	0	+	0	+	+	0	+	2	+	R					
Neutropenia	R	0	0	+	R	+	+	+	+	6	+	0	+	+		+					
Eosinophilia	+	+	+	22	22	2	+	2	+	+	+	+	5	+		8					
Thrombocytopenia	R	0	0	R	R	R	R	R	R	+	+	R	R	+	+	+					
↑ PT/PTT	R	0	0	+	0	+	0	+	0	+	+	+	+	R		R					
GI																					
Nausea/vomiting		+	+	0	0	2	3	2	+	+	7	+	1	2	4	R					
Diarrhea		+	+	0	0	**5**	**9**	**10**	**2**	2	11	3	1	2	5	R					
AAC		R	R	R	R	R	+	R	+	+	+	+	+	+		+					
Hepatic, LFTs	R	R	R	0	+	R	+	R	6	+	+	0	+	4	4	2				15	
Hepatic failure	0	0	0	0	0	0	0	0	0	0	0	0	0	0	1						
Renal: ↑ BUN, Cr	R	0	0	0	0	R	0	R	R	+	+	0	0	+	0	0	**8**	**8**	**+**	**9**	**10**
CNS																					
Headache	R	0	0	R	R	0	+	R	R	R	8	R	R	+	3	+	+				
Confusion	R	0	0	R	R	0	0	R	R	R	R	R	R	+		+					
Seizures	R	0	0	0	+	0	R	R	0	0	R	R	+	**1**	**0.4**	+					
Special Senses																					
Ototoxicity	0	0	0	0	0	0	0	0	0	0	0	0	0	R		0	**5**	**+**	**2**	**+**	**R**
Vestibular	0	0	0	0	0	0	0	0	0	0	0	0	0	0		0	**+**	**2**	**+**	**R**	**+**
Cardiac																					
Dysrhythmias	R	0	0		0	0	0	0	0	0	0	0	0	0		+					
Miscellaneous, Unique (Table 9B)	+		+	+	+	+	+	+	+			+		+		+					
Drug/drug interactions, common (Table 21)	0	0	0	0	0	0	0	0	0	0	0	0	0	0		0	+	+	+	+	+

CEPHALOSPORINS/CEPHAMYCINS

ADVERSE REACTIONS	Cefazolin	Cephapirin	Cefotetan	Cefoxitin	Cefuroxime	Cefoperazone	Cefotaxime	Ceftazidime	Ceftizoxime	Ceftriaxone	Cefepime	Cefpirome[NUS]	Cefaclor/Cef.ER[1]	Cefadroxil	Cefdinir	Cefixime	Cefpodoxime	Cefprozil	Ceftibuten	Cefuroxime-ax.	Cephalexin	Loracarbef
Local, phlebitis	+	+	R	R	2	1	5	1	4	2	1											
Hypersensitivity	5		1						2		+		2									
Fever	+	+	+	+		R		R	+	R		+				R	+		R		+	
Rash	+	+		2	R	2	2	2	2	2	2	1	1	+	R	1	1	1	R	R	1	1
Photosensitivity	0	0	0	0	0	0	0	R	0	0												
Anaphylaxis	R	R	+						R				R				R			R		
Serum sickness													≤0.5	+							+	+
Hematologic																						
Anemia					10	5		R					+						2			
+ Coombs	3	+	+	2	R	2	6	8			14	3	R							R	+	
Neutropenia	+	+		2	R	2	+	1	+	2	1		+	+	R	R	R	R			3	+
Eosinophilia		+	+	3	7	10	1	8	4	6	1				R	R	3	2	5	1	9	1
Thrombocytopenia	+	+						+	+		+		2			R	R	+	R			+
↑ PT/PTT		+	++	+		++	+	+	+	+	+											
GI				2									3	3	13			6		2		
Nausea/vomiting			1		R		R	R		R	1	+			7	4	4	2	3			2
Diarrhea			4		R	3	1	1		3	1	+	1		16	16	7	3	3	4		4
AAC	+	+	+	+	+	+	+	+	+	+	+	+	+	+	+	+	+	+	+	+	+	+
Hepatic, ↑ LFTs	+	+	1	3	4	8	1	6	4	3	+	+	3	+	1	R	4	2	R	2	+	R
Hepatic failure	0	0	0	0	0	0	0	0	0	0	0	0										
Renal: ↑ BUN, Cr	+	R		3		6		R		1	+		+		R	+	4	R	R		+	+
CNS						R																
Headache	0								2		2				2		1	R	R	R	+	3
Confusion	0												+					R		+		
Seizures	0	+																				
Special Senses																						
Ototoxicity	0	0	0	0		0	0	0	0	0			0	0	0	0	0	0	0	0	0	0
Vestibular	0	0	0	0		0	0	0	0	0			0	0	0	0	0	0	0	0	0	0
Cardiac																						
Dysrhythmias	0	0	0	0		0	0	0	0	0			0	0	0	0	0	0	0	0	0	0
Miscellaneous, Unique (Table 9B)						+				+			+									
Drug/drug interactions, common (Table 21)	0	0	0	0	0	0	0	0	0	0			0	0		0	0	0	0	0	0	0

[1] Cefaclor extended release tablets

TABLE 9A* (3)

ADVERSE REACTIONS (AE)	MACROLIDES				QUINOLONES[1]									OTHER AGENTS								
	Azithromycin	Clarithromycin	Dirithromycin	Erythromycin	Ciprofloxacin	Gatifloxacin	Levofloxacin	Lomefloxacin	Moxifloxacin	Norfloxacin	Ofloxacin	Sparfloxacin	Trovafloxacin	Chloramphenicol	Clindamycin	Metronidazole	Minocycline	Quinupristin/dalfopristin[2]	Rifampin	Tetracycline/Doxycycline	TMP/SMX	Vancomycin
Rx stopped due to AE	1	3	3		3.5	2.9	4	3	3.8	1	4	6.6	5									
Local, phlebitis				+	5										+		++			+		13
Hypersensitivity																		1	R	++	8	
Fever					R	R	R			1				+	+				+	+	+	1
Rash	R		R	+	3	R	1.7	R	R	1	2		1	+	+	+	+	R		+	+	3
Photosensitivity	R				R				**2**		R	**7.9**	R	4			R			+	+	0
Anaphylaxis				+	R			R	R		R	R	R									R
Serum sickness															+							
Hematologic					R					R		R								R		
Anemia														++							+	
Neutropenia	R	1			R	R				2	1			+	+	+	+			+	+	2
Eosinophilia			1		R					2	1				+		+			+	+	+
Thrombocytopenia	R	R	R		R					R				+	+		R	+		+	+	+
↑ PT/PTT		1																				0
GI			6	++											+					3		
Nausea/ vomiting	3	3	8	20-25	**5**	**8/2**	**1.2**	**4**	**8/2**	**3**	**7**	**7**	**7**			12	+			+	+	+
Diarrhea	5	3	8	**8**	2	4	1.2	1	6		4	3	2	+	**7**	+	+		+	3		
AAC		+		+	**R**	**R**	**R**	**R**		**R**	**R**	**R**	**R**	++					R	+		+
Hepatic, LFTs	R	R	R	+	2	R	+		R	<2	2	2	≥1		+		2		+	+		0
Hepatic failure	0	0	0										**R**						+	+		0
Renal																						
↑ BUN, Cr	+	4	1		1					R	R			0					+	+	+	5
CNS																++						
Dizziness, light-headedness					R	3	**2.5**	**2.3**	**3**	**2.6**	**3**	**2**	**4**									
Headache	R	2	4		1	4	5.4	6	2	2		4	5	+	+	+				+	+	
Confusion				+	+			+	R	R	+	2		+		+	+		+	+		
Seizures				+	+			+	+		+	R	R			+						
Special senses																						
Ototoxicity	+			+	0						R							+				R
Vestibular																	21					
Cardiac																						
Dysrhythmias				+	R							R	+[3]	R								0
Miscellaneous, Unique (Table 9B)	+			+				+	+		+	+	+	+	+	+	+	+	+	+	+	+
Drug/drug interactions, common (Table 21)	+	+	+	+	+	+	+	+	+	+	+	+	+						++	+		+

[1] Concern expressed that quinolones may be associated with episodes of tendonitis.
[2] Quinupristin/dalfopristin = Synercid
[3] Can cause prolongation of QT_c interval

See note at head of table, page 60

TABLE 9B: SUMMARY OF CURRENT ANTIBIOTIC DOSAGE* AND SIDE-EFFECTS

CLASS, AGENT, GENERIC NAME (TRADE NAME)	USUAL ADULT DOSAGE (Cost)	ADVERSE REACTIONS, COMMENTS (See Table 9A for Summary)
NATURAL PENICILLINS		
Benzathine penicillin G (Bicillin)	600,000–1.2 million u. Cost: 1.2 mu $16.14	**Most common adverse reactions are hypersensitivity.** Anaphylaxis in up to 0.05%, 5–10% fatal. Commercially available skin test antigen (penicilloyl polylysine) does not predict anaphylactic reactions. Hematologic, renal, CNS (seizures) reactions usually seen with high dose (>20 million units/day) and renal failure. With procaine pen G and benzathine pen G, an immediate but transient (5–30 min. after injection) toxic reaction with bizarre behavior and neurologic reactions can occur (Hoignes syndrome). Coombs test positive hemolytic anemias are rare but typically severe; in contrast, the Coombs test is often positive with cephalosporin therapy, but clinically significant hemolysis is rare.
Penicillin G	Low: 600,000–1.2 million u/d IM High: ≥20 million u qd IV (=12 gm) Cost: 10 mu $6.66	Penicillin allergy ref.: *JAMA 278:1895, 1997*
Penicillin V	0.25–0.5 gm bid, tid, qid post. Cost: 500 mg G $0.08, NB $0.13	
PENICILLINASE-RESISTANT PENICILLINS (PRSP)		
Cloxacillin (Cloxapen)	0.25–0.5 gm q6h ac, po. Cost: 500 mg NB $0.73, G $0.29	
Dicloxacillin (Dynapen)	0.125–0.5 gm q6h ac, po. Cost: 500 mg G $0.66	Blood levels ~2x greater than cloxacillin. Acute hemorrhagic cystitis reported. Acute abdominal pain with GI bleeding without antibiotic-associated colitis also reported.
Flucloxacillin[NUS] (Floxapen, Lutropin, Staphcil)	0.25–0.5 gm q6h po 1.0–2.0 gm q4h IV	In Australia, cholestatic hepatitis [women predominate, age >65, rx mean 2 weeks, onset 3 weeks from starting rx (*Ln 339:679, 1992*)], 16 deaths since 1980: recommendation: use only in severe infection (*Ln 344:676, 1994*).
Nafcillin (Unipen, Nafcil)	1.0–2.0 gm q4h IV, IM. Cost: 1.0 gm $2.27	Extravasation can result in tissue necrosis. With dosages of 200–300 mg/kg/d hypokalemia may occur. **Reversible neutropenia (over 10% with ≥21-day rx, occasionally WBC <1000/mm³).**
Oxacillin (Prostaphlin)	1.0–2.0 gm q4h IV, IM. Cost: 1.0 gm $2.68	**Hepatic dysfunction with ≥12 gm/d.** LFTs usually ↑ 2–24 days after start of rx, reversible. ↑ SGOT in 9/11 HIV+ pts (*AnIM 120:1048, 1994*).
AMINOPENICILLINS		
Amoxicillin (Amoxil, Polymox)	0.5 gm q8h po or 0.875 gm q12h. Cost: 500 mg G $0.31, NB $0.40, 0.875 gm $0.97	IV available in UK, Europe. IV amoxicillin rapidly converted to ampicillin. Rash with infectious mono—see *Ampicillin*.
Amoxicillin/clavulanate (Augmentin)	875/125 mg bid po **(note new dosage)**. Cost: 875/125 mg NB $4.65 500/125 mg tid po. Cost: $3.48	With bid regimen and less clavulanate, less diarrhea (*PIID 16:463, 1997*). Cholestatic hepatitis reported, esp. men >60 yrs, on rx >2 weeks. Jaundice resolved in 1–8 weeks (risk <1:100,000) (*Gut 33:368, 1992; ArIM 156:1327, 1996*). 2 cases anaphylactic reaction to clavulanic acid (*J All Clin Immun 95:748, 1995*).
Ampicillin (Omnipen, Principen)	0.25–0.5 gm q6h po. Cost: 500 mg G $0.13, NB $0.26 150–200 mg/kg/d IV. Cost: 1.0 gm G $1.64	A maculopapular rash occurs (not urticarial), **not true penicillin allergy**, in 65–100% pts with infectious mono, 90% with chronic lymphocytic leukemia, and 15–20% with allopurinol rx.
Ampicillin/sulbactam (Unasyn)	1.5–3.0 gm q6h IV. Cost: 3.0 gm NB $15.26 (see Comment)	Supplied in vials: ampicillin 1.0 gm, sulbactam 0.5 gm or amp 2.0 gm, sulbactam 1.0 gm. Antibiotic is not active vs pseudomonas. Total daily dose sulbactam ≤4 gm.
Bacampicillin (Spectrobid)	400 mg q12h po. Cost: 400 mg NB $2.39	↑ po absorption compared to ampicillin.
ANTIPSEUDOMONAL PENICILLINS: Ureidopenicillins (piperacillin, mezlocillin) (congeners of aminopenicillins) have better activity vs enterococci & klebsiella than carboxypenicillins (ticarcillin)		
Mezlocillin (Mezlin)	3.0 gm q4h IV. Cost: 3.0 gm $14.13	1.85 mEq Na⁺/gm
Piperacillin (Pipracil)	3.0–4.0 gm q4–6h IV (200–300 mg/kg/d up to 500 mg/kg/d). Cost: 3.0 gm NB $19.12	1.85 mEq Na⁺/gm

(See page 69 for footnotes and abbreviations)   ** NOTE: all dosage recommendations are for adults (unless otherwise indicated) and assume normal renal function.*

TABLE 9B (2)

CLASS, AGENT, GENERIC NAME (TRADE NAME)	USUAL ADULT DOSAGE (Cost)	ADVERSE REACTIONS, COMMENTS (See Table 9A for Summary)
ANTIPSEUDOMONAL PENICILLINS *(continued)*		
Piperacillin tazobactam (Zosyn)	3.375 gm q6h IV. Cost: 3.375 gm NB $16.21 PIP/TZ 3.375 gm q6h 4.5 gm prep available mid-2000	Supplied in vials: piperacillin 3.0 gm, tazobactam (TZ) 0.375 gm. In Europe, studied mostly as 4.0 gm pip/0.5 gm tazo. TZ is similar to clavulanate and more active than sulbactam as β-lactamase inhibitor. Has ↑ activity over pip alone vs gram-negatives and anaerobes. OK when combined with an aminoglycoside as monotherapy **not** adequate for serious pseudomonas infections; (tobramycin).
Ticarcillin disodium (Ticar)	3.0 gm q4-6h IV. Cost: 3.0 gm NB $12.92	Coagulation abnormalities common with large doses, interferes with platelet function, ↑ bleeding times; may be clinically significant in pts with renal failure. (4.7-5.0 mEq Na⁺/gm)
Ticarcillin/clavulanate (Timentin)	3.1 gm q4-6h IV. Cost: 3.1 gm NB $15.40	Supplied in vials: ticarcillin 3.0 gm, clavulanate 0.1 gm/vial. 4.7-5.0 mEq Na⁺/gm. Diarrhea due to clavulanate.
CARBAPENEMS		
Imipenem + cilastatin (Primaxin)	0.5 gm q6h IV. Cost: 500 mg NB $30.32	Seizure incidence with 0.5 gm q6h is 0.2-1.0%; with 1.0 gm q6h increases to ~10%. In elderly pts with ↓ renal function, cerebrovascular disease or seizure disorders, dosage needs to be decreased. Cross-reactivity in ½ pts with anaphylaxis to penicillin (*J All Clin Imm 82:213, 1988*). Resistance of P. aeruginosa reported (*see Table 5*).
Meropenem (Merrem)	0.5-1.0 gm q8h IV. Cost: 1.0 gm NB $51.84	In animals, less likely than IMP to cause seizures. Comments: Does not require a dehydropeptidase inhibitor (cilastatin). Activity vs aerobic gm-neg. slightly ↑ over IMP, activity vs staph & strep slightly ↓; anaerobes = to IMP. B. ovatus, B. distasonis more resistant to meropenem.
MONOBACTAMS		
Aztreonam (Azactam)	1.0 gm q8h-2.0 gm q6h IV. Cost: 1.0 gm NB $16.97	Can be used in pts with allergy to penicillins/cephalosporins. Animal data and a letter raise concern about cross-reactivity with ceftazidime (*Rev Inf Dis 7:613, 1985*); side-chains of aztreonam and ceftazidime are identical.
CEPHALOSPORINS (1st parenteral, then oral drugs).	NOTE: Prospective data demonstrate correlation between use of cephalosporins (esp. 3rd generation) and ↑ risk of C. difficile toxin-induced diarrhea. May also ↑ risk of colonization with vancomycin-resistant enterococci.	
1st Generation, Parenteral		
Cefazolin (Ancef, Kefzol)	0.25 gm q8h-1.5 gm q6h IV, IM. Cost: 1.0 gm G $1.74, NB $4.17	Do not give into lateral ventricles—seizures!
Cephapirin (Cefadyl)	0.5 gm q6h-2.0 gm q4h IV,IM. Cost: 1.0 gm NB $1.64	Cephalothin no longer available in the U.S.
2nd Generation, Parenteral		
Cefamandole (Mandol)	0.5 gm q6h-2.0 gm q4h IV, IM. Cost: 1.0 gm NB $9.06	Mild ↑ in BUN, creatinine esp. in pts >50 yrs. Concurrent furosemide may ↑ reaction rates (34%). Rare disulfiram-like reactions after alcohol.
Cefotetan (Cefotan)	1-3 gm q12h IV, IM. (Max. dose not >6 gm qd). Cost: 1.0 gm NB $11.58	3 cases anaphylaxis after 2.0 gm IV over 15 min. (*Am J Ob Gyn 59:125, 1988*). Active vs B. fragilis, Prevotella bivius, Prevotella disiens (most common in pelvic infections).
Cefoxitin (Mefoxin)	1.0 gm q8h-2.0 gm q4h IV, IM. Cost: 1.0 gm NB $10.48	In vitro may induce ↑ β-lactamase, esp. in Enterobacter sp.; clinical significance ?.
Cefuroxime (Zinacef)	0.75-1.5 gm q8h IV,IM. Cost: 1.5 gm NB $13.93	More stable vs staphylococcal β-lactamase than cefazolin.
3rd Generation, Parenteral—One study correlated use of P Ceph 3 drugs with incidence of C. difficile toxin diarrhea (*Am J Gastro 89:519, 1994*)		
Cefoperazone (Cefobid)	2.0 gm q12h-4 gm q6h IV. Pyelonephritis: 1.0 gm q12h IV. Cost: 2.0 gm NB $32.83	Maximum dose 8.0 gm qd. Q6h dosage required for Pseudomonas sp. Disulfiram-like reactions after alcohol, up to 48 hrs after completion of antibiotic rx.
Cefotaxime (Claforan)	1.0 gm q8-12h to 2.0 gm q4h IV. Cost: 2.0 gm NB $21.16	Maximum daily dose: 12 gm

(See page 69 for footnotes and abbreviations)   * *NOTE: all dosage recommendations are for adults (unless otherwise indicated) and assume normal renal function.*

(See page 69 for footnotes and abbreviations)   * *NOTE: all dosage recommendations are for adults (unless otherwise indicated) and assume normal renal function.*

TABLE 9B (3)

CLASS, AGENT, GENERIC NAME (TRADE NAME)	USUAL ADULT DOSAGE (Cost)	ADVERSE REACTIONS, COMMENTS (See Table 9A for Summary)
CEPHALOSPORINS, 3rd Generation, Parenteral *(continued)*		
Ceftazidime (Fortaz, Tazicef, Tazidime)	1.0–2.0 gm q8–12h IV, IM. Cost: 2.0 gm NB $28.45–41.17	Excessive use may result in ↑ incidence of C. difficile-assoc. diarrhea and/or selection of vancomycin-resistant E. faecium. Ceftaz is susceptible to extended-spectrum cephalosporinases (CID 27:76 & 81, 1998).
Ceftizoxime (Cefizox)	1.0 gm q8–12h to 4.0 gm q8h IV. Cost: 2.0 gm NB $21.14	Maximum daily dose: 12 gm. In vitro active vs B. fragilis, dependent on testing method.
Ceftriaxone (Rocephin)	Commonly used IV dosage in adults: < Age 60: 2.0 gm once daily > Age 60: 1.0 gm once daily Purulent meningitis: 2.0 gm q12h. Can give IM in 1% lidocaine. Cost: 1.0 gm NB $42.00	Dosage: 2.0 gm IV qd gives better tissue levels than 1.0 gm q12h (overcomes protein binding). "Pseudocholelithiasis" 2° to sludge in gallbladder by ultrasound (50%), symptomatic (9%) (NEJM 322:1821, 1990). More likely with ≥2 gm/d with pt on total parenteral nutrition and not eating (AnIM 115:712, 1991). Clinical significance still unclear but has led to cholecystectomy (JID 17:356, 1995) and gallstone pancreatitis (Ln 17:662, 1998).
4th Generation, Parenteral		
Cefepime (Maxipime)	1.0–2.0 gm q12h IV. Cost: 2.0 gm NB $31.63	Active vs P. aeruginosa and many strains of Enterobacter, serratia, C. freundii resistant to ceftazidime, cefotaxime, aztreonam (CID 20:56, 1995). More active vs S. aureus than 3rd generation cephalosporins.
Cefpirome^NUS (HR 810)	1.0–2.0 gm q12h IV	Similar to cefepime: ↑ activity vs enterobacteriaceae, P. aeruginosa, Gm + organisms. Anaerobes: less active than cefoxitin, more active than cefotax or ceftaz
Oral Cephalosporins—Also see footnote, Table 1, page 10		The oral cephalosporins are generally safe. **Patients with a history of IgE-mediated allergic reactions to a penicillin (e.g., anaphylaxis, angioneurotic edema, immediate urticaria) should not receive a cephalosporin.** If the history is a "measles-like" rash to a penicillin, available data suggest a 5–10% risk of rash in such patients; there is no enhanced risk of anaphylaxis. Any of the cephalosporins can result in C. difficile toxin-mediated diarrhea/enterocolitis. The reported frequency of nausea/vomiting and non-C. difficile toxin diarrhea is summarized in Table 9A. There are few drug-specific adverse effects, e.g., Cefaclor: Serum sickness-like reaction 0.1–0.5%—arthralgia, rash, erythema multiforme but no adenopathy, proteinuria or demonstrable immune complexes. Anecdotal reports of similar reaction to loracarbef. Cefpodoxime: There are rare reports of acute liver injury, bloody diarrhea, pulmonary infiltrates with eosinophilia.
1st Generation, Oral		
Cefadroxil (Duricef)	0.5–1.0 gm q12h po. Cost: 0.5 gm NB $3.05	
Cephalexin (Keflex, Keftab, generic)	0.25–0.5 gm q6h po. Cost: 0.5 gm NB $2.96, G $1.07	
Cephradine (Velosef, generic)	0.25–0.5 gm q6h po. Cost: 0.5 gm NB $1.68, G $1.05	
2nd Generation, Oral		
Cefaclor (Ceclor)	0.25–0.5 gm q8h po. Cost: 0.5 gm NB $3.83, G $2.39	
Cefaclor-ER (Ceclor CD)	0.375–0.5 gm q12h po. Cost: 0.5 gm NB $3.66	
Cefprozil (Cefzil)	0.25–0.5 gm q12h po. Cost: 0.5 gm NB $6.53	
Cefuroxime axetil (Ceftin)	0.125–0.5 gm q12h po. Cost: 0.5 gm NB $7.45, 0.25 gm $4.07	
Loracarbef (Lorabid)	0.4 gm q12h po. Cost: 0.4 gm NB $4.05	
3rd Generation, Oral	See Comments, above	
Cefixime (Suprax) 0.2–0.4 gm q12–24h po. Cost: 0.4 gm NB $7.20	Cefpodoxime proxetil (Vantin) 0.1–0.2 gm q12h po. Cost: 0.2 gm NB $3.91	Ceftibuten (Cedax) 0.4 gm qd po. Cost: 0.2 gm NB $7.41	Cefdinir (Omnicef) 300 mg q12h. Cost: 300 mg $3.36

(See page 69 for footnotes and abbreviations)   * NOTE: all dosage recommendations are for adults (unless otherwise indicated) and assume normal renal function.

TABLE 9B (4)

CLASS, AGENT, GENERIC NAME (TRADE NAME)	USUAL ADULT DOSAGE (Cost)—See Table 9C, page 70, and Table 17, page 121	ADVERSE REACTIONS, COMMENTS (See Table 9A for Summary)
AMINOGLYCOSIDES AND RELATED ANTIBIOTICS—See Table 9C, page 70		
CHLORAMPHENICOL, CLINDAMYCIN(S), ERYTHROMYCIN GROUP, QUINUPRISTIN/DALFOPRISTIN (SYNERCID), VANCOMYCIN/TEICOPLANIN		
Chloramphenicol (Chloromycetin)	50 mg/kg IV. Cost: 1.0 gm $6.65	No oral drug distributed in U.S. Hematologic (↓ RBC ~1/3 pts, aplastic anemia 1:21,600 courses). Gray baby syndrome in premature infants, anaphylactoid reactions, optic atrophy or neuropathy (very rare), digital paresthesias, minor disulfiram-like reactions.
Clindamycin (Cleocin)	0.15–0.45 gm po q6h. 600–900 mg q8h IV, IM. Cost: 150 mg po NB $1.36 600 mg IV NB $13.88 / Lincomycin (Lincocin) 0.5 gm q6–8h po. 0.6 gm q8h IV, IM. Cost: 500 mg po $2.00, 300 mg IV $3.37	Based on number of exposed pts, these drugs are the most frequent cause of C. difficile toxin-mediated diarrhea. In most severe form can cause pseudomembranous colitis/toxic megacolon.
Erythromycin Group (Review drug interactions before use) Ref: *Mayo Clin Proc 74:613, 1999*		Motilin is gastric hormone that activates duodenal/jejunal receptors to initiate peristalsis. Erythro (E) and E esters, both po and IV, activate motilin receptors and cause uncoordinated peristalsis with resultant 20–25% incidence of anorexia, nausea or vomiting (*Gut 33:397, 1992*). Less binding and GI distress with azithromycin/clarithromycin.
Azithromycin (Zithromax)	po: 0.5 gm on day 1, then 0.25 gm qd on days 2–5 po. Cost: 250 mg $6.50 IV: 0.5 gm/d. Cost: $23.70	Frequent drug-drug interactions: see *Table 21, page 131*. Ex: Astemizole (non-sedating antihistamine) + erythro or clarithro can result in ↑ Q-T intervals, torsades de pointes, or ventricular tachycardia. Erythro alone an prolong QT_c interval (*Chest 115:983, 1999*), esp. in women (*JAMA 280:1774, 1998*).
Base and esters (Erythrocin, Ilosone) IV names: E. gluceptate (Ilotycin)	0.25 gm q6h–0.5 gm q6h po. IV: 15–20 mg/kg up to 4.0 gm qd. Infuse over 30 or more minutes. Cost: po 250 mg base G $0.18, stearate $0.18, estolate $0.29, ESS 400 $0.23. IV 1.0 gm NB $22.16	Cholestatic hepatitis in approx. 1:1000 adults (not children) given E estolate. Transient reversible tinnitus or deafness with ≥4 gm/d of erythro IV in pts with renal or hepatic impairment. Reported with ≥600 mg/d of azithro (*CID 24:76, 1997*). Dosages of oral erythro preparations expressed as base equivalents. With differences in absorption/biotransformation, variable amounts of erythro esters required to achieve same free erythro serum level, e.g., 400 mg E ethyl succinate = 250 mg E base.
Clarithromycin (Biaxin) or clarithro extended release (Biaxin XL)	0.5 gm q12h po. Cost: 500 mg $3.28 Extended release: Two 0.5 gm tabs po/d.	Macrolide-induced Churg-Strauss syndrome reported in an atopic pt (*Ln 350:563, 1997*).
Quinupristin + dalfopristin (Synercid) Teicoplanin[NUS] (Targocid)	Dosage: 7.5 mg/kg q8h IV x21–72 d. For septic arthritis—maintenance dose 12 mg/ kg/d; S. aureus endocarditis—trough serum levels >20 µg/ml required (12 mg/kg q12h x3 loading dose, then 12 mg/kg qd)	Venous irritation (5%), none with central venous line. Asymptomatic ↑ in unconjugated bilirubin. Arthralgia 2%. Hypersensitivity: fever (at 3 mg/kg 2.2%, at 24 mg/kg 8.2%), skin reactions 2.4%. Marked ↓ platelets (high dose ≥15 mg/kg/d). Red neck syndrome less common than with vancomycin (*JAC 32:792, 1993*).
Vancomycin (Vancocin)	15 mg/kg q12h IV; 125 mg q6h po; intrathecal 5–10 mg q48–72h. Cost: 500 mg IV G $13.24, NB $7.80. Oral "pulvule" 125 mg: Cost $5.38	Measure serum levels if: planned dose ≥2.0 gm/d, rapidly changing renal function, chronic renal failure. Target levels: peak 20–50 µg/ml, trough 5–10 µg/ml. Rapid infusion (over <1 hr) can cause non-specific histamine release manifest as angioneurotic edema, flushed skin ("red neck syndrome"), or hypotension. Can continue vanco but infuse over 1–2 hrs. Ototoxicity and nephrotoxicity now rare unless vanco given with an aminoglycoside; aminoglycoside amplifies the risk of nephrotoxicity. Neutropenia, rash occur. Rarely, association with linear IgA bullous dermatosis (*AnIM 129:507, 1998*).
TETRACYCLINES (*Mayo Clin Proc 74:727, 1999*)		
Doxycycline (Vibramycin, Doryx, Monodox)	0.1 gm po or IV q12h. Cost: 100 mg po G $0.08–0.11, NB $3.96; 100 mg IV NB $21.07	Similar to other tetracyclines. ↑ nausea on empty stomach. Erosive esophagitis, esp. if taken hs. Phototoxicity + but less than with tetracycline. Deposition in teeth less. Can be used in patients with renal failure. *Comments*: Effective in treatment and prophylaxis for malaria, leptospirosis, typhus fevers.

(See page 69 for footnotes and abbreviations) * NOTE: all dosage recommendations are for adults (unless otherwise indicated) and assume normal renal function.

TABLE 9B (5)

CLASS, AGENT, GENERIC NAME (TRADE NAME)	USUAL ADULT DOSAGE (Cost)	ADVERSE REACTIONS, COMMENTS (See Table 9A for Summary)
TETRACYCLINES *(continued)*		
Minocycline (Minocin)	0.1 gm q12h po. Cost: 100 mg G $0.80, NB $3.33	Similar to other tetracyclines. Vestibular symptoms (30–90% in some groups, none in others). (Vertigo 33%, ataxia 43%, nausea 50%, vomiting 3%), women more frequently than men. Hypersensitivity pneumonitis, reversible, ~34 cases reported *(BMJ 310:1520, 1995)*. **Comments:** More effective than other tetracyclines vs staph and in prophylaxis of meningococcal disease. P. acnes: many resistant to other tetracyclines, not to mino. Active vs Nocardia asteroides, Mycobacterium marinum.
Tetracycline, Oxytetracycline (Terramycin)	0.25–0.5 gm q6h po, 0.5–1.0 gm q12h IV. Cost: 250 mg po $0.06	GI (oxy 19%, terra 4), anaphylactoid reaction (rare), deposition in teeth, negative N balance, hepatotoxicity, enamel agenesis, pseudotumor cerebri/encephalopathy. Outdated drug: Fanconi syndrome. See *drug-drug interactions, Table 21*. **Contraindicated in pregnancy, hepatotoxicity in mother, transplacental to fetus.** **Comments:** IV dosage over 2.0 gm/d may be associated with fatal hepatotoxicity.
FLUOROQUINOLONES. Review Drug/Drug Interactions (Table 21, page 130) before prescribing. Major concerns have been drug-drug interactions, CNS toxicity (varies from lightheadedness to seizures), phototoxicity (see *Tables 7 & 9A*), nausea/vomiting, and potential adverse effect on joint cartilage. Potential cartilage injury based on animal studies; no unequivocal FQ-induced arthropathy in humans *(CID 25:1196, 1997)*. Use of FQs in children summarized in *PIDJ 18:467, 1999*; none approved under 16 yrs of age.		
Ciprofloxacin (Cipro)	500-750 mg bid po. Urinary tract infection: 250 mg bid po. Parenteral rx 200–400 mg q12h IV. Cost: 500 mg po $4.15, 400 mg IV $30.00	CNS: 0.4%; headache, restlessness, insomnia, nightmares, toxic psychosis (VR); convulsions (VR) *(AAC 37:1764, 1993)*. (See *drug interactions, esp. with caffeine, Table 21, page 130*). With alkaline urine, ≥1.0 gm/d, crystalluria in ⅓ pts. See *Cystic Fibrosis, Table 1, page 31, for discussion*. (400 mg IV = 750 mg po).
Gatifloxacin (Tequin)	400 mg IV or po qd. Cost: Not available *(12/99)*	Stopped for adverse events related to drug in 3% of pts: Nausea 8%, vaginitis 6%, diarrhea 4%, headache/dizziness 3%; all others <3%. Only drug interaction with multivalent cations other than Ca++ *(Table 21, page 130)*.
Levofloxacin (Levaquin)	250–500 mg qd po or IV. Cost: 500 mg po $8.06; 500 mg IV $39.60	Ofloxacin is a racemic mixture of L- and D- optical isomers. The D-isomer has little to no antibacterial activity. Levofloxacin is the pure L-isomer of ofloxacin. Levo has enhanced activity against Gm-pos. cocci and perhaps less toxicity.
Lomefloxacin (Maxaquin)	400 mg qd po. Cost: 400 mg $6.93	Overall 2.6% Photosensitivity 2.4% may be severe, avoid direct or indirect sunlight (tanning lamps). Evening dosing ↓ reactions *(Clin Pharm Therap 56:587, 1994)*. NOT indicated vs S. pneumoniae. No drug interactions with theophylline or caffeine.
Moxifloxacin (Avelox)	400 mg po qd. Cost: Not available *(12/99)*	Adverse events GI (nausea 8%, vomiting 2%, diarrhea 6%) CNS (headache, dizziness 3%, drowsiness). 3.8% pts stopped rx due to adverse events. Possible ↑ QT interval if concomitant use of quinidine, procainamide, amiodarone, sotalol or if hypokalemic.
Norfloxacin (Noroxin)	400 mg bid po ac. Cost: 400 mg $3.39	Does not have antipseudomonal activity. See *Comments, Fluoroquinolones, above*. Crystalluria if dose exceeded, force fluids.
Ofloxacin (Floxin)	200–400 mg bid po; 200–400 mg q12h IV. Cost: 400 mg po $4.67, 400 mg IV $26.40	Seizures in 4 elderly pts *(CID 21:1504, 1995)*.
Sparfloxacin (Zagam)	400 mg po x1, then 200 mg qd. Cost: 200 mg $6.72	Torsade de pointes reported in pts given sparfloxacin with disopyramide or amiodarone. Contraindicated in pts receiving any drug known to prolong Q-T interval. **The overall incidence of drug-related phototoxicity is 7.9%** (mild in 4.1%, moderate in 3.3%, severe in 0.6%). 1.1% stopped drug due to phototoxicity. Reactions have occurred after exposure to direct/indirect (through window glass) sunlight or sunlamps. Sunscreens may not protect. At risk for up to 5 days after last dose.

(See page 69 for footnotes and abbreviations)   *NOTE: all dosage recommendations are for adults (unless otherwise indicated) and assume normal renal function.*

67

TABLE 9B (6)

CLASS, AGENT, GENERIC NAME (TRADE NAME)	USUAL ADULT DOSAGE (Cost)	ADVERSE REACTIONS, COMMENTS (See Table 9A for Summary)
FLUOROQUINOLONES (continued)		
Trovafloxacin Trovafloxacin mesylate tabs po (Trovan) & alatrofloxacin mesylate IV (Trovan IV) **See Comment**	Adult IV dosage is 200–300 mg/d. NOTE: Reduce dose in pts with chronic liver disease (see package insert). Cost: 200 mg IV $36.88, 200 mg po $7.20	In a small number of pts, trova associated with serious liver injury leading to liver transplant and/or death. Reported after both short- & long-term treatment. Rx over 2 wks assoc. with ↑ risk liver injury. Recommended that trova use be reserved for serious life- or limb-threatening infection in pts in hospital or nursing care facility.
MISCELLANEOUS AGENTS		
Fosfomycin (Monurol)	3.0 gm mixed with water po x1 dose. Cost $27.00	Generally well-tolerated. Diarrhea in 9% of study population compared to 6% of pts given nitrofurantoin and 2.3% given TMP/SMX. If given with metoclopramide (Reglan), ↓ serum level.
Fusidic acid[NUS] (Fucidin)	500 mg tid po. IV (Leo Laboratories, Denmark)	Mild GI, occ. skin rash, jaundice (17% with IV, 6% with po). (None in CSF; <1% in urine)
Immune globulin IV therapy	Dosage, frequency vary with the indication. At least 7 manufacturers. Cost by trade name: Sandoglobulin 12 gm $609; Gammar 10 gm $800; Gamimune-N 10 gm $900; Gammagard S/D 10 gm $870; Panglobulin 12 gm $990; Venoglobulin 10 gm $900; Iveegam 10 gm $800	At present, 6 FDA-approved indications: primary immune-def., immune thrombocytopenia, Kawasaki syndrome, recent bone marrow transplant, B-cell lymphocytic leukemia, pediatric HIV. Many other endorsed uses (MMWR 48:159, 1999). Reported adverse reactions range from 1–15%. Fever, headache, myalgia, N/V relate to rate of infusion, mild, & self-limited. Less common/more serious: anaphylactoid reactions, thromboemboli, aseptic meningitis, & perhaps renal injury (MMWR 48:518, 1999).
Methenamine hippurate (Hiprex, Urex)	1.0 gm q6h po. Cost: 1.0 gm $1.21 1.0 gm = 480 mg methenamine	Nausea and vomiting, skin rash or dysuria. Overall ~3%. Methenamine requires (pH ≤5) urine to liberate formaldehyde. Limited place in therapy; useful in suppressive therapy when original infecting organisms have been cleared. Do not use for pyelonephritis. *Comment:* Fluids should not be forced, as concentration of formaldehyde may fall below inhibitory concentrations. Of no value in pts with continuously draining urethral catheter. If urine pH >5.0, co-administer ascorbic acid (1–2 gm q4h) to acidify the urine. Cranberry juice (1200–4000 ml/day) has been used, results ±.
Methenamine mandelate (Mandelamine)	1.0 gm q6h po (480 mg methenamine). Cost: 1.0 gm NB $0.60	
Metronidazole (Flagyl) Ref.: Mayo Clin Proc 74:825, 1999	Anaerobic infections: usually IV, 7.5 mg/kg (~500 mg) q6h (not to exceed 4.0 gm qd). With long T½, can use IV at 15 mg/kg q12h. If life-threatening, use loading dose of 15 mg/kg IV. Oral dose: 500 mg qid. Cost: 250 mg tab G $0.21, NB $1.55; 500 mg IV $19.03; 70 gm vaginal gel $32.28. Ext. release 750 mg $5.70	Can be given rectally (enema or suppository). In pts with decompensated liver disease (manifest by ≥2 L of ascites, encephalopathy, ↑ prothrombin time, ↓ serum albumin) t½ prolonged; unless dose ↓ by approx. ½, side-effects ↑. Absorption with vaginal gel. Neurol.: headache, rare paresthesias or peripheral neuropathy, ataxia, seizures, aseptic meningitis. **Avoid alcohol during & 48 hrs after (disulfiram-like reaction).** Very dark urine (common but harmless). Skin: urticaria. Mutagenic in Ames test. Tumorigenic in animals (high dose over lifetime). No evidence of risk in man. No teratogenicity.
Mupirocin (Bactroban)	tid x5 d., topical ointment; cost: 15 gm $22. Topical cream, cost: 15 gm $25	Burning, stinging 1.5%; itching 1% rash, contact dermatitis <1%.
Nitrofurantoin macrocrystals (Macrodantin)	100 mg q6h po. Cost: 100 mg G $1.16, NB $1.52. Dose for long-term UTI suppression: 50–100 mg at bedtime	Absorption ↑ with meals. Increased activity in acid urine, much reduced at pH 8 or over. Not effective in endstage renal disease [JAC 33(Suppl. A):121, 1994]. Nausea and vomiting, hypersensitivity, peripheral neuropathy. Pulmonary reactions (with chronic rx): acute ARDS type, **chronic desquamative interstitial pneumonia with fibrosis.** Intrahepatic cholestasis & hepatitis similar to chronic active hepatitis. Hemolytic anemia in G6PD deficiency. Contraindicated in renal failure. Should not be used in infants <1 month of age.
monohydrate/macrocrystals (Macrobid)	100 mg bid po. Cost: 100 mg $1.42	Efficacy of Macrobid 100 mg bid = Macrodantin 50 mg qid. Adverse effects 5.6%, less nausea than with Macrodantin.

(See page 69 for footnotes and abbreviations)   * NOTE: all dosage recommendations are for adults (unless otherwise indicated) and assume normal renal function.

TABLE 9B (7)

CLASS, AGENT, GENERIC NAME (TRADE NAME)	USUAL ADULT DOSAGE (Cost)	ADVERSE REACTIONS, COMMENTS (See Table 9A for Summary)
MISCELLANEOUS AGENTS (continued)		
Sulfonamides [e.g., sulfisoxazole (Gantrisin), sulfamethoxazole (Gantanol)]	Sulfisoxazole (Gantrisin): Cost 500 mg G $0.08, NB $0.53	**Short-acting are best:** high urine concentration and good solubility at acid pH. More active in alkaline urine. **Allergic reactions:** skin rash, drug fever, pruritus, photosensitization. Periarteritis nodosa & SLE. Stevens-Johnson syndrome, serum sickness syndrome, myocarditis. Neurotoxicity (psychosis, neuritis). Blood dyscrasias, usually agranulocytosis. Crystalluria. Nausea & vomiting, headache, dizziness, lassitude, mental depression, acidosis, sulf-hemoglobin. Hemolytic anemia in G6PD deficient & unstable hemoglobins (Hb Zurich). Do not use in newborn infants or in women near term, ↑ frequency of kernicterus (binds to albumin, blocking binding of bilirubin to albumin).
Trimethoprim (Trimpex and others)	100 mg tab po q12h or 200 mg (2 tabs) po q24h. Cost: 100 mg NB $0.70, G $0.15	Frequent side-effects are rash and pruritus. Rash in 3% pts at 100 mg bid; 6.7% at 200 mg qd. Rare reports of photosensitivity, exfoliative dermatitis, Stevens-Johnson syndrome, toxic epidermal necrosis, and aseptic meningitis (CID 19:431, 1994). Check drug interaction with phenytoin. Increases serum K⁺ (see TMP/SMX Comments). TMP can ↑ homocysteine blood levels (Ln 352:1827, 1998).
Trimethoprim (TMP)/ Sulfamethoxazole (SMX) (Bactrim, Septra) Single-strength (SS) is 80 TMP/400 SMX, double-strength (DS) 160 TMP/800 SMX	Standard po rx (UTI, otitis media): 1 DS tablet bid. P. carinii: see Table 12, page 90. **IV rx** (base on TMP component): standard 8–10 mg/kg/d divided q6h, q8h, or q12h. For shigellosis: 2.5 mg/kg IV q6h. Cost: 160/800 po G $0.09, NB $1.30–1.60; 160/800 IV $16.42	Adverse reactions in 10% or more of pts: GI and skin. GI: nausea, vomiting, anorexia. Skin: Rash, urticaria, photosensitivity. Less often but more serious (1–10%): Stevens-Johnson syndrome and toxic epidermal necrolysis. Skin adverse reactions may represent toxic metabolites of SMX and ↓ glutathione rather than allergy (An Pharm 32:381, 1998). See other sulfonamide adverse reactions above. TMP competes with creatinine for tubular secretion and serum creatinine can ↑; TMP also blocks distal renal tubule reabsorption of Na⁺ and secretion of K⁺. ↑ serum K⁺ in 21% of pts (AnIM 124:316, 1996). TMP/SMX suspected etiology of aseptic meningitis, esp. TMP component (CID 19:431, 1994). TMP/SMX contains sulfites and may trigger asthma in sulfite-sensitive pts. One of most frequent drugs to cause thrombocytopenia (AnIM 129:886, 1998).

* Cost to pharmacist according to manufacturer's listing in Oct. 1998 Medi-Span Hospital Formulary Pricing Guide (average wholesale price).

Abbreviations: **G** = generic, **NB** = name brand, **MRSA** = methicillin-resistant Staph. aureus, **APAG** = antipseudomonal aminoglycoside, **NUS** = not available in the U.S.

NOTE: All dosage recommendations are for adults (unless otherwise indicated) and assume normal renal function.

TABLE 9C
AMINOGLYCOSIDE ONCE-DAILY AND MULTIPLE DAILY DOSING REGIMENS
(See Table 17, page 121, if estimated creatinine clearance <90 ml/min.)

General: Dosage given as both once-daily (OD) and multiple daily dose (MDD) regimens.
Pertinent formulae:

(1) Estimated creatinine clearance (CrCl): $\dfrac{(140-\text{age})(\text{ideal body weight in kg})}{(72)(\text{serum creatinine})[1]}$ = CrCl for men in ml/min; multiply answer × 0.85 for CrCl of women

(2) Ideal body weight (IBW)—Females: 45.5 kg + 2.3 kg per inch over 5' = weight in kg
Males: 50.0 kg + 2.3 kg per inch over 5' = weight in kg

(3) Obesity adjustment: use if actual body weight (ABW) is ≥30% above IBW. To calculate adjusted dosing weight in kg: IBW + 0.4(ABW–IBW) = adjusted weight (CID 25:112, 1997)

DRUG	MDD AND OD IV REGIMENS/ TARGETED PEAK (P) AND TROUGH (T) SERUM LEVELS	COST Name Brand (NB), Generic (G)	COMMENTS For more data on once-daily dosing, see AJM 105:182, 1998, and Table 17, page 121

Gentamicin (Garamycin),
Tobramycin (Nebcin)
	MDD: 2 mg/kg load, then 1.7 mg/kg q8h
	P 4–10 µg/ml, T 1–2 µg/ml
	
	OD: 5.1 (7 if critically ill) mg/kg q24h
	P 16–24 µg/ml, T <1 µg/ml
		Gentamicin: 80 mg NB $5.35, G $1.14
		Tobramycin: 80 mg NB $7.28, G $3.82
			All aminoglycosides have potential to cause tubular necrosis and renal failure, deafness due to cochlear toxicity, vertigo due to damage to vestibular organs, and rarely neuromuscular blockade. Risk minimal with oral or topical application due to small % absorption unless tissues altered by disease.
			  Risk of nephrotoxicity ↑ with concomitant administration of cyclosporin, vancomycin, ampho B, radiocontrast.
			  Risk of nephrotoxicity ↓ by concomitant AP Pen and perhaps by once-daily dosing method (especially if baseline renal function normal).

Kanamycin (Kantrex), **Amikacin** (Amikin), Streptomycin	MDD: 7.5 mg/kg q12h P 15–30 µg/ml, T 5–10 µg/ml OD: 15 mg/kg q24h P 56–64 µg/ml, T <1 µg/ml	Kanamycin: 500 mg NB $3.36 Amikacin: 500 mg NB $32.89, G $17.50 Streptomycin: 1.0 gm NB $5.95	In general, same factors influence risk of ototoxicity. **NOTE: There is no known method to eliminate risk of aminoglycoside nephro/ototoxicity. Proper rx attempts to ↓ the % risk.** The clinical trial data of OD aminoglycosides have been reviewed extensively by meta-analysis (CID 24:816, 1997).
Netilmicin (Netromycin)	MDD: 2.0 mg/kg q8h P 4–10 µg/ml, T 1–2 µg/ml OD: 6.5 mg/kg q24h P 22–30 µg/ml, T <1 µg/ml	Netilmicin: 100 mg NB $15.70	**Serum levels:** Collect serum for a peak serum level (PSL) exactly 1 hr after the start of the infusion of the 3rd dose. In critically ill pts, it is reasonable to measure the PSL after the 1st dose as well as later doses as volume of distribution and renal function may change rapidly. Other dosing methods and references: For once-daily 7 mg/kg/d of gentamicin—Hartford Hospital method, see AAC 39:650, 1995.
Isepamicin[NUS]	Only OD: Severe infections 15 mg/kg q24h, less severe 8 mg/kg q24h		
Spectinomycin (Trobicin)	2.0 gm IM x1—gonococcal infections	2 gm NB $24.69	
Neomycin—oral	Prophylaxis GI surgery: 1.0 gm po x3 with erythro, see Table 15B, page 117 For hepatic coma: 4–12 gm/d. po	500 mg G $0.37	

Tobramycin—inhaled: See Cystic fibrosis, Table 1, page 31. Adverse effects few: transient voice alteration (13%) and transient tinnitus (3%). Cost: 300 mg $40.60

Paromomycin—oral: See Entamoeba and Cryptosporidia, Table 12, page 87. Cost: 500 mg $4.66

[1] Estimated CrCl invalid if serum creatinine <0.6 mg/dl. Consultation suggested.

TABLE 10A: TREATMENT OF FUNGAL, ACTINOMYCOTIC, AND NOCARDIAL INFECTIONS—ANTIMICROBIAL AGENTS OF CHOICE[*]
(See Table 10B for Amphotericin B Preparations and Adverse Effects)

TYPE OF INFECTION/ORGANISM/ SITE OF INFECTION	ANTIMICROBIAL AGENTS OF CHOICE		COMMENTS
	PRIMARY	ALTERNATIVE	
Actinomycosis (CID 26:1255, 1998) (A. israelii most common, also A. naeslundii; A. viscosus, A. odontolyticus, A. meyeri, A. gerencseriae) Cervicofacial, pulmonary, abdominal, cerebral	Ampicillin 50 mg/kg/d IV x 4–6 wks, then 0.5 gm amoxicillin tid po x 6 mos. or Penicillin G 10–20 million u/d IV x 4–6 wks. then penicillin V 2–4 gm/d po for 6–12 mos.	Doxycycline or ceftriaxone or clindamycin or erythromycin. Chloramphenicol 50–60 mg/kg/d div. q6h IV or po has been recommended for CNS infection in pen-allergic pts.	Tuboovarian abscesses may complicate IUDs. Removal of IUD is primary rx. With abscesses or fistulae, surgery often required. While penicillin G and ampicillin IV have been traditional, with home IV therapy, agents which can be given qd, e.g., ceftriaxone, may prove useful (CID 19:161, 1994).
Aspergillosis (A. fumigatus most common, also A. flavus and others) Allergic bronchopulmonary	Antifungal agents not recommended (see Comments)		Corticosteroids primary rx. Itraconazole (200 mg po bid) ↑ pulmonary function in 6/6 pts (Chest 100:813, 1991)
Aspergilloma (fungus ball)	Efficacy of antimicrobial agents not proven but in one study itraconazole (po) of benefit in 10/14 pts (J Am Acad Derm 23:607, 1990). Another case responded to itra 200 mg/d x3 mos. (IDCP 7:122, 1998).		Surgery if hemoptysis becomes massive (post-op complications 25%)
Invasive, pulmonary or extrapulmonary. Occurs post-transplantation and post-chemotherapy in neutropenic (PMN <500/mm³). Usually a late diagnosis (AJM 1125:197, 1996). Median survival 36 days, but overall mortality rates vary from 78–94% (CID 28:322, 1999). See CID 26:781, 1998, for excellent review.	**Ampho B:** Rapid increase to 1.0 mg/kg (1–1.25 mg/kg if neutropenic) qd IV. Total dose of 2.0–2.5 gm rec. by some but data to support this lacking. If response good may switch to itra after 2–3 wks. or **Itraconazole.** 200 mg tid[1] x 4 d. followed by 200 mg bid po. This oral alternative attractive if pt is eating, has good intestinal function and not on drugs that induce cytochrome P450 (RIF, phenytoin, barbiturates, etc.: see Table 27) or cyclosporin. IV prep now available (200 mg IV bid x4 doses followed by 200 mg IV qd) (See Table 10B).	See footnote[2] Ampho B lipid complex (ABLC) (Abelcet) or Ampho B cholesteryl complex (Amphotec) or Liposomal Ampho B (AmBisome) or Amphotericin colloidal dispersion (ABCD)	**Ampho B overall success rate 34%** (CID 26:781, 1998). Response rate in pts with pulmonary aspergillosis rx ≥14 days: 83% heart/kidney transplants, 54% neutropenic leukemia pts, 33% bone marrow transplant, 20% liver transplant (CID 23:608, 1996). Combination of ampho + itra antagonistic in vitro and in vivo (Drug Res Update 1:89, 1998). ABLC approved for aspergillosis refractory or intolerant to ampho B. 40% of 151 pts rx with ABLC had clinical responses vs 23% of 122 pts rx with ampho B with less nephrotoxicity [CID 22(Suppl 2):S133, 1996]. ABCD gave 50% response and survival rates with less nephrotoxicity (8.2 vs 43.1%) than ampho B, lipid formulations appear to be **equally efficacious but not more so than ampho B.**
Blastomycosis (Blastomyces dermatitidis) Cutaneous, pulmonary or extrapulmonary	**Itraconazole** 200–400 mg/d po for 6 mos. or **Ampho B** 0.5 mg/kg/d to a total dose of ≥1.5 gm for very sick pts	Fluconazole 400–800 mg/d for at least 6 mos. 85%+ effective for non-lifethreatening disease (CID 25:200, 1997)	Itra: in patients treated for ≥ 2 months, 95% cure (AJM 93: 489, 1992). Ampho B successful in >90% when ≥1.5 gm total dose used (CID 22:S102, 1996).
Candidiasis [Major pathogens: C. albicans, C. tropicalis, C. parapsilosis & C. pseudotropicalis: **Both C. lusitaniae & C. guilliermondi are resistant to ampho B. Candida glabrata & C. krusei and C. norvegensis (AAC 41:1375, 1997) are relatively resistant to fluconazole.** C. glabrata associated with highest mortality in cancer pts (CID 28:1071, 1999).]			
Bloodstream with or without venous catheter (no metastatic lesions), non-neutropenic. In recent years there has been a shift to bloodstream infections caused by non-Candida albicans isolates that are more drug-resistant (AJM 100: 67, 1996). **All positive blood cultures require therapy!**	**Fluconazole** 400 mg qd IV x7 d. then po for 14 d. after last + blood culture or **Ampho B** 0.5–0.6 mg/kg IV, total dose 5–7 mg/kg	In pts who fail to respond or deteriorate, higher dose of either drug may be used (ampho B 0.8–1.0 mg/kg IV or fluconazole 800 mg po/IV) (CID 25:43, 1997)	**Remove & replace venous catheters** (not "over a wire"!). Mortality 21% vs 41% if catheter not removed (ArIM 155:2429, 1995). Observe for metastatic lesions (endophthalmitis). In a multicenter trial fluconazole = ampho B but less toxicity with flu (NEJM 331:1325, 1994; ArIM 155: 2429, 1995), microbiologic failure 10–14% in both. Similar results found in cancer pts (AJM 101:170, 1996).

[1] Oral solution preferred to tablets because of ↑ absorption (see Table 10B, page 78)
[2] May be as effective and less nephrotoxic than standard ampho B **but much more expensive. Dosages: ABLC** 5.0 mg/kg/d IV over 2 hrs; **Ampho B cholesteryl complex** 3–4 mg/kg/d IV given as 1 mg/kg/hr; **Liposomal ampho B** 3–5 mg/kg/d IV given over 1–2 hrs; **ABCD** 2–6 mg/kg/d IV [doses up to 8 mg/kg have been given to bone marrow transplant recipients (CID 24:636, 1997)].

See page 76 for abbreviations   * All dosage recommendations are for adults (unless otherwise indicated) and assume normal renal function

TABLE 10A (2)

TYPE OF INFECTION/ORGANISM/ SITE OF INFECTION	ANTIMICROBIAL AGENTS OF CHOICE		COMMENTS
	PRIMARY	ALTERNATIVE	
Candidiasis (continued)			
Bloodstream: neutropenic but stable See Results of 1997 Consensus Conference (CID 25:43, 1997)	**Fluconazole** 400 mg qd x7 d. IV then po until neutropenia resolved	**Ampho B** 0.5–0.6 mg/kg/d to total dose 5–7 mg/kg IV, then switch to fluconazole 400 mg po. Continue flu until neutropenia resolved	Some authorities recommend combination ampho B + flucon for failures (AAC 39:1907, 1995). Although in vitro antagonism has been observed (AAC 42:1382, 1998) with flu and ampho, in vivo studies suggest additive or no interaction (Drug Res Update 1:89, 1998). ABLC successful in some who had failed ampho B (CID 21:1184, 1995; CID 22:S95, 1996). Non-albicans candidemia (therefore more likely to be fluconazole-resistant) more likely in pts with leukemia, neutropenia, and those receiving antifungal prophylaxis (CID 28:1071, 1999).
Bloodstream: unstable, deteriorating, or with metastatic lesions (pulmonary or hepatosplenic) ± neutropenia For endophthalmitis, see Table 1, page 10	**Ampho B:** 0.8–1.0 mg/kg/d IV ± 5FC 37.5[1] mg/kg q6h (adjust for renal failure) **or** **Fluconazole** 800 mg qd IV If start ampho "B", switch to fluconazole 400 mg po/d for 14 d. after last positive blood culture, resolution of neutropenia and disappearance of signs/symptoms of candidal infection.	**Ampho B lipid complex** (ABLC) 5 mg/kg/d (of up to 1.1 gm total dose has been used)	
Chronic mucocutaneous	**Ketoconazole** 400 mg/d po (as single dose with food) for 3–9 months	Usually children: Peds dose of fluconazole 3–6 mg/kg/d as single dose	Respond to ampho B but relapse is usual. Fluconazole used and may be less toxic, but experience limited.
Cutaneous (including paronychia, Table 1, page 19)	Apply topical ampho B, clotrimazole, econazole, miconazole, or nystatin 3–4x daily for 7–14 days or ketoconazole 400 mg po once daily x14 d. Ciclopirox olamine 2x daily 7–14 d.		Cost (30 gm tube cream): AB $29.21, Clo $13.40, Eco $19.44, MIC $21.00, Nys $3.58. Clc $18.20
Endocarditis	**Ampho B** 0.6 mg/kg/d IV for 7 days, then 0.8 mg/kg qod IV. Continue 6–10 weeks after surgery + **Flucytosine** 100–150 mg/kg/d po divided qid.	**Fluconazole** 200–400 mg/d for chronic suppression may be of value when valve not replaced	Adjust flucyt dose and interval to produce serum levels; peak 70–80 mg/L, trough 30–40 mg/L. With nephrotoxicity, dosage of flucyt needs to be ↓. Surgery may not always be required (CID 22:262, 1996).
Oral (thrush)—not AIDS patient	**Fluconazole** 200 mg single dose or 100 mg/d x5–14 days **or** **Itraconazole** oral solution 200 mg (20 ml) qd without food x7 days	Nystatin pastilles (200,000 u) lozenge qid, 500,000 u (swish & swallow) qid or 2 (500,000 u) tabs tid for 14 d. **or** Clotrimazole 1 troche (10 mg) 5x/d x14d.	**Fluconazole: Single dose 100 mg po; 16/16 clinical cure,** 75% mycologic at 2 weeks (AAC 34:2267, 1990). Maintenance not required in non-AIDS pts. Usually improves in 3–4 days, longer rx ↓ relapse. C. krusei fungemia reported in flucon-rx pts (NEJM 325: 1315, 1991).
AIDS patient: stomatitis, esophagitis, vaginitis Marked reduction in frequency in era of highly active antiretroviral therapy (J AIDS 21:20, 1999) Flu prophylaxis associated with ↓ vaginal C. albicans but ↑ C. glabrata (CID 28:1025, 1999)	**Fluconazole** 200 mg po 1st day then 100 mg qd x14 days **or** **Itraconazole** oral solution 200 mg po qd or 100 mg po bid x14 days (see Table 10B, page 78) then consider chronic suppression with fluconazole 100 mg po qd or 100–150 mg po q wk (suppression not associated with ↑ resistance—AJM 105:7, 1998) vs rx of clinical exacerbations.	**For fluconazole-refractory disease:** Options include: 1. Fluconazole 400–800 mg po qd or bid **or** 2. Itraconazole solution 100–200 mg po bid **or** 3. Parenteral ampho B 0.5 mg/kg IV qd **or** 4. Ampho B oral solution 100 mg/ml (1 ml) po 4x/d.	Fluconazole resistance ↑ frequency and associated with ↑ use of flu but clinical relevance difficult to establish; >50% of resistant isolates respond to flu. **Fluconazole-refractory disease remains low** (4% in ACTG 816) and is seen in pts with low CD4 counts (<50/ mm³). Most have prior exposure to flu and exhibit in vitro resistance. Some have acquired new candida species resistant to flu: C. tropicalis, C. parapsilosis, C. glabrata, but most have C. dubliniensis, C. Christ, C. glabrata (Drug Res Update 1:11, 1998; CID 26:557, 1998). **Flu similar to itra in 3 studies** (JID 176:227, 1997; CID 24:1204, 1997; AJM 104:33, 1998). Itra oral solution superior to tablets (J Clin Path 50:477, 1997). Flu superior to oral suspension of nystatin (CID 24:1204, 1997).

[1] Some experts reduce dose of 5FC to 100 mg/kg/d divided q6h

See page 76 for abbreviations

* All dosage recommendations are for adults (unless otherwise indicated) and assume normal renal function

TABLE 10A (3)

TYPE OF INFECTION/ORGANISM/ SITE OF INFECTION	ANTIMICROBIAL AGENTS OF CHOICE		COMMENTS
	PRIMARY	ALTERNATIVE	

Candidiasis *(continued)*

Peritonitis (Chronic Ambulatory Peritoneal Dialysis)
Based on *Peritoneal Dialysis International 16:557, 1996*
- Primary: [**Flucytosine** 2 gm po (loading dose) then 1.0 gm qd po + (**fluconazole** 200 mg po or IP daily)] x4–6 weeks.
- Alternative: Ampho B, continuous IP dosing at 1.5 mg/L of dialysis fluid x4–6 weeks.
- Comments: If no clinical improvement in 4–7 d., remove catheter. Oral flucytosine not available in Canada.

Cystitis
References: *CID 16:145, 1993; 20:1152, 1995; 20:1570, 1995; 21:960, 1995; J Urol 154:2032, 1995*
- Primary: **Fluconazole** 200 mg po 1st day, then 100 mg po qd x4 days
- Alternative: Ampho B (bladder irrigation) with 5 mg/ 100 ml H₂O at 42 ml/hr x1–2 d. or ampho B 0.3 mg/kg IV single dose (*J Urol 154:2032, 1995*)
- Comments: If poor response, consider fungus "ball" in renal pelvis. If possible, remove urethral catheter.

Vaginitis—Non-AIDS patients
Review article: NEJM 337:1896, 1997 (Candida vaginitis in AIDS patients: see above)
- Primary: Oral: **Fluconazole** 150 mg po x1 or **Itraconazole** 200 mg po bid x1
- Alternative: Intravaginal: Multiple imidazoles with 85–95% cure rates. See doses in footnote[1]
- Comments: **In general, oral and vaginal rx are similarly effective.** Rx aided by avoiding tight clothing, e.g., pantyhose. In pregnancy double rx duration. Oral drugs ↓ rectal candida and may ↓ relapses. Fluconazole resistance reported in both HIV+ and HIV– pts (*CID 22:726, 1996*) but incidence of flu-refractory disease remains low (*CID 26:557, 1998*). Boric acid solution intravaginally has also been used (*CID 24:649, 1997*).

"Candida syndrome"
- In a double-blind study, nystatin did not reduce systemic or psychological symptoms vs placebo (*NEJM 323:1717, 1990*).

Chromomycosis (Cladosporium or Fonsecaea); Cutaneous (usually feet, legs).
- Primary: If lesions small and few, surgical excision or cryosurgery with liquid nitrogen. If lesions chronic, extensive, burrowing: itraconazole.
- Alternative: Itraconazole: 100 mg po qd x 18 months (until response).[NFDA1] Fluconazole experience disappointing.
- Comments: 13/13 patients rx Itra responded, 2 relapses (18, 24 mos.) (*CID 15:553, 1992*). Terbinafine[NFDA1] impressive in a small number of pts (*AJTMH 55:45, 1996*).

Coccidioidomycosis (Coccidioides immitis) (see *AnIM 130:293, 1999; IDCP 8:21, 1999*)

Primary pulmonary (San Joaquin or Valley Fever)
Uncomplicated in normal host. Influenza-like illness of 1–2 wks duration
- Primary: **Antifungal rx not generally recommended** but pt should be monitored periodically and rx if fever, wt loss and/or fatigue do not resolve within several wks to 2 months *(see below)*
- Comments: **Cure rate (ampho B) 50–70%. Responses to azoles are similar.** Itra may have slight advantage esp. in soft tissue infection. Relapse rates after rx 40%. Relapse rate ↑ if ↑ CF titer ≥1:256 (RR= 4.7), or neg. coccidioidin skin test (RR=4.8) (*CID 25:1205, 1997*). Following CF titers after completion of rx important and rising titers should probably warrant readministration of rx (*CID 25: 1217, 1997*). Lifetime suppression in HIV+ patients: flucon 200 mg po qd or itra 200 mg po bid.

Primary pulmonary in pts with ↑ risk for complications or dissemination. Rx indicated:
- Immunosuppressive disease (AIDS) or therapies (steroids)
- Pregnancy in 3rd trimester
- Diabetes
- ↑ complement fixation antibody titer (titer >1:16)
- pulmonary infiltrates
- Documented extrapulmonary involvement —dissemination (identification of spherules or culture of organism from ulcer, joint effusion, pus from abscess or bone bx, etc.)

- Primary:
  - Mild to moderate severity: **Itra** 200 mg po bid (IV form now available) OR **Fluconazole** 400 mg po qd for 3–12 months
  - Locally severe or extensive disease: **Ampho B** 0.6–1.0 mg/kg/d. then 0.8 mg/kg/qod. Total dose 2.5 gm or more, followed by itra or flu
  - Consultation with specialist recommended; surgery may be required
- Alternative: Itraconazole: 100 mg po qd x 18 months (until response).[NFDA4] Fluconazole experience disappointing.

---

[1] **Butoconazole** 2% cream (5 gm) qd hs x3 d or **clotrimazole** 100 mg vaginal tabs (2 qd hs x3 d) or 1% cream (5 gm) qd hs x7 d (14 d may ↑ cure rate) or **miconazole** 200 mg vaginal tabs (1 qd hs x3 d) or 2% cream (5 gm) qd hs x7 d or **terconazole** 80 mg vaginal tab (1 qd hs x3 d) or 0.4% cream (5 gm) qd hs x7 d or **tioconazole** 6.5% vag. ointment x1 dose
See page 76 for abbreviations   * *All dosage recommendations are for adults (unless otherwise indicated) and assume normal renal function*

TABLE 10A (4)

TYPE OF INFECTION/ORGANISM/ SITE OF INFECTION	ANTIMICROBIAL AGENTS OF CHOICE		COMMENTS
	PRIMARY	ALTERNATIVE	
Coccidioidomycosis (continued)			
Meningitis: occurs in ⅓ to ½ of pts with disseminated coccidioidomycosis			
Adult	**Fluconazole** 400–800 mg qd po indefinitely	Ampho B IV as for pulmonary (above) + 0.1–0.3 mg daily intrathecal (intraven-tricular) via reservoir device.	**37/47 patients responded to flucon (median rx 3 yrs)** (AnIM 119:28, 1993). 14/18 pts rx with azoles relapsed when drug discontinued, therefore recommended that **fluconazole be continued indefinitely** (AnIM 124:305, 1996).
Child	**Fluconazole** (po) (Pediatric dose not estab-lished, 6 mg/kg qd used)		
Cryptococcosis (Cryptococcus neoformans)			
Non-meningeal (non-AIDS)	**Ampho B** 0.5–0.8 mg/kg/d IV till response then change to fluconazole 400 mg qd po for 8–10 week course OR **Fluconazole** 400 mg/d IV or po for 8 wks	Ampho B 0.3 mg/kg/d IV + flucytosine 37.5 mg/kg' qid po x6 wks.	Adjust flucyt dose and interval to produce serum levels of peak 70–80 mg/L, trough 30–40 mg/L. **Fluconazole alone 90% effective for meningeal and non-meningeal forms** (74% on steroid rx). French study suggests fluconazole equally as effective as ampho B (CID 22:S154, 1996).
Meningitis (non-AIDS)	**Ampho B** 0.5–0.8 mg/kg/d IV + **flucytosine** 37.5 mg/kg' q6h po until pt afebrile and cultures negative (~ 6 weeks) (NEJM 301:126, 1979), then stop ampho B/flucyt, start fluconazole 200 mg po qd (AnIM 113:183, 1990) OR **Fluconazole** 400 mg qd po x8–10 weeks (for relapse see Comment). Some recommend continuing flu for 2 yrs to reduce relapse rate (CID 28:297, 1999).	Ampho B 0.5–0.8 mg/kg/d IV + flucytosine 37.5 mg/kg' qid po x6 wks. Some (for controlled data available)	**Flucytosine levels must be measured**: adjust dose and interval to give serum levels: peak 70–80 mg/L, trough 30–40 mg/L. **Fluconazole alone has been used successfully**, comparative clinical trials lacking (NEJM 330:263, 1994). Hydrocephalus may be successfully rx with VP or VA or VA[2] shunt-ing (CID 28:629, 1999).
HIV+/AIDS (usually meningitis) >90% have positive serum cryptococcal antigen. Mortality still high: 12% in 1st 2 wks, 26% within 10 wks (CID 28:82, 1999)	**Ampho B** 0.7–1.0 mg/kg/d IV ± **5FC** 25 mg/kg q6h po for 2 wks or until clinically stable, then switch to fluconazole 400 mg qd po for 10 wks total, then switch to 200 mg qd (suppressive rx) **indefinitely** (even if CD4 count rises with effective antiretroviral rx). Itra not as effective as flu for maintenance rx (CID 28:291, 1999).	**Fluconazole** 400 mg po qd x6–10 wks, then suppressive rx (for pt with mild disease—see Comment) OR Ampho B lipid complex IV 5 mg/kg/d x2 wks, then 3x/wk x4 wks (CID 22:315, 1996)	For mild disease (normal mental status, CSF >20 cells/mm³, CSF crypto antigen <1:1024) some use fluconazole alone. **Some authorities add 5FC to ampho B for initial rx since recent study demonstrates ↑ rate of clearance of fungus from CSF** but without evidence of clinical benefit (NEJM 337:15, 1997). ↑ CSF pressure is associated with poor out-come (blindness, death): recommend ↓ pressure by removal of CSF (↓ pressure by 50% and maintain at <300 cm).
Dermatophytosis			
Erythrasma (Corynebacterium minutissimum)	Erythromycin 250 mg qid po for 14 days	2% aqueous clindamycin topically	Diff. dx with Tinea versicolor, Tinea cruris. Erythrasma coral red fluorescence with Woods light.
Onychomycosis (Tinea unguium) (see CID 23:305, 1996; Lancet 351:541, 1998)	**Fingernail Rx Options:** Terbinafine 250 mg po qd (children <20 kg: 67.5 mg/d, 20–40 kg: 125 mg/d, >40 kg: 250 mg/d) x6 wks (79% effective)[NFDA-I] or Itraconazole 200 mg po qd x3 mos.[NFDA-I] or Fluconazole 150–300 mg po q wk x3–6 mos.[NFDA-I]	**Toenail Rx Options:** Terbinafine 250 mg po qd (children <20 kg: 67.5 mg/d, 20–40 kg: 125 mg/d, >40 kg: 250 mg/d) x12 wks (70–81% effective) or Itraconazole 200 mg po bid x1 wk/mo. x3–4 mos. (46–84% effective)[NFDA-I] or Fluconazole 150–300 mg po q wk x6–12 mos. (90% effective)[NFDA-I]	

[1] Some experts would reduce to 25 mg/kg/d.
[2] **VP** = ventriculoperitoneal, **VA** = ventriculoatrial

See page 76 for abbreviations   * All dosage recommendations are for adults (unless otherwise indicated) and assume normal renal function

TYPE OF INFECTION/ORGANISM/ SITE OF INFECTION	ANTIMICROBIAL AGENTS OF CHOICE		COMMENTS
	PRIMARY	ALTERNATIVE	
Dermatophytosis (continued)			
Tinea capitis ("ringworm") (Trichophyton tonsurans, Microsporum canis, N. America; other sp. elsewhere) (PIDJ 18:191, 1999)	**Terbinafine** 250 mg tab qd x2–3 wks for T. tonsurans, 4–8 wks for Microsporum canis[NFDA-I]	Ketoconazole: adults 200 mg po qd, children 3.3–6.6 mg/kg po qd for 4 wks Itraconazole 3–5 mg/kg/d for 30 days Griseofulvin: adults 500 mg po qd x4–6 wks, children 10–20 mg/kg/d until hair regrows, usually 6–8 wks	In an open study, 8/10 cured with terbinafine (Br J Derm 126/S39:47, 1995). Addition of topical antifungal shampoo (selenium sulfate) daily results in negative cultures by 2 weeks (Rep Ped ID 5:8, 1995).
Tinea corporis, cruris, or pedis (Trichophyton rubrum, T. mentagrophytes, Epidermophyton floccosum)	Topical rx: Generally applied 2x/d. Available as creams, ointments, sprays, by prescription & 'over the counter'. Apply 2v/d for 2–3 wks. See footnote[*] for names and prices.	Terbinafine 250 mg po qd x2 wks[NFDA-I] OR ketoconazole 200 mg po qd x4 wks OR fluconazole 150 mg po 1x/wk for 1–4 wks[NFDA-I]	Keto po often effective in severe recalcitrant infection. Follow for hepatotoxicity. Terbinafine: 87% achieved mycological cure in double-blind study (32 pts) (J Med Assn Thai 76:388, 1993; Brit J Derm 130(S43):22, 1994).
Tinea versicolor (Malassezia furfur or Pityrosporum orbiculare)	Ketoconazole (400 mg po single dose)[NFDA-I] or (200 mg qd x7 days) or (2% cream applied 1x qd x2 wks)	Fluconazole 400 mg po single dose or itraconazole 400 mg po qd x3–7 days	Keto (po) x1 97% effective in 1 study. Another alternative: Selenium sulfide (Selsun), 2.5% lotion, apply as lather, leave on 10 min then wash off, 1x/d x7d or 3–5x/week x2–4 weeks
Histoplasmosis (Histoplasma capsulatum): Best diagnostic test is urinary antigen (ELISA) (CID 22:S102, 1996). Historeference Lab (1-800-HISTO DG)			
Immunocompetent patient: Pulmonary, localized, disseminated	**Minimal disease: No rx Moderate: Itraconazole** 200 mg/d po for 9 months. **Severe: Ampho B** 0.5–1.0 mg/kg/d IV x7 d. followed by 0.8 mg/kg qod IV.	[2] **Itra** not recommended for meningitis. IV prep now available. Dose 200 mg IV bid x4 doses followed by 200 mg IV qd (see Table 10B).	**With ≥2 months itra rx, 86% success in chronic pulmonary & extrapulmonary** (AJM 93:489, 1992). Antifungal rx not useful for histo fibrous mediastinitis. Clinical: Temp >39.5°C, Karnofsky <60, albumin <3 gm/dl, hepatic enzymes >5x normal, WBC <500, platelets <50,000, creatinine >6 mg/dl (CID 19(Suppl 1):S19, 1994). Flu less effective than itra (CID 23:996, 1996).
Immunocompromised patient (AIDS) (CID 24:1195, 1997)	**Ampho B** (80–85% response rate) 0.5–1.0 mg/kg/d IV x7 d. followed by 0.8 mg/kg/d IV (or 3x/week) IV to total dose of 10–15 mg/kg. Then begin suppressive rx: itraconazole 200 mg/d po	**Itraconazole:** (300 mg bid po x3 d, then 200 mg bid po x12 wks) or (400 mg qd x12 wks (85–90% response)) then 200 mg qd. **Not recommended for meningitis.**	**Itra (ACTG 120) 50/59 (85%)** pts responded, cleared fungemia with only 5% toxicity. 1 pt with meningitis failed, 2 failed because of low serum levels. Avoid rifampin, reduces itra serum concentration (AJM 98:336, 1995). **Itra best drug for suppression at 200 mg qd** but 3/46 had probable hepatic toxicity (J AIDS & Human Retro 16:100, 1997). Flu less effective than itra (AJM 103:223, 1997).
Madura foot (See Comments) (See Nocardia, Pseudallescheria boydii, below)	None, unless Nocardia	In U.S., usually Pseudallescheria boydii (Petrolidium spp.). Miconazole IV agent of choice.[NUS] In Mexico, usually Nocardia brasiliensis, in Japan, N. asteroides.	
Mucormycosis (Rhizopus sp.)—zygomycoses Rhinocerebral, pulmonary (ArM 159:1301, 1999)	**Ampho B:** Increase rapidly to 0.8–1.5 mg/kg/d IV; when improving, then qod. Total dose usually 2.5–3.0 gm	Treatment requires control of underlying condition, esp. diabetic ketoacidosis. Surgical debridement usually required and discontinue deferoxamine if applicable.	

[1] Drug name (trade name) and wholesale price for 15 gm. All are applied to affected area bid. **Prescription drugs:** butenafine (Mentax) $27.12, ciclopirox (Loprox) $11.58, clotrimazole (Lotrimin $12.86, Mycelex $10.03), econazole (Spectazole) $12.60, ketoconazole (Nizoral) $15.24, miconazole (Micatin, Monistat-Derm) NB $5–13, G $2.43, naftifine (Naftin) $16.79, oxiconazole (Oxistat) $14.38, fluconazole (Exelderm) $10.15, terconazole (Terazol) $8.74. **Non-prescription (over-the-counter):** Tolnaftate (Tinactin $5.28, Ting $1.99, Tolnate $1.70), undecylenic acid (Cruex $5.28, Desenex $5.28), and others.
[2] Oral solution preferred to tablets because of ↑ absorption (see Table 10B, page 78).
See page 76 for abbreviations   * All dosage recommendations are for adults (unless otherwise indicated) and assume normal renal function

TABLE 10A (6)

TYPE OF INFECTION/ORGANISM/ SITE OF INFECTION	ANTIMICROBIAL AGENTS OF CHOICE		COMMENTS
	PRIMARY	ALTERNATIVE	
Nocardiosis (Nocardia asteroides). Culture & sensitivities may be valuable in refractory cases: Reference Labs, R.J. Wallace (903) 877-7680 or CDC (404) 639-3158 *(IDCP 8:27, 1999)*			
Brain abscess and/or overwhelming disease	**Sulfisoxazole** 2 gm po q6h) or (**TMP/SMX**-DS 1 tab po bid) for 6 mos. (lifelong if pt has AIDS).	For acutely ill: cefotaxime 1–2 gm IV q8h + imipenem 500 mg IV q6h. Switch to po rx when possible. Another rx alternative in toxic pt: (imipenem or cefotaxime) + amikacin 7.5 mg/kg IV q12h.	Survival may be improved when sulfa-containing regimen used *(Medicine 68:38, 1999)*. Measure sulfonamide blood levels early to ensure absorption of po rx. Desire peak level of 100–150 µg/ml 2 hrs post-po dose.
Nodular lymphangitides (Nocardia brasiliensis). Abscess formation with ulcerations common		Minocycline 200 mg po bid x6 mos.	Duration of rx generally 3 mos. for immunocompetent host (38%) and 6 mos. for immunocompromised (62% organ transplant, malignancy, chronic lung disease, diabetes, ETOH use, steroid rx, and AIDS).
Pulmonary, not critically ill Cavitation common, pleural effusions in ⅓, may form sinus tract			
Paracoccidioidomycosis (South American blastomycosis)/P. brasiliensis	**Itraconazole** 200 mg po x 6 months or Ketoconazole 400 mg/d po for 6–18 months	Ampho B 0.4–0.5 mg/kg/d IV to total dose of 1.5–2.5 gm or sulfonamides *(dose. see Comment)*	Improvement in >90% pts on itra or keto.[NFDA-I] Sulfa: 4-6 gm/d for several weeks, then 500 mg/d for 3-5 yrs *(CID 14(Suppl.):S-68, 1992)*. HIV+: TMP/SMX suppressive rx indefinitely *(CID 21:1275, 1995)*.
Lobomycosis (keloidal blastomycosis)/P. loboi	Surgical excision, clofazimine or ampho B		
Penicilliosis (Penicillium marneffei). Common disseminated fungal infection in AIDS pts in SE Asia (esp. Thailand & Vietnam) *(CID 24:1080, 1997; Intl J Inf Dis 3:48, 1998)*	**Ampho B** 0.5–1.0 mg/kg/d x2 wks followed by itraconazole 400 mg/d for 10 wks followed by 200 mg/d po indefinitely for HIV-infected pts *(CID 26:1107, 1998)*. See Comment	Itra 200 mg po tid x3 d, then 200 mg bid po x12 wks.	3rd most common OI in AIDS pts in SE Asia following TBc and cryptococcal meningitis. May resemble histoplasmosis or TBc *(CID 23:125, 1996)*. Skin nodules are umbilicated (mimic cryptococcal infection or molluscum contagiosum). In AIDS pts long-term suppression with itra was effective in **preventing relapses in 36/36 pts,** whereas 20/35 pts receiving placebo relapsed within 6 mos. *(NEJM 339:1739, 1998)*.
Phaeohyphomycosis (black molds) Sinuses, skin, brain abscess	Surgery + itraconazole 400 mg/d po, probably 6 months[NFDA-I]	Genera include Drechslera, Bipolaris, Curvularia, Alternaria, Exophiala. May be manifestation of allergic sinusitis.	
Pseudallescheria boydii (Scedosporium apiosporum) Skin, subcutaneous (madura foot), brain abscess	Surgery + itraconazole 200 mg po bid until clinically well.[NFDA-I]	Miconazole[NUS] 600 mg IV q8h	Not an FDA-approved indication (itra). Resistant to ampho-tericin.
Sporotrichosis *(Ref.: CID 29:231, 1999)*			Itra ref.: *CID 17:210, 1993.*
Cutaneous/Lymphonodular	**Itraconazole** 100–200 mg/d po x6 mos. (then 200 mg po bid long-term[1] for HIV-infected pts[NFDA-I])	Sat. soln. potassium iodide (SSKI). 1 gm of KI in 1 ml of H₂O is SSKI. Start with 5–10 drops tid, gradually ↑ to 40–50 drops tid for 3–6 mos. Take after meals.	Some authorities use ampho B as primary therapy. Ampho B resistant strains reported *(AJM 95:279, 1993)*. Itra rx for up to 24 months effective in multifocal osteoarticular infection *(CID 23:394, 1996)*. SSKI side-effects: nausea, rash, fever, metallic taste, salivary gland swelling.
Extracutaneous: Osteoarticular, pulmonary, disseminated, meningeal	**Osteoarticular, pulmonary: Itraconazole** 300 mg po bid x6 mos., then 200 mg po bid (long-term for HIV-infected pts)	**Disseminated, meningeal: Ampho B** 0.5 mg/kg/d to total of 1–2 gm	

Abbreviations: AM/CL = amoxicillin clavulanate; **Ampho B** = amphotericin B; **Clot** = clotrimazole; **dc** = discontinue; **Flu** = fluconazole; **G** = generic; **Griseo** = griseofulvin; **I** = investigational; **IMP** = imipenem; **IT** = intrathecal or intraventricular; **Itra** = itraconazole; **IUD** = intrauterine contraceptive device; **Keto** = ketoconazole; **NB** = name brand; **NFDA-I** = not FDA-approved indication; **NUS** = not available in the U.S.; **PSL** = peak serum level; **R/O** = rule out; **TMP/SMX** = trimethoprim/sulfamethoxazole; **vag. oint.** = vaginal ointment

1 Oral solution preferred to tablets because of ↑ absorption *(see Table 10B, page 78)*.
* AI dosage recommendations are for adults *(unless otherwise indicated) and assume normal renal function*

TABLE 10B
ANTIFUNGAL DRUGS: ADVERSE EFFECTS, COMMENTS, COST

DRUG NAME, GENERIC (TRADE)/ USUAL DOSAGE/COST*	ADVERSE EFFECTS/COMMENTS
Non-lipid amphotericin B (Fungizone): 0.3–1 mg/kg/d as single infusion 50 mg $17.30 to $38.55	**Non-lipid amphotericin B (Fungizone):** **Admin.:** Commercial amphotericin B is a colloidal suspension that must be prepared in electrolyte-free D5W at 0.1 mg/ml to avoid precipitation. No need to protect drug suspensions from light. Ampho B infusions often cause chills/fever, myalgia, anorexia, nausea, rarely hemodynamic collapse/hypotension. Postulated due to release of proinflammatory cytokines; hypersensitivity reaction cannot be excluded. Manufacturer recommends a test dose of 1 mg, but often not done (1st few ml of 1st dose is a test dose). Duration of infusion usually 4 or more hrs. No difference found in 1- vs 4-hr infusions *(AAC 34:1402, 1992; AJM 93:123, 1992)* except chills/fever occurred sooner with 1-hr. infusion. Frequency and severity of febrile reactions decrease with repeated doses. Severe rigors respond to meperidine (25–50 mg IV). Premedication with acetaminophen, diphenhydramine, hydrocortisone (25–50 mg) and heparin (1000 units) had no influence on rigors/fever *(CID 70:755, 1995)*. If cytokine postulate correct, NSAIDs or high-dose steroids may prove efficacious but their use may risk worsening infection under rx or increased risk of nephrotoxicity (i.e., NSAIDs). Clinical side effects ↓ with ↑ age *(CID 26:334, 1998)*. **Toxicity:** Major concern is nephrotoxicity (15% of 102 pts surveyed, *CID 26:334, 1998*), ↓ in renal erythropoietin and anemia, and rising BUN/serum creatinine. Hypomagnesemia may occur. Manifest initially by kaliuresis and hypokalemia, then fall in serum bicarbonate (may proceed to renal tubular acidosis), ↓ in renal erythropoietin and anemia, and rising BUN/serum creatinine. Can reduce risk of renal injury by (a) pre- and post-infusion hydration with 500 ml saline (if clinical status will allow salt load), (b) avoidance of other nephrotoxins, e.g., radiocontrast, aminoglycosides, cis-platinum, (c) perhaps use of lipid prep of ampho B. Use of low-dose dopamine did not significantly reduce renal toxicity *(AAC 42:3103, 1998)*
Lipid ampho B products:[1] Amphotericin B lipid complex (ABLC) (Abelcet): 5 mg/kg/d as single infusion 100 mg IV $173.33 to $194.00 *(CID 26:1383, 1998)*	**Ampho B lipid complex (ABLC) (Abelcet):** **Admin.:** Indicated for rx of invasive fungal infections in pts refractory or intolerant to non-lipid ampho B. Consists of ampho B complexed with 2 lipids. Compared to standard ampho B, larger volume of distribution, rapid blood clearance and high tissue concentrations (liver, spleen, lung). Dosage: 5 mg/kg once daily; infuse at 2.5 mg/kg/hr; adult and ped. dose the same. Do NOT dilute with saline solution or mix with other drugs or electrolytes *(AAC 41:2201, 1997)*.[2] **Toxicity:** Fever and chills in 14–18%; nausea 9%, vomiting 8%; serum creatinine ↑ in 11%; renal failure 5%; anemia 4%, ↓ K 5%; rash 4%.
Amphotericin B cholesteryl complex (Amphotec): 3–4 mg/kg/d as single infusion 100 mg $160.00	**Ampho B cholesteryl complex (Amphotec):** **Admin.:** Approved for rx of aspergillosis in pts who either failed or are intolerant to standard ampho B. Consists of ampho B deoxycholate stabilized with cholesteryl sulfate resulting in a disc-shaped colloidal complex. Compared to standard ampho B, larger volume of distribution, high tissue concentrations. Dosage: Initial dose for adults & children: 3–4 mg/kg/day. If necessary, can ↑ to 6 mg/kg/day. Dilute in D5W & infuse at 1 mg/kg/hr. Do NOT use in-line filter. **Toxicity:** Chills 50%, fever 33%, ↑ serum creatinine 12–20%; ↓ Ca 6%, ↓ K 17%.
Amphotericin B colloidal dispersion (ABCD) (Amphocil) (I) *(JID 173:1208, 1996; CID 27:296, 1998)* 1–5 mg/kg/d as single infusion 50 mg $188.00	
Ampho B oral suspension available (Fungizone) *(AAC 42:606, 1998)* Dose: 100 mg (1 ml) po 4x/d 100 mg $1.50	**Liposomal amphotericin B (AmBisome):** **Admin.:** Approved for empirical rx for presumed fungal infections in febrile neutropenic pts; rx of pts with aspergillus, candida and/or cryptococcus infections refractory to conventional ampho B, or in pts where renal impairment or unacceptable toxicity precludes the use of conventional ampho B; and rx of visceral leishmaniasis. Dosage: 3–5 mg/kg IV as single dose infused over a period of approx. 120 min. If infusion is well tolerated, infusion time can be reduced to 60 min.[2] 1 mg/kg/d was as effective as 4 mg/kg/d (6 mos. survival rates 43% vs 37%, respectively) in pts with invasive aspergillosis complicating bone marrow tx and/or neutropenia from malignancy *(CID 27:1406, 1998)*. **Major toxicity:** Generally less than ampho B. Nephrotoxicity 18.7% vs 33.7% for ampho B, chills 47% vs 75%, nausea 39.7% vs 38.7%, vomiting 31.8% vs 43.9%, rash 24% for both, ↓ Ca 18.4% vs 20.9%, ↓ K 20.4% vs 25.6%, ↓ Mg 20.4% vs 25.6%.

---

[1] Published data from patients intolerant of or refractory to conventional ampho B deoxycholate (Amp B d). None of the lipid ampho B preps has shown superior efficacy compared to Ampho B in prospective trials. Nephrotoxicity ↓ with all lipid ampho B preps *(IDCP 7:516, 1998; CID 27:603, 1998; NEJM 340:764, 1999)*.

[2] Comparisons between Abelcet and AmBisome suggest a higher infusion associated toxicity (rigors) and febrile episodes with Abelcet (70% vs 36%) but a higher frequency of mild hepatic toxicity with AmBisome (59% vs 38%, p=0.05). Mild elevations in serum creatinine were observed in ⅓ of both *(BJ Hemat 103:198, 1998; Focus on Fungal Inf #9, 1999; Bone Marrow Tx 20:39, 1997; CID 26:1383, 1998)*.

* From 1998 Red Book, Medical Economics Data and Hospital Formulary Pricing Guide (5/99). Price is average wholesale price (AWP).
All dosage recommendations are for adults (unless otherwise indicated) and assume normal renal function

TABLE 10B (2)

DRUG NAME, GENERIC (TRADE)/ USUAL DOSAGE/COST*	ADVERSE EFFECTS/COMMENTS
Fluconazole (Diflucan) 100 mg tabs $7.00 200 mg tabs $11.70 400 mg IV $125.00 Oral suspension: 10 mg/ml ($30/35 ml) or 40 mg/ml ($108/35 ml)	Maximum tolerated dose: 2000 mg/d. **Pharmacology:** absorbed po, water solubility enables IV. Peak serum levels (see *Table 8B, page 59*). t/2 22 hrs. 12% protein bound. **CSF levels 50–60% of serum in normals.** ↑ in normals. Up to 85% of plasma concentrations have been found in breast milk (*PIDJ 14:235, 1995*). No effect on mammalian steroid metabolism. **Drug-drug interactions common,** see *Table 21.* Side-effects overall 16% [more common in HIV+ pts (21%)]. Nausea 3.7%, headache 1.9%, skin rash 1.8%, abdominal pain 1.7%, vomiting 1.7%, diarrhea 1.5%, ↑ SGOT 20%. Alopecia (scalp, pubic crest) in 12–20% pts on ≥400 mg po qd after median of 3 months (reversible in approx. 6 mos.) (*AnIM 123:354, 1995*). Rare: severe hepatotoxicity, exfoliative dermatitis. Anaphylaxis (*CID 13:81, 1993*), thrombocytopenia, leucopenia. Good reference: *NEJM 330:263, 1994.* ? congenital anomalies (*CID 22:336, 1996*).
Flucytosine (Ancobon) 500 mg $5.52	AEs: Overall 30%. GI 6% (diarrhea, anorexia, nausea, vomiting); hematologic 22% [leucopenia, thrombocytopenia, when serum level > 100 µg/ml (esp. in azotemic pts)]; hepatotoxicity (asymptomatic ↑ SGOT, reversible); skin rash 7%; aplastic anemia (rare--2 or 3 cases). False ↑ in serum creatinine on EKTACHEM analyzer.
Griseofulvin (Fulvicin, Grifulvin, Grisactin) 500 mg G $1.40, NB $10.50	Photosensitivity, urticaria, GI upset, fatigue, leucopenia (rare). Interferes with warfarin drugs. Increases blood and urine porphyrins, should not be used in patients with porphyria. Minor disulfiram-like reactions. Exacerbation of systemic lupus erythematosus.
Imidazoles, topical: for vaginal and/or skin use	Not recommended in 1st trimester of pregnancy. Local reactions: 0.5–1.5%: dyspareunia, mild vaginal or vulvar erythema, burning, pruritus, urticaria, rash. Rarely similar symptoms in sexual partner. Expense of treating vaginitis topically: Butoconazole x3 d $20.16, clotrimazole x7 d $14.71, miconazole x3 d $23.34, tioconazole x1 dose $24.20.
Itraconazole (Sporanox), 30s ea. $194.38 100 mg tabs $6.80 (with cola or food) --- 10 mg/ml oral solution (fasting state) 100 mg of oral solution $7.00 (AAC 42:1862, 1998) --- 10 mg/ml solution for IV infusion available late 1999. Usual dose 200 mg bid x4 doses followed by 200 mg qd, each dose infused over 1 hr.	**Itraconazole now available in tablet and solution forms—the 2 are not interchangeable.** To obtain the highest plasma concentration, the tablet is given with food and acidic drinks (e.g., cola) while the solution is taken in the fasted state; under these conditions, the peak conc. of the capsule is approx. 3.0 µg/ml and of the solution 5.4 µg/ml. Peak plasma concentrations after IV injection (200 mg) similar to oral capsule (200 mg): 2.8 µg/ml (on day 7 of rx) vs 2.0 µg/ml (on day 36 of rx). Protein-binding is over 99%, the latter explains the virtual absence of penetration into the CSF **(do not use to treat meningitis)**. **Oral solutions more desirable if taste and increased expense are acceptable.** Most common adverse effects are dose-related nausea 10% and abdominal discomfort 5.7%. Allergic rash 8.6%, edema 3.5%, and hepatitis 2.7% reported. ↑ doses may produce hypokalemia 2% and ↑ blood pressure 3.2%. Thrombocytopenia and leucopenia reported (*AnIM 125:757, 1996*). Other concern, as with fluconazole and ketoconazole, is **drug-drug interactions; see Table 21. WARNING: Co-administration with terfenadine, astemizole, cisapride, oral triazolam and oral midazolam contraindicated. Itra will ↑ serum levels of these drugs and life-threatening arrhythmias have resulted.**
Ketoconazole (Nizoral) 100 mg $3.40	Gastric acid required for absorption—cimetidine, omeprazole, antacids block absorption. In achlorhydria, dissolve tablet in 4 ml 0.2N HCl, drink with a straw. Coca-Cola ↑ absorption by 65% (*AAC 39:1671, 1995*). CSF levels "none". **Drug-drug interactions important, see Table 21. Some interactions can be life-threatening.** Liver toxicity of hepatocellular type reported in about 1:10,000 exposed pts—usually after weeks to weeks of exposure. At doses of ≥800 mg/d serum testosterone and plasma cortisol levels fall. With high doses, adrenal (Addisonian) crisis reported.
Miconazole (Monistat IV) 200 ml—*not available in U.S.*	IV miconazole indicated in patient critically ill with Pseudallescheria boydii. Used in some centers as prophylaxis or in initial rx regimens in febrile neutropenic pts (*AJM 83:1103, 1987; J Clin Onc 8:280, 1990*). Very toxic due to vehicle needed to get drug into solution.
Nystatin (Mycostatin) 30 gm cream $27.00, 500,000 u oral tab $0.67	Topical: virtually no adverse effects. Less effective than imidazoles and triazoles. PO: large doses give occasional GI distress and diarrhea.
Terbinafine (Lamisil) 250 mg tabs $7.30	Rare cases of symptomatic cholestatic hepatitis reported. In controlled trials, changes in ocular lens and retina reported—clinical significance unknown. Major drug-drug interaction is 100% ↑ in rate of clearance by rifampin. AEs: All mild, transient and rarely caused discontinuation of rx. % with AE, terbinafine vs placebo: nausea/diarrhea 2.6–5.6 vs 2.9; rash 5.6 vs 2.2; taste abnormality 2.8 vs 0.7.

* From 1998 Red Book, Medical Economics Data and Hospital Formulary Pricing Guide (5/99). Price is average wholesale price (AWP).
All dosage recommendations are for adults (unless otherwise indicated) and assume normal renal/renal function

TABLE 11A: TREATMENT OF MYCOBACTERIAL INFECTIONS*

Tuberculin skin test (abbreviation TST). The standard is the Mantoux test, 5 TU PPD in 0.1 ml diluent stabilized with Tween 80. Read at 48-72 hrs measuring maximum diameter of induration. A reaction of ≥5 mm is defined as + in the following: + HIV or risk factors, recent close case contacts, pts with medical conditions which ↑ risk (see above, preventive rx). ≥10 mm is + in: foreign-born in countries of high prevalence, injection drug users, low income populations, nursing home residents, health care workers. **Two-stage TST:** use in individuals in whom TST is to be tested regularly, i.e. health care workers. If 1st TST is reactive but <10 mm, if then ≥10 mm is +, ↓ next conversion (ARRD 119:587, 1979). TBn reactivity may ↓ over time but be boosted by skin testing. If unrecognized, individual may be incorrectly diagnosed as recent converter (ARRD 119:587, 1979). **BCG vaccination** may produce a PPD reaction but a reaction of ≥10 mm in an adult who was vaccinated as a child and who is from a country with a high prevalence of TB should be attributed to M. tbc infection (JAMA 253: 3438, 1985). For TST in children, see Pediatrics 97:282, 1996. Currently available PPD preparations are of comparable specificity (JAMA 281:169, 1999).

CAUSATIVE AGENT/DISEASE	MODIFYING CIRCUMSTANCES	SUGGESTED REGIMENS	
		INITIAL THERAPY	CONTINUATION PHASE OF THERAPY
I. Mycobacterium tuberculosis exposure but TST negative (household members & other close contacts of potentially infectious cases)	Neonate—Rx essential	INH (10 mg/kg/day for 3 months)	Repeat tuberculin skin test (TST) in 3 mos. If mother's smear negative & infant's TST negative & chest x-ray (CXR) normal, stop INH. In UK, BCG is then given (Ln 2:1479, 1990), unless mother HIV+. If infant's repeat TST positive & CXR abnormal (hilar adenopathy &/or infiltrate), ↑ risk (see above, preventive rx) (or SM). Total rx 6 months. If mother is being rx, separation of infant from mother not indicated.
	Children <5 years of age—Rx indicated	As for neonate for 1st 3 months	If repeat TST at 3 months is negative, stop. If repeat TST positive, continue INH for total of 9 months. If INH not given initially, repeat TST at 3 mos., if positive rx with INH for 9 mos. (see Category II below).
	Older children and adults—Risk 2-4% 1st year	No rx	Repeat TST at 3 months; if positive, rx with INH for 9 mos. (see Category II below). With heavy exposure (hospitals/nursing homes), active TB can occur by time of TST conversion (19%). Start rx with known exposure, discontinue if TST negative at 3 mos. (AnIM 122:906, 1995).

CAUSATIVE AGENT/DISEASE	MODIFYING CIRCUMSTANCES		
II. Prophylaxis for M. tuberculosis	(1) + tuberculin reactor & HIV+ (risk of active disease 10%/yr, AIDS 170x ↑, HIV+ 113x ↑)*		
	(2) Newly infected persons (TST conversion in past 2 yrs— risk 3.3% 1st yr)		
	(3) Past tuberculosis, not rx with adequate chemotherapy (INH, RIF or alternatives) (risk 0.5– 5.0%/yr)		
	(4) + tuberculin reactors with CXR consistent with non-progressive tuberculous disease		
	(5) + tuberculin reactors with specific predisposing conditions: illicit injection drug use (MMWR 38:236, 1989), silicosis, diabetes mellitus, prolonged adrenocorticoid rx (>15 mg prednisone/day), immunosuppressive rx, hematologic diseases (Hodgkin's), leukemia), endstage renal disease, clinical condition with substantial rapid weight loss or chronic under-nutrition, previous gastrectomy (AARD 134: 355, 1986)		
	* **NOTE: For HIV, see SANFORD GUIDE TO HIV/AIDS THERAPY and/or MMWR 48:RR-10, 1999**		

		SUGGESTED REGIMENS	
		INITIAL THERAPY	ALTERNATIVE
A. INH indicated due to high-risk Assumes INH susceptibility likely, INH 54–88% effective in preventing active TB for ≥20 years.		INH (5 mg/kg/day, maximum 300 mg/day for adults; 10 mg/kg/day for children) not to exceed 300 mg/day for children). Results with 6 mos. effective as 12 mos. (65% vs 75% reduction in disease). Am. Thoracic Soc. 6 mos., Am. Acad. Pediatrics 1994 9 mos. If CXR abnormal, rx minimum of 12 mos. In HIV+ pt, rx minimum of 12 mos. [MMWR 43:(RR-13):65, 1994].	If compliance problem: INH by DOT† 18 mg/kg 2x/wk x12 mos. If INH not possible, no proven regimen, but reasonable options: [(ETB 15 mg/kg/d po to a max. of 1.0 gm/d + RIF 600 mg/d po) x9-12 mos.] OR [(PZA 20 mg/kg/d po to max. of 2.0 gm/d + RIF 600 mg/d po) x6-12 mos.] Recent studies suggest 2-month regimen of (RIF 600 mg/d po + PZA 15-20 mg/kg/d po) or (RIF 600 mg 2x/wk + PZA 50 mg/kg 2x/wk) effective in preventing TBc in HIV+ pts (Ln 351:786, 1998).

CAUSATIVE AGENT/DISEASE	MODIFYING CIRCUMSTANCES	SUGGESTED REGIMENS	
		INITIAL THERAPY	ALTERNATIVE
B. TST positive (organisms likely to be INH-susceptible)	**Age <35 years,** not in Risk Category A above **(Age ≥35,** see Comments)	INH (5 mg/kg/d, max. 300 mg/d for adults; 10 mg/kg/d, max not to exceed 300 mg/d for children). Results with 6 mos. rx nearly as effective as 12 mos. (65% vs 75% reduction in disease). Am. Thoracic Soc. 6 mos., Am. Acad. Peds. 1994 9 months. If CXR abnormal, rx 12 mos. See II.A above for alternative rx.	**COMMENTS:** Reanalysis of earlier studies favors INH prophylaxis (if INH related, hepatitis case fatality rate <1% and TB case fatality ≥6.7%, which appears to be the case) (AnIM 150: 2577, 1990). Recent data suggest INH prophylaxis has positive risk-benefit ratio in pts ≥35 if monitored for hepatotoxicity (AIM 127: 1051, 1997). Overall risk of hepatotoxicity 0.1–0.15% (JAMA 281:1014, 1999).
	Pregnancy—Any risk factors (II.A above)	Treat with INH as above	Risk of INH hepatitis may be ↑ (Ln 346:199, 1995)
	Pregnancy—No risk factors	No initial rx (see Comment)	Delay rx until after delivery (AJRCCM 149:1359, 1994)

See page 84 for all footnotes and abbreviations   * Dosages are for adults unless otherwise indicated and assume normal renal function.   † **DOT** = directly observed therapy

TABLE 11A (2)

CAUSATIVE AGENT/DISEASE	MODIFYING CIRCUMSTANCES	SUGGESTED REGIMENS	COMMENTS
II. Prophylaxis for M. tuberculosis (cont'd) and drug resistance likely (For data on world-wide prevalence of drug resistance, see NEJM 338:1641, 1998)	INH-resistant (or adverse reaction to INH), RIF-sensitive organisms likely	RIF 10 mg/kg up to 600 mg/d po x6-12 months[1] OR (RIF 600 mg/d po[1] + ETB 15 mg/kg/d to max. of 1.0 gm) x6-12 months.	IDSA guideline lists rifabutin in 600 mg/d dose as another alternative; however, current recommended max. dose of rifabutin is 300 mg/d.
		PZA 20 mg/kg/d to max. of 2.0 gm/d + RIF 600 mg/d po[1] x2 months, then INH + RIF daily until sensitivities of index case (if available) known, then if INH-CR, dc INH & continue RIF for 9 mos.	Estimate RIF alone has protective effect of 56%; 26% of pts reported adverse effects (only 2/157 did not complete 6 mos. rx) (AJRCCM 155:1735, 1997).
	INH- and RIF-resistant organisms likely	Efficacy of all regimens unproven. (PZA 25-30 mg/kg/d to max. of 2 gm/d + ETB 15-25 mg/kg/d po) x6-12 mos.	If ETB used in dose above 15 mg/kg/d, monitor pt for retrobulbar neuritis. (Visual acuity and red/green color test, ≥10% loss considered significant.) PZA + oflox has been associated with asymptomatic hepatitis (CID 24:1264, 1997).
		[(PZA 25 mg/kg/d to max. of 2.0 gm/d) ± (ETB 15-25 mg/kg/d) + (CIP 750 mg bid or oflox 400 mg bid)], all po, x6-12 mos.	

SUGGESTED REGIMENS

CAUSATIVE AGENT/DISEASE	MODIFYING CIRCUMSTANCES	INITIAL THERAPY	CONTINUATION PHASE OF THERAPY (In vitro susceptibility known)	COMMENTS
III. Mycobacterium tuberculosis A. Pulmonary TB (General reference on rx in adults & children: CID 21:9, 1995; CID 28:130, 1999)		SEE COMMENTS FOR DOSAGE AND DIRECTLY OBSERVED THERAPY (DOT) REGIMENS		
	• Rate of INH resistance known to be <4%	INH + RIF (or RFB) + PZA daily x2 mos.	INH + RIF (or RFB) daily x4 mos. (total 6 mos.)	See separate dosage table below.
Isolation essential! Pts with active TB should be isolated in single rooms, not cohorted. Older observations on infectivity of susceptible & resistant M. tbc before and after rx (ARRD 85:511, 1962) may not be applicable to MDR M. tbc or to the HIV+ individual. Extended isolation may be appropriate.		Authors add pyridoxine 25-50 mg po daily to regimens that include INH NOTE: For pts with sputa + for AFB, continue isolation for a minimum of 2 weeks of therapy and longer for cavitary/laryngeal tbc.		
	• Rate of INH resistance not known or ≥4% —Compliant pt	INH + RIF (or RFB) + PZA + either SM or ETB daily until susc. data available. Even if susc. INH + RIF (or RFB) + PZA for total of 2 mos.	INH + RIF (or RFB) daily to complete 6 months of therapy	
	—Non-compliant or unreliable pt DOT rx effective in this setting (JAMA 279:943, 1998)	Directly observed therapy (DOT): 1. INH + RIF (or RFB) + PZA + either SM or ETB daily for 2 wks and then 2-3x/wk for 6 wks OR 2. INH + RIF (or RFB) + PZA + either SM or ETB 3x/wk for 6 months	INH + RIF (or RFB) 2-3x/wk to complete 6 months of therapy	
	• Known resistance (or intolerance) to INH	DOT recommended for all drug-resistant tuberculosis: RIF (or RFB) + ETB + PZA daily x18 months (≥12 months post-negative sputum cultures).		Risk factors for drug-resistant TB: Recent immigration from Latin America or Asia or living in area of ↑ resistance (≥4%) or previous rx without RIF: exposure to known MDR TB. Incidence of MDR TB in U.S. appears to have stabilized and may be slightly decreasing in early 1990s (JAMA 278:833, 1997).
	• Resistance (or intolerance) to RIF	INH + ETB + PZA daily x18 months (≥12 months post-negative sputum cultures)		

Dosage Table

Regimen[1]	Dose in mg/kg (max. daily dose)					
	INH	RIF	PZA	ETB	SM	RFB
Daily:						
Child	10-20 (300)	10-20 (600)	15-30 (2000)	15-25	20-40 (1000)	10-20 (300)
Adult	5 (300)	10 (600)	15-30 (2000)	15-25	15 (1000)	5 (300)
2x/wk (DOT):						
Child	20-40 (900)	10-20 (600)	50-70 (4000)	50	25-30 (1500)	10-20 (300)
Adult	15 (900)	10 (600)	50-70 (4000)	50	25-30 (1500)	5 (300)
3x/wk (DOT):						
Child	20-40 (900)	10-20 (600)	50-70 (3000)	25-30	25-30 (1500)	NA
Adult	15 (900)	10 (600)	50-70 (3000)	25-30	25-3 (1500)	NA

Second-line anti-TB agents can be dosed as follows to facilitate DOT: Cycloserine 500-750 mg qd (5x/wk) po
Ethionamide 500-750 mg qd (5x/wk) po
Kanamycin or capreomycin 15 mg/kg qd (3-5x/wk) IM/IV
Ciprofloxacin 750 mg qd (5x/wk) po
Ofloxacin 600-800 mg qd (5x/wk) po
Levofloxacin 750 mg qd (5x/wk) po (CID 21:1245, 1995)

(continued on next page)

[1] See page 81 for options regarding concomitant use of protease inhibitors and RIF or rifabutin.

* Dosages are for adults unless otherwise indicated and assume normal renal function.   † DOT = directly observed therapy

See page 84 for all footnotes and abbreviations

TABLE 11A (3)

CAUSATIVE AGENT/DISEASE	MODIFYING CIRCUMSTANCES	SUGGESTED REGIMENS		COMMENTS
		INITIAL THERAPY	CONTINUATION PHASE OF THERAPY (in vitro susceptibility known)	
(continued from previous page) REFERENCE: CID 22:683, 1996 **Multidrug-Resistant Tuberculosis (MDR TB):** Defined as resistant to at least 2 drugs. Pt clusters with high mortality (*AnIM 118:17, 1993*).	• Resistance to both INH and RIF = Multiple drug-resistant tuberculosis (MDR TB)	Want ≥3 drugs active vs MDR TB strains: INH + RIF (or RFB) + PZA + ETB or SM + additional second-line drug (AMK) + quinolone (CIP or sparfloxacin or levofloxacin)	Continue ≥3 drugs shown active in vitro vs patient's strain of MDR TB. Appropriate duration if susceptibility is not known. Less effective of intensive regimens have ↑ failure rates (*Ln 353:969, 1999*).	*(continued from previous page)* For MDR TB, consider rifabutin (~30% RIF-resistant strains are rifabutin-susceptible). Note that CIP not as effective as PZA + ETB in multidrug regimen for susceptible TB (*CID 22:287, 1996*). Sparfloxacin and levofloxacin have enhanced activity compared with CIP against M. tuberculosis. Mortality reviewed: *Ln 349:71, 1997.* Rapid (24-hr) diagnostic tests for M. tuberculosis: (1) the Amplified Mycobacterium tuberculosis Direct Test amplifies and detects Mycobacterium tuberculosis ribosomal RNA; (2) the AMPLICOR Mycobacterium tuberculosis Test amplifies and detects M. tuberculosis DNA. Both tests have sensitivities and specificities >95% in sputum samples that are AFB-positive. In negative smears, specificity remains >95% but sensitivity is 40–77% (*Am J Crit Care Med 155:1497, 1997*).

CAUSATIVE AGENT/DISEASE: MODIFYING CIRCUMSTANCES	SUGGESTED REGIMENS		COMMENTS
	INITIAL THERAPY	CONTINUATION PHASE OF THERAPY (in vitro susceptibility known)	
III. **Mycobacterium tuberculosis** *(cont')* **B. Extrapulmonary TB**	INH + RIF (or RFB) + PZA daily x2 months (Authors add pyridoxine 25–50 mg po daily to regimens that include INH)	INH + RIF (or RFB) daily x4–10 months (total 6–12 months)	6-month regimens probably effective. Most experience with 9–12 month regimens. Am Acad Ped (1994) recommends 6 mos. rx for isolated cervical adenitis, renal and 12 mos. for meningitis, miliary, bone/joint. DOT useful here as well as for pulmonary tuberculosis.
C. **Tuberculous meningitis** For critical appraisal of adjunctive steroids: *CID 25:872, 1997*	INH + RIF + ETB + PZA	May omit ETB when susceptibility to INH and RIF established. Treat total of 12 months. See *Table 8C, page 59, for CSF drug penetration.*	3 drugs often recommended for initial rx. we prefer 4. May substitute ethionamide for ETB. Dexamethasone (for 1st month) has been shown to ↓ complications (*Pediatrics 99: 26, 1997*). PCR of CSF markedly increases diagnostic sensitivity and provides rapid dx (*Neurol 45:2228, 1995; Arch Neurol 53:771, 1996*).
D. **Tuberculosis during pregnancy**	INH + RIF + ETB for 9 months		PZA not recommended: teratogenicity data inadequate. Because of potential ototoxicity to fetus throughout gestation (16%), SM should not be used unless other drugs contraindicated.
E. **Treatment failure or relapse:** Usually due to poor compliance or resistant organisms (*AJM 102:164, 1997*)	Directly observed therapy (DOT). Check susceptibilities. (See *section III.A, page 80*)		Patients whose sputum has not converted after 5–6 mos. = treatment failures. Failures may be due to non-compliance or resistant organisms. Check susceptibilities of original isolates and obtain susceptibility on current isolates. Non-compliance common, therefore institute DOT. If isolates show resistance, modify regimen to include at least 2 active agents, preferably ones which patient has not received. Surgery may be necessary. In HIV+ patients, reinfection a possible explanation for "failure".
F. **HIV infection or AIDS—pulmonary or extrapulmonary** (NOTE: 60–70% of HIV+ pts with TB have extrapulmonary disease)	INH + RIF (or RFB) + PZA daily x2 months. (Authors add pyridoxine 25–50 mg po daily to regimens that include INH)	INH + RIF (or RFB) daily x4 mos (total 6 mos.). May treat up to 9 mos. in pts with delayed response.	1. Clinical and microbiologic response same as in HIV-negative patient. 2. Post-treatment suppression not necessary for drug-susceptible strains. 3. Rate of INH resistance known to be <4% (for ↑ rates of resistance, see *Section III.A*). 4. For more information, see *MMWR 47(RR-20):1, 1998 & CID 28:139, 1999.* **Alternative regimen:** INH + SM + PZA + ETB x2 mos.; then INH + SM + PZA 2–3 times/wk for 7 mos. May be used with any PI regimen. May be prolonged up to 12 mos. in pts with delayed response.
Concomitant protease inhibitor (PI) therapy (3 options) (Modified from *MMWR 47:54, 1998*)	**Initial & cont. therapy:** Use (nelfinavir 750 mg q8h) or (indinavir 800 mg q8h) as the PI component of antiretroviral rx. (INH 300 mg + rifabutin 150 mg + PZA 25 mg/kg + ETB 15 mg/kg) po daily for 2 mos., then INH + rifabutin for 4–7 mos.		**Comments:** Rifamycins induce cytochrome CYP450 enzymes (RIF > RFP > RFB) & reduce serum levels of concomitantly administered PIs. Conversely, PIs (ritonavir > amprenavir > indinavir = nelfinavir > saquinavir) inhibit CYP450 & cause ↑ serum levels of RIF, RFP & RFB. If dose of RFB is not reduced, toxicity ↑. **Do not use RIF + PI.**

* Dosages are for adults unless otherwise indicated and assume normal renal function.   † **DOT** = directly observed therapy

See page 84 for all footnotes and abbreviations

TABLE 11A (4)

CAUSATIVE AGENT/DISEASE	MODIFYING CIRCUMSTANCES	SUGGESTED REGIMENS PRIMARY/ALTERNATIVE	COMMENTS
Other Mycobacterial Disease ("Atypical") (See ATS Consensus: AJRCCM 152:51, 1997)			
A. M. bovis		INH + RIF + ETB	The M. tuberculosis complex includes M. bovis. **All isolates resistant to PZA.** 9–12 months of rx used by some authorities. Isolation not required.
B. Bacillus Calmette-Guerin (BCG) (derived from M. bovis)	Only fever (>38.5°C) for 12–24 hrs	INH 300 mg qd x3 months	Intravesical BCG effective in superficial bladder tumors and carcinoma in situ. Adverse effects: fever 2.9%, granulomatosis, pneumonitis, hepatitis 0.7%, sepsis 0.4% (J Urol 147:596, 1992). With sepsis, consider initial adjunctive prednisolone. Resistant to PZA.
	Systemic illness or sepsis	(INH 300 mg) + (RIF 600 mg) + (ETB 1200 mg) qd po x6 months	
C. M. avium-intra-cellulare complex (MAC, MAI, or Battey bacillus) [Excellent review: AJM 102 (5C):1, 1997] ATS Consensus: AJRCCM 156:51, 1997	**Immunocompetent patients** with chronic pulmonary, disseminated disease (subcutaneous, bone)	Clarithro 500 mg po bid + ETB (25 mg/kg po x2 mos, then 15 mg/kg po) + CLO[1] 100–200 mg qd (until tan, then 50 mg qd or 100 mg tiw) + streptomycin or amikacin 15 mg/kg tiw for 2–6 mos. Rx until culture-neg x1 yr. **Alternative:** (Clarithro 500 mg po bid + ETB 15–25 mg/kg po qd + rifabutin 300 mg po qd) for up to 24 mos.	"Classic" pulmonary MAC: Men 50–75, smokers, COPD. "New" pulmonary MAC: Women 30–70, scoliosis, mitral valve prolapse, (bronchiectasis), pectus excavatum. Susceptibility testing of MAC not recommended except clarithro testing of isolates from pts who have failed prior clarithro rx. Clarithro + rifabutin shown effective for cervical adenitis in children (J Peds 128:383, 1996). Preliminary studies suggest 3x/wk azithromycin (600 mg po), ETB (25 mg/kg po), rifabutin (600 mg po), and initial 2x/wk SM may be effective in immunocompetent patients (JID 178:121, 1998).
	HIV+/AIDS patients: Primary prophylaxis—Pts CD4 count <50–100/mm³	Azithro 1200 mg po weekly OR Clarithro 500 mg po bid OR Rifabutin 300 mg po qd	Rifabutin reduces MAC infection rate by 55% (no survival benefit); clarithro by 68% (30% survival benefit); azithro by 59% (no survival benefit demonstrated in studies to date). Many drug-drug interactions, see Table 21. Rifabutin ↑ metabolism of ZDV with 32% ↓ in AUC. Clarithro ↑ blood levels of non-sedating antihistamines with attendant risk of arrhythmias. Need to be sure no active M. tbc; rifabutin used for prophylaxis may promote selection of rifamycin-resistant M. tbc (NEJM 335:384 & 428, 1996).
	HIV+/AIDS patients: Treatment Either presumptive dx or after positive culture of blood, bone marrow, or other usually sterile body fluids, e.g., liver	Clarithro 500 mg po bid + ETB 15–25 mg/kg/d ± RFB 300 mg po qd. **Alternative:** Azithro 500 mg po qd + ETB 15–25 mg/kg/d ± RFB 300 mg po qd or [(clarithro or azithro) + ETB ±RFB] + one or more of: (CIP 750 mg po bid or Ofloxacin 400 mg po bid or Amikacin 7.5–15 mg/kg IV qd	Median time to negative blood culture: clarithro + ETB 4.4 weeks vs azithro + ETB >16 weeks. At 16 weeks clearance of bacteremia seen in 37.5% of azithro & 85.7% of clarithro treated pts (CID 27:1278, 1998). **Adding CLO of no value** (AIDS 11:311, 1997). One study suggests adding AMK also of no value. Addition of RFB to clarithro + ETB regimen had no impact on bacterial response or survival but may ↓ clarithro resistance (CID 28:1080, 1999). Drug toxicity: With clarithro, 23% pts had to stop drug 2° to dose-limiting adverse reaction (AnIM 121:905, 1994). Doses of >500 mg bid assoc. with ↑ mortality (CID 29:125, 1999). Combination of clarithro, ETB and rifabutin led to uveitis and pseudojaundice (NEJM 330:438, 1994); result is reduction in max. dose of rifabutin to 300 mg. Treatment failure rate is high. Reasons: drug toxicity, development of drug resistance, and inadequate serum levels. Serum levels of clarithro ↓ in pts also given RIF or rifabutin (JID 171: 747, 1995). If pt not responding to initial regimen after 2–4 weeks, add one or more drugs. Anecdotal report of 5 pts not responding to usual primary regimen who gained weight and became afebrile with dexamethasone 2 mg/d po (AAC 38:2215, 1994).
	HIV+/AIDS patients: Chronic post-treatment suppression— secondary prophylaxis always necessary	[(Clarithro or azithro) + ETB (lower dose to 15 mg/kg/d (dosage above) **Alternative:** Clarithro or azithro or rifabutin (dosage above)	Recurrences almost universal without chronic suppression. In patients on HAART who have a robust CD4 cell response, it may be possible to discontinue chronic suppression, but insufficient data at present to make firm recommendation (JID 178:1446, 1998).
D. Mycobacterium celatum	Treatment	Not defined; see Comments	Isolated from pulmonary lesions and blood in AIDS patients (CID 24:144, 1997). Easily confused with M. xenopi (and MAC). Susceptibilities similar to MAC, but highly resistant to RIF (CID 24:140, 1997).

[1] CLO = clofazimine   * Dosages are for adults unless otherwise indicated and assume normal renal function.   † DOT = directly observed therapy

See page 84 for all footnotes and abbreviations

TABLE 11A (5)

CAUSATIVE AGENT/DISEASE	MODIFYING CIRCUMSTANCES	SUGGESTED REGIMENS	COMMENTS

Other Mycobacterial Disease ("Atypical") (continued)

CAUSATIVE AGENT/DISEASE	MODIFYING CIRCUMSTANCES	SUGGESTED REGIMENS	COMMENTS
E. **Mycobacterium chelonae ssp. abscessus** **Mycobacterium chelonae ssp. chelonae**	Treatment; Surgical excision may facilitate cure in subcutaneous abscess and is important adjunct to rx (CID 24:1147, 1997)	Clarithro 500 mg po bid x6 mos. (AnIM 119:482, 1993; CID 24:1147, 1997)	M. abscessus susceptible to AMK[1] (70%), clarithro (100%), cefoxitin (70%), clofazimine, cefmetazole[NUS]. Single isolates of M. abscessus often not associated with disease. M. chelonae susceptible to AMK (80%), clarithro, azithro, tobramycin (100%). Resistant to cefoxitin, FQ (CID 24:1147, 1997; AJRCCM 156:S1, 1997).
F. **Mycobacterium fortuitum**	Treatment; optimal regimen not defined. Surgical excision of infected areas.	AMK[1] + cefoxitin + probenecid 2–6 weeks, then po TMP/SMX, or doxycycline 2–6 mos. (JID 152:50, 1985). Usually responds to 6–12 mos. of oral rx with 2 drugs to which it is susceptible (AJRCCM 156:S1, 1997).	**Resistant to all standard anti-TBc drugs.** Sensitive in vitro to doxycycline, minocycline, cefoxitin, IMP, AMK[1], TMP/SMX, CIP, oflox, azithro, clarithro. Trials with neomacrolides (clarithro, azithro) indicated (AAC 36:180, 1992), but may be resistant to azithromycin, rifabutin (JAC 39:567, 1997).

CAUSATIVE AGENT/DISEASE; MODIFYING CIRCUMSTANCES	SUGGESTED REGIMENS		COMMENTS
	PRIMARY	**ALTERNATIVE**	
G. **Mycobacterium haemophilum**	Regimen(s) not defined. In animal model, clarithro + rifabutin effective (AAC 39:2316, 1995). Combination of CIP + RFB + clarithro reported effective but clinical experience limited (CMR 9:435, 1996). Surgical debridement may be necessary (CID 26:505, 1998).		Clinical: Ulcerating skin lesions, synovitis, osteomyelitis. Lab: Requires supplemented media to isolate. Sensitive in vitro to: CIP, cycloserine, rifabutin. Over ½ resistant to: INH, RIF, ETB, PZA (AnIM 120:118, 1994).
H. **Mycobacterium genavense**	Regimen(s) not defined. Regimens used include ≥2 drugs: ETB, RIF, RFB, CLO[2], clarithro. In animal model, clarithro & RFB (& to lesser extent amikacin & ETB) shown effective in reducing bacterial counts; CIP not effective (JAC 42:483, 1998).		Clinical: CD4 <50. Symptoms of fever, weight loss, diarrhea. Lab: Growth in BACTEC vials slow (mean 42 days). Subcultures grow only on Middlebrook 7H11 agar containing 2 μg/ml mycobactin J—growth still insufficient for in vitro sensitivity testing (Ln 340:76, 1992; AnIM 117:586, 1992). Survival ↑ from 81 to 263 days in pts rx for at least 1 month with ≥2 drugs (Arch Int Med 155:400, 1995).
I. **Mycobacterium gordonae**	Regimen(s) not defined, but consider INH + RIF + ETB for 6 weeks with surgical excision.		In vitro: sensitive to ETB, RIF, AMK, CIP, clarithro. Resistant to INH (CID 14:1229, 1992). Surgical excision.
J. **Mycobacterium kansasii**	Daily po: INH (300 mg) + RIF (600 mg) + ETB (25 mg/kg x2 mos, then 15 mg/kg) Rx for 18 mos. (until culture-neg. sputum x12 mos; 15 mos. if HIV+ pt.	If RIF-resistant, daily po: INH (900 mg) + pyridoxine (50 mg) + ETB (25 mg/kg) + sulfamethoxazole (1.0 gm tid). Rx until pt culture-neg. x12–15 mos.	Susceptibility testing: Test only RIF. Testing INH and streptomycin give misleading results. **All isolates are resistant to PZA.** If HIV+ pt taking protease inhibitor, substitute either clarithromycin (500 mg bid) or rifabutin (150 mg/d) for RIF (AJRCCM 156:S1, 1997). However, resistance to clarithromycin has been reported (DMID 37:369, 1998).
K. **Mycobacterium marinum**	(Clarithro 500 mg bid) or (minocycline 100 mg qd), or (TMP/SMX 160/800 mg po bid), or (RIF + ETB) for 3 mos.	or (doxycycline 100 mg qd) or (RIF + ETB) for 3 mos.	Resistant to INH and PZA (AJRCCM 156:S1, 1997)
L. **Mycobacterium scrofulaceum**	Surgical excision. Chemotherapy seldom indicated. Although regimens not defined, clarithro + CLO[2] with or without ETB, INH, RIF, step + cycloserine have also been used.		In vitro resistant to INH, RIF, ETB, PZA, AMK[1], CIP (CID 20:549, 1995). Susceptible to clarithro, strep, erythromycin.
M. **Mycobacterium simiae**	Regimen(s) not defined. Start 4 drugs as for disseminated MAI.		Most isolates resistant to all 1st-line anti-tbc drugs. Isolates often not clinically significant (CID 26:625, 1998).
N. **Mycobacterium ulcerans** (Buruli ulcer)	RIF + AMK[1] (7.5 mg/kg IM q12h bid) or (ETB + TMP/SMX (160/800 mg po q8h tid)) for 4–6 weeks. Surgical excision.		Susceptible in vitro to RIF, strep, CLO[2], clarithro (AAC 42:2070, 1998). Treatment generally disappointing—see review, Ln 354:1013, 1999.

[1] **AMK** = amikacin; [2] **CLO** = clofazimine

See page 84 for all footnotes and abbreviations   * Dosages are for adults unless otherwise indicated and assume normal renal function.   † **DOT** = directly observed therapy

TABLE 11A (6)

CAUSATIVE AGENT/DISEASE; MODIFYING CIRCUMSTANCES	SUGGESTED REGIMENS		COMMENTS
	PRIMARY	ALTERNATIVE	
O. **Mycobacterium xenopi**	Regimen(s) not defined (CID 24:226 & 233, 1997). Some recommend a macrolide + (RIF or rifabutin) + ETB ± SM (A/RCCM 156:S1, 1997).		In vitro: sensitive to clarithro (AAC 36:2841, 1992) and rifabutin (JAC 39:567, 1997) and many standard antimycobacterial drugs.
Mycobacterium leprae(leprosy) Paucibacillary (tuberculoid or indeterminate)	Dapsone 100 mg daily unsupervised + RIF 600 mg 1x/month supervised for 6 months		Side-effects overall 0.4%. Single lesion paucibacillary disease may be treated with single-dose rx (RIF 600 mg + oflox 400 mg + minocycline 100 mg) (Ln 353:655, 1999).
Multibacillary (lepromatous or borderline) **See Comment for erythema nodosum leprosum**	[Dapsone 100 mg daily + CLO 50 mg daily unsupervised] + [RIF 600 mg + CLO 300 mg 1x/month supervised for 24 months (WHO Tech Rpt 874:1, 1998). Recent data suggest 12 mos. rx effective (Ln 353:655, 1999)]	Ethionamide (250 mg daily) or prothionamide (375 mg daily) may be substituted for CLO	Side-effects overall 5.1%. For erythema nodosum leprosum: prednisone 60–80 mg/d or thalidomide 300 mg/d (BMJ 44: 775, 1998). CLO available from Ciba-Geigy [(908) 277-3572]. Pefloxacin 800 mg qd po, oflox 400 mg qd po, sparfloxacin 200 mg qd bactericidal and effective clinically with 4 log ↓ in organisms in small trials (Int J Leprosy 58:281, 1990; AAC 38:662, 1994; AAC 38:61, 1994). Clarithro also rapidly bactericidal (AAC 38:515, 1994). (Good reference: Ln 345:4, 1995.) 1 recent study suggests dapsone monotherapy as effective as combination rx for multibacillary leprosy (AAC 38:2249, 1994). Regimens incorporating clarithro, minocycline, RIF and/or oflox also show promise (AAC 41:1953, 1997). High relapse rate in pts treated with daily RIF + oflox for 4 wks (AAC 41:1618, 1997). Resistance to dapsone, RIF & oflox reported (Ln 349:103, 1997).

Abbreviations: **AMK** = amikacin; **ATS** = American Thoracic Society; **Azithro** = azithromycin; **BL/BLI** = β-lactam/β-lactamase inhibitors; **CIP** = ciprofloxacin; **Clarithro** = clarithromycin; **CLO** = clofazimine; **CXR** = chest x-ray; **dc** = discontinue; **ddC** = zalcitabine; **DOT** = directly observed therapy; **ETB** = ethambutol; **FQ** = fluoroquinolones; **IDSA** = Infectious Diseases Society of America; **IMP** = imipenem cilastatin; **INH** = isoniazid; **INH-CR** = complete INH resistance; **KM** = kanamycin; **Neomacrolides** = azithromycin, clarithromycin, roxithromycin; **NUS** = not available in the U.S.; **Oflox** = ofloxacin; **pts** = patients; **PZA** = pyrazinamide; **RFB** = rifabutin; **RFP** = rifapentine; **RIF** = rifampin; **rx** = treatment; **SM** = streptomycin; **sens** = sensitive; **TBc** = tuberculosis; **TMP/SMX** = trimethoprim/sulfamethoxazole

TABLE 11B: DOSAGE, PRICE AND SELECTED ADVERSE EFFECTS OF ANTIMYCOBACTERIAL DRUGS[1]

AGENT (TRADE NAME)	USUAL DOSAGE	ROUTE/[1] DRUG RESISTANCE (RES) US/COST*	SIDE-EFFECTS, TOXICITY AND PRECAUTIONS	SURVEILLANCE
FIRST LINE DRUGS				
Ethambutol (Myambutol)	25 mg/kg/day for 2 months & then 15 mg/kg/d qd as 1 dose [Bacteriostatic to both extracellular & intracellular organisms]	po RES:[2] 0.3% (0–0.7%) 400 mg tab $1.89	**Optic neuritis** with decreased visual acuity, central scotomata, and loss of green and red perception; peripheral neuropathy and headache (~ 1%), rashes (rare), arthralgia (rare), hyperuricemia (rare). Anaphylactoid reaction (rare). *Comment:* Primarily used to inhibit resistance. Disrupts outer cell membrane in M. avium with ↑ activity to other drugs.	Monthly visual acuity & red/green with dose >15 mg/kg/day. ≥10% loss considered significant. Usually reversible if drug discontinued
Isoniazid (INH) (Nydrazid, Laniazid, Teebaconin)	Daily dose: 5–10 mg/kg/day up to 300 mg/kg/day as 1 dose. Twice weekly dose: 15 mg/kg (900 mg maximum dose) [Bactericidal to both extracellular and intracellular organisms]	po RES: 4.1% (2.6–8.5%) 300 mg tab $0.02 IM (IV route not FDA-approved but has been used, esp. in AIDS 100 mg/ml 10 ml vials (IM) $16.64	Overall ~1% Liver: **Hepatitis** (children 10% mild ↑ SGOT, normalizes with continued rx, age <20 years rare, 20–34 years 1.2%, ≥50 years 2.3%) (also ↑ with daily alcohol). May be fatal. With **Peripheral neuropathy** (17% on 6 mg/kg/d, low incidence if dose <5 mg/kg/d, reduce risk with pyridoxine 10 mg daily will ↓ incidence; other neurologic sequelae, convulsions, optic neuritis, toxic encephalopathy, psychosis, muscle twitching, dizziness, coma (all rare); allergic skin rashes, fever, minor disulfiram-like reaction, flushing after Swiss cheese; blood dyscrasias (rare); + anticholinergic (20%). **Drug-drug interactions** common, see Table 21.	Pre-rx liver functions. Repeat if symptoms (fatigue, weakness, malaise, anorexia, nausea or vomiting) >3 days (A/RCCM 152:1705, 1995). Some recommend SGOT at 2, 4, 6 months esp. if age >50 years. Clinical evaluation every month.
Pyrazinamide	25 mg/kg/day (maximum 2.5 gm/d) qd as 1 dose [Bactericidal for intracellular organisms]	po 500 mg tab $1.12	**Arthralgia; hyperuricemia** (with or without symptoms); hepatitis (not over 2% if recommended dose not exceeded); gastric irritation; photosensitivity (rare).	Pre-rx liver functions. Monthly SGOT, uric acid. Measure serum uric acid if symptomatic gouty attack occurs.
Rifamate®—combination tablet	2 tablets single dose qd	po (1 hr before meal) 1 tab $2.43	1 tablet contains 150 mg INH, 300 mg RIF	As with individual drugs

[1] Note: Malabsorption of antimycobacterial drugs may occur in patients with AIDS enteropathy.

[2] **RES** = % resistance of M. tuberculosis

See page 84 for all footnotes and abbreviations

Dosages are for adults unless otherwise indicated and assume normal renal function. † **DOT** = directly observed therapy

* *Dosages are for adults unless otherwise indicated and assume normal renal function*

* *See page 84 for all footnotes and abbreviations*

TABLE 11B (2)

AGENT (TRADE NAME)	USUAL DOSAGE	ROUTE/[1] DRUG RESISTANCE (RES) US[1]/COST[1]	SIDE-EFFECTS, TOXICITY AND PRECAUTIONS	SURVEILLANCE
Rifampin (Rifadin, Rimactane, Rifocin)	10.0 mg/kg/day up to 600 mg/day qd as 1 dose (60–90% protein binding) [Bactericidal to all populations of organisms]	po RES:[1] 0.2% (0–0.3%) 300 mg Cap $2.11 (IV available, Merrell-Dow, Cost 600 mg $79.38)	INH/RIF dcd in ~3% for toxicity; gastrointestinal irritation, antibiotic-associated colitis, drug fever (1%), pruritus with or without skin rash (1%), anaphylactoid reactions in HIV+ pts, mental confusion, thrombocytopenia (1%), leucopenia (1%), hemolytic anemia, transient **abnormalities in liver function. "Flu syndrome"** (fever, chills, headache, bone pain, shortness of breath) seen if RIF taken irregularly or if daily dose restarted after an interval of no rx. **Discolors urine, tears, sweat, contact lens an orange-brownish color.** May cause drug-induced lupus erythematosus (Ln 349:1521, 1977).	Pre-rx liver function. Repeat if symptoms. **Multiple significant drug-drug interactions, see Table 21.**
Rifater® combination tablet (See Side-Effects)	Wt ≥55 kg, 6 tablets single dose qd	po (1 hr before meal) 1 tab $1.80	1 tablet contains 50 mg INH, 120 mg RIF, 300 mg PZA. Used in 1st 2 months of rx (PZA 25 mg/kg). Purpose is convenience in dosing, ↑ compliance (AnIM 122: 951, 1995) but cost 1.58 more. Side-effects = individual drugs.	As with individual drugs. PZA 25 mg/kg
Streptomycin	15 mg/kg IM qd, 0.75–1.0 gm initially for 60–90 days; then 1.0 gm 2–3 times/week (15 mg/kg/day) qd as 1 dose	IM (or IV) RES: 3.9% (2.7–7.6%) 1.0 gm $0.30	Overall 8%. **Ototoxicity:** vestibular dysfunction (vertigo); paresthesias; dizziness & nausea (all less in pts receiving 2–3 doses/week); tinnitus and high frequency loss (1%); nephrotoxicity (rare); peripheral neuropathy (rare); allergic skin rashes (4–5%); drug fever. Available at no charge for treatment of new pts with labeled use from Pfizer/Roerig, 1-800-254-4445. Reference re: IV—CID 19:1150, 1994.	Monthly audiogram. In older pts, serum creatinine or BUN at start of rx and weekly if pt stable

SECOND LINE DRUGS (more difficult to use and/or less effective than first line drugs)

AGENT (TRADE NAME)	USUAL DOSAGE	ROUTE/[1] DRUG RESISTANCE (RES) US[1]/COST[1]	SIDE-EFFECTS, TOXICITY AND PRECAUTIONS	SURVEILLANCE
Amikacin (Amikin)	7.5–10.0 mg/kg qd [Bactericidal for extracellular organisms]	IV or IM RES: (est. 0.1%) 500 mg NB $33, G $18.75	See Table 9, pages 60 & 70	Monthly audiogram. Serum creatinine or BUN weekly if pt stable
Capreomycin sulfate (Capastat sulfate)	1 gm/day (15 mg/kg/day) qd as 1 dose	IM or IV RES: 0.1% (0–0.9%) 1 gm $24.33	**Nephrotoxicity** (36%), **ototoxicity** (auditory 11%), eosinophilia, leucopenia, skin rash, fever, hypokalemia, neuromuscular blockade.	Monthly audiogram, biweekly serum creatinine or BUN
Ciprofloxacin (Cipro)	750 mg bid	po, IV 750 mg (po) $3.89	TB not an FDA-approved indication for CIP. Desired CIP serum levels 4–6 μg/ml, requires median dose 800 mg (AJRCCM 151:2006, 1995). Discontinuation rates 6–7%, CIP well tolerated (AJRCCM 151:2006, 1995). FQ-resistant M. Tb identified in New York (Ln 345:1148, 1995). See Table 9, pages 62 & 67 for adverse effects.	None
Clofazimine (Lamprene)	50 mg/d (unsupervised) + 300 mg 1x/month supervised or 100 mg/d	po (with meals) 50 mg $0.13	Skin: **pigmentation (pink-brownish black)** 75–100%, dryness 20%, pruritus 5%. GI: abdominal pain 50% (rarely severe leading to exploratory laparoscopy), splenic infarction (VR), bowel obstruction (VR), GI bleeding (VR). Eye: conjunctival irritation, retinal crystal deposits.	None
Cycloserine (Seromycin)	750–1000 mg/day (15 mg/kg/day) 2–4 doses/day [Bacteriostatic for both extracellular & intracellular organisms]	po RES: 0.1% (0–0.3%) 250 mg cap $3.82	Convulsions, **psychoses** (5–10% of those receiving 1.0 gm/day); headache; somnolence; hyperreflexia; increased CSF protein and pressure, **peripheral neuropathy.** 100 mg pyridoxine (or more) daily should be given concomitantly. Contraindicated in epileptics.	None
Dapsone	100 mg/day	po 100 mg $0.20	Blood: ↓ **hemoglobin** (1–2 gm) & ↑ retics (2–12%) in most pts. Hemolysis in G6PD deficiency, **Methemoglobinemia.** CNS: peripheral neuropathy (rare). GI: nausea, vomiting. Renal: albuminuria, nephrotic syndrome. Erythema nodosum leprosum in pts rx for leprosy (½ pts 1st year).	None

[1] **RES** = % resistance to M. tuberculosis   ***** Dosages are for adults unless otherwise indicated and assume normal renal function.   **† DOT** = directly observed therapy

See pages 84 & 86 for all footnotes and abbreviations

TABLE 11B (3)

AGENT (TRADE NAME)	USUAL DOSAGE	ROUTE/1° DRUG RESISTANCE (RES) US$/COST*	SIDE-EFFECTS, TOXICITY AND PRECAUTIONS	SURVEILLANCE
Ethionamide (Trecator-SC)	500–1000 mg/day (10–15 mg/kg/day) 1–3 doses/day [Bacteriostatic for extracellular organisms only]	po RES: 0.8% (0–1.5%) 250 mg tab $1.70	**Gastrointestinal irritation** (up to 50% on large dose); goiter; peripheral neuropathy (rare); convulsions (rare); changes in affect (rare); difficulty in diabetes control; rashes; hepatitis; purpura; stomatitis; gynecomastia. Give drug with meals or antacids; 50–100 mg pyridoxine per day concomitantly; SGOT monthly. Possibly teratogenic.	Liver functions monthly
Ofloxacin (Floxin)	400 mg bid	po, IV 400 mg (po) $4.45	Not an FDA-approved indication. Overall adverse effects 11%, 4% discontinued due to side-effects. GI: nausea 3%, diarrhea 1%, headache 1%. **CNS:** insomnia 3%, dizziness 1%.	None
Para-aminosalicylic acid (PAS, Paser) (Na+ or K+ salt)	4–6 gm bid (200 mg/kg/day) [Bacteriostatic for extracellular organisms only]	po RES: 0.8% (0–1.5%) 450 mg tab $0.08 (see Comment)	**Gastrointestinal irritation** (10–15%); goitrogenic action (rare): depressed prothrombin activity (rare); G6PD-mediated hemolytic anemia (rare), drug fever, rashes, hepatitis, myalgia, arthralgia. Retards hepatic enzyme induction, may ↓ INH hepatotoxicity. Available from CDC, (404) 639-3670, Jacobus Pharm. Co. (609) 921-7447.	None
Rifabutin (Mycobutin)	300 mg/day (prophylaxis or treatment)	po 150 mg $4.08	Polymyalgia, polyarthralgia, leucopenia, granulocytopenia. Anterior uveitis when given with concomitant clarithromycin; avoid 600 mg dose (NEJM 330:438, 1994). Uveitis reported with 300 mg/d (AnIM 12:510, 1994). Reddish urine, orange skin (pseudojaundice).	None
Rifapentine (Priftin)	600 mg twice weekly for 1st 2 mos., then 600 mg q week	po 150 mg $2.75	Similar to other rifabutins. (See RIF, RFB). Hyperuricemia seen in 21%. Causes red-orange discoloration of body fluids. Note ↑ prevalence of RIF resistance in pts on weekly rx (Ln 353:1843, 1999).	None
Sparfloxacin (Zagam)	400 mg loading dose, then 200 mg po qd	po 200 mg $6.69	Not approved by FDA for mycobacterial disease, but most active of current fluoroquinolones against mycobacteria. Major adverse effects: phototoxicity 7.9%, diarrhea 4.6%, nausea 4.3%, QTc prolongation 1.3%	None
Thalidomide (Thalomid)	100–300 mg po qd (may use up to 400 mg po qd for severe erythema nodosum leprosum)	po	**Contraindicated in pregnancy. Causes severe life-threatening birth defects. Both male and female patients must use barrier contraceptive methods (Pregnancy Category X). Frequently causes drowsiness or somnolence. May cause peripheral neuropathy.**	Available only through pharmacists participating in System for Thalidomide Education and Prescribing Safety (S.T.E.P.S.)

* Adult dosage only; § Mean (range) (higher in Hispanics, Asians, and patients <10 years old); ** Average wholesale price according to 10/98 Medispan Hospital Formulary Pricing Guide

Abbreviations: **VR** = very rare; **esp.** = especially; **dc** = discontinue

‡ **RES** = % resistance to M. tuberculosis

* *Dosages are for adults unless otherwise indicated and assume normal renal function.* † **DOT** = directly observed therapy

See page 84 for all footnotes and abbreviations

TABLE 12A: TREATMENT OF PARASITIC INFECTIONS

Many of the drugs suggested are not licensed in the United States. The following are helpful resources available through the Center for Disease Control and Prevention (CDC) in Atlanta. Website is www.cdc.gov. General advice for parasitic diseases other than malaria: (770) 488-7760 or (770) 488-7775.
For parasitic disease drug service[1] EST: 8:00 a.m.–4:30 p.m. EST: (404) 639-3670 (or -3356); emergency after hours: (404) 639-2888; fax: (404) 639-3717.
For malaria: Prophylaxis advice (770) 488-7788 or (888) 232-3228; treatment (770) 488-7788; website: www.cdc.gov.
NOTE: All dosage regimens are for adults with normal renal function unless otherwise stated.
For licensed drugs, suggest checking package inserts to verify dosage and side-effects. Occasionally, post-licensure data may alter dosage as compared to package inserts.
For abbreviations of journal titles, see *Table 1, page 47.* **Reference with pediatric dosages:** *Medical Letter 40:1, 1998.*

INFECTING ORGANISM	SUGGESTED REGIMENS		COMMENTS
	PRIMARY	**ALTERNATIVE**	
PROTOZOA—INTESTINAL (non-pathogenic: E. hartmani, E. dispar, E. coli, Iodamoeba butschlii, Endolimax nana, Chilomastix mesnili)			
Balantidium coli	Tetracycline 500 mg po qid x10 d.		*See Table 9B for side-effects.*
Blastocystis hominis	Role as pathogen controversial. No controlled rx trials.	Metronidazole 750 mg po tid x5 d.	Metronidazole suggested, 750 mg po tid x10 d., if present in high numbers and only pathogen found.
Cryptosporidium parvum No therapy proven efficacious. Self-limited in immunocompetent pts. Chronic diarrhea in AIDS pts. *EIN 3:51, 1997*	In AIDS pts, can try paromomycin 500–750 mg tid or qid. Others suggest 1.0 gm po bid.	In AIDS pts, CD4 <100 cells/µl, oral combination of paromomycin (1.0 gm 2x/d.) + azithro (600 mg 1x/d.) x4 wks and then paromomycin alone ↓ oocyst excretion with some clinical benefit (*JID 178:900 & 915, 1998*).	Nitrazoxamide (Cryptaz) 2.0 gm/d. promising; drug not FDA-approved. To obtain on investigational basis, contact Unimed Co.: 1-800-864-6330. Supplemental benefit from Imodium, diphenoxylate, or tincture of opium (may need in combination). Octreotide (Sandostatin) may help, but expensive.
Cyclospora cayetanensis	Immunocompetent pts: TMP/SMX-DS tab 1 po bid x7 d.	AIDS pts: TMP/SMX-DS tab 1 po qid x10 d.; then tab 1 po 3x/week	Ref.: *CID 23:429, 1996*
Dientamoeba fragilis	Iodoquinol[NUS] 650 mg po tid x20 d.	Tetracycline 500 mg po qid x10 d.	Other alternatives: doxy 100 mg po bid x10 d; paromomycin 500 mg po tid x7 d.
Entamoeba histolytica: Distinguish between E. histolytica and non-pathogenic E. dispar (*CID 29:1117, 1999*)			
Asymptomatic cyst passer	Paromomycin (aminosidine in U.K.) 500 mg po tid x7 d. OR iodoquinol[NUS] 650 mg po tid x20 d.	Diloxanide furoate[NUS] (Furamide) 500 mg po tid x10 d.	Metronidazole not effective vs cysts.
Patient with diarrhea/dysentery	Metronidazole 750 mg po tid x10 d., followed by:	(Tinidazole[NUS] 1.0 gm po q12h x3 d.) or (ornidazole[NUS] 500 mg po q12h x5 d.) followed by:	Drug side-effects in Table 9B. Colitis can mimic ulcerative colitis; ameboma can mimic adenocarcinoma of colon.
	Either [paromomycin 500 mg po tid x7 d.] or [iodoquinol[NUS] 650 mg po tid x20 d.]	[iodoquinol[NUS] (was diiodohydroxyquin) 650 mg po tid x20 d.]	Dx: trophs or cysts in stool. Watch out for non-pathogenic but morphologically identical E. dispar (*Ln 351:1672, 1998*).
Extraintestinal infection, e.g., hepatic abscess	Metronidazole 750 mg IV/PO tid x10 d. followed by paromomycin 500 mg po tid x7 d. Outside U.S., may substitute tinidazole (600 mg bid or 800 mg tid) po x5 d. for metro.		Serology positive with extraintestinal disease.
Giardia lamblia Ref.: *CID 25:545, 1997*	Metronidazole 250 mg po tid x5 d. OR albendazole 400 mg po qd x5 d.	(Tinidazole[NUS] 2.0 gm po x1) OR (quinacrine[NUS] 100 mg po tid after meals x5 d.)	Treat asymptomatic cyst passers. Dx: detect antigen in stool.
Isospora belli	TMP/SMX-DS tab 1 po qid x10 d., then bid x3 weeks	(Pyrimethamine 75 mg/d po + folinic acid 10 mg/d po) x14 d.	Chronic suppression in AIDS pts; either 1 TMP/SMX-DS tab 3x/wk OR (pyrimethamine 25 mg/d + folinic acid 5 mg/d po)

[1] **Drugs available from Parasitic Disease Service as of 9/19/99: Bithionol, dehydroemetine, diethylcarbamazine, melarsoprol, nifurtimox, stibogluconate, suramin.**

NOTE: All dosage recommendations are for adults (unless otherwise indicated) and assume normal renal function. See page 98 for abbreviations.

TABLE 12 (2)

INFECTING ORGANISM	SUGGESTED REGIMENS		COMMENTS
	PRIMARY	ALTERNATIVE	
PROTOZOA—INTESTINAL *(continued)*			
Microsporidiosis *(Ref.: CID 27:1, 1998)*			
Ocular: Encephalitozoon hellum or cuniculi, Vittaforma corneae or Nosema sp.	Albendazole 400 mg po bid	In HIV+ pts, reports of response of E. hellum to fumagillin eyedrops. For V. corneae, may need keratoplasty	To obtain fumagillin: 1-800-547-1392. Thrombocytopenia when fumagillin used to rx E. bieneusi. Dx: Most labs use modified trichrome stain. Need electron micrographs for species identification. FA and PCR methods in development.
Intestinal (diarrhea): Enterocytozoon bieneusi; Encephalitozoon (Septata) intestinalis	Albendazole 400 mg po bid	Oral fumagillin reported effective for E. bieneusi (AIDS 11:603, 1997)	
Disseminated: E. hellum, cuniculi or intestinalis; Pleistophora sp.	Albendazole 400 mg po bid	No established rx for Pleistophora sp.	
PROTOZOA—EXTRAINTESTINAL			
Amebic meningoencephalitis			
Naegleria fowleri	Ampho B 1 mg/kg/d IV + 0.1–1.0 mg into lateral ventricle via an Omaya reservoir		>95% mortality. *See Table 10B for ampho B side-effects.*
Acanthamoeba sp.—no proven rx		One pt successfully treated with IV pentamidine, topical chlorhexidine & 2% ketoconazole cream & then po itra (NEJM 331:85, 1994).	*For treatment of keratitis, see Table 1, page 9*
Babesia microti *(CID 22:611, 1996)*	(Clindamycin 600 mg po tid) + (quinine 650 mg po tid) x7 d.	For adults, can give clinda IV as 1.2 gm bid. For children: clinda is 20–40 mg/kg/d in 3 div. doses and quinine is 25 mg/kg/d po in 3 div. doses. Other alternatives: (TMP/SMX + pentamidine) or (quinine + azithro).	
Ehrlichiosis—See Table 1, page 41			
Leishmaniasis (see CID 25:677, 1997 & 27:1457, 1998; Ln 354:1191, 1999). NOTE: Responses of various species differ—see references.			
Visceral—Kala-azar L. donovani: India/Africa L. infantum: Mediterranean L. chagasi: New World **WARNING: Avoid combined antimony & ampho B** (Ln 351:1928, 1998)	Antimony (stibogluconate or meglumine antimoniate) 20 mg/kg/d (in 2 div. doses) IM or IV x28 d. Not marketed in U.S. Contact CDC Parasitic Drug Service: (404) 639-3670.	[AmB IV (1.0 mg/ kg/d x20 d.) or (0.5 mg/kg/d x14 doses)] or (L-AmB IV 3 mg/kg/d on days 1–5 & 10) or (ABCD IV 2 mg/kg/d x10 d.) or (ABLC IV 3 mg/ kg qod x5 doses) See abbreviations below[1]	Antimony resistance a problem in India (JID 180:564, 1999); an ampho B regimen should be used. Other alternative regimens with approx. cure rate (%): 1. Pentamidine 4 mg/kg IV 3x/wk x15–25 doses (75) 2. Paromomycin 15 mg/kg/d IV x20 d. (80) 3. Interferon 100 μg/M² qod IV + antimony as in primary rx (90) Ampho B lipid complex success: AnIM 127:133, 1997; CID 24,684, 1997
Mucosal: nasal mucosa & mouth	Antimony, as for Visceral	AmB1 1 mg/kg IV qod x20–30 doses	Approx. cure rates (%) antimony 60, AmB >75
Cutaneous: Most resolve spontaneously L. mexicana and L. braziliensis in New World L. tropia and L. major in Old World	Antimony, as for Visceral, or Pentamidine (2 mg/kg IV qod x7 doses) or (3 mg/kg IV qod x4 doses) (See Comment)	Topical 15% paromomycin + 15% methylbenzethonium chloride in paraffin bid x10 d. did not work & was painful (CID 26:56, 1998; 29:466, 1999). More options—see Comment.	For L. mexicana, ketoconazole 600 mg po qd x28 d. IV antimony x20 d. + intralesional GM-CSF (200 μg at day 1 and day 10) healed faster than IV antimony alone, p < 0.05 (JID 180:1735, 1999).
Malaria (Plasmodia species)—NOTE: CDC Malaria info—prophylaxis (888) 232-3228; treatment (770) 488-7788; website: www.cdc.gov. Also, see JAMA 278:1767, 1997			
Prophylaxis—Drugs plus personal protection: screens, nets, 30–35% DEET skin repellent (avoid 95% products in children), permethrin spray on clothing and nets (AnIM 128:931, 1998)			
For areas **free** of chloroquine (CQ)-resistant P. falciparum: Haiti, Dominican Republic, Central America west and north of the Panama Canal, and parts of the Middle East	CQ² 500 mg (300 mg base) po per week starting 1–2 wks before travel, during travel, & 4 wks post-travel.	CQ Peds dose: 8.3 mg/kg (5 mg/kg of base) po 1x/wk up to 300 mg (base) max. dose	CQ safe during pregnancy. **The areas free of CQ-resistant falciparum malaria continue to shrink:** Central America north of Panama Canal, Haiti, and parts of Middle East. CQ-resistant falciparum malaria reported from Saudi Arabia (AJTMH 56:573, 1997).

1 **AmB** = amphotericin B; **L-AmB** = liposomal ampho B; **ABCD** = ampho B colloidal dispersion; **ABLC** = ampho B lipid complex

2 **CQ** = chloroquine phosphate; **MQ** = mefloquine

NOTE: All dosage recommendations are for adults (unless otherwise indicated) and assume normal renal function. See page 98 for abbreviations.

TABLE 12 (3)

INFECTING ORGANISM	SUGGESTED REGIMENS		COMMENTS
	PRIMARY	ALTERNATIVE	

PROTOZOA—EXTRAINTESTINAL/Malaria/Prophylaxis *(continued)*

INFECTING ORGANISM	PRIMARY	ALTERNATIVE	COMMENTS
For areas with **CQ-resistant P. falciparum** CDC voice info on prophylaxis at (888) 232-3228 or website: www.cdc.gov Ref.: *JAMA 278:1767, 1997*	**Mefloquine (MQ)**[2] 250 mg (228 mg base) po per week, 1 wk before, during, and for 4 wks after travel. Peds dose in footnote[1]	**Doxycycline** 100 mg po daily for adults & children >12 years of age[1] **OR** **Atovaquone** 250 mg—proguanil 100 mg (Malarone) comb. tablet, 1/day. Peds dose in footnote[1]. (Ref.: *Ln 351:709, 1998*) Another option for adults: primaquine tab 1, 26.3 mg, po daily while in endemic area and x1 wk after leaving: *AnIM 129:241, 1998.*	**Pregnancy: No MQ (esp. 1st trimester)** unless only option. Atovaquone + proguanil pregnancy category C *(see Table 6)*. May be used if potential benefit exceeds potential risk. Not teratogenic in animals. Primaquine: Used only if prolonged exposure to endemic area (e.g., Peace Corps). Give 15 mg of base po daily for last 2 wks of exposure to eradicate hepatic forms of P. vivax and P. ovale.

Treatment *(NEJM 335:800, 1996)* **(P. falciparum, P. vivax, P. malariae, P. ovale).** Tylenol prolonged time to clear parasitemia *(Ln 350:704, 1997).*

INFECTING ORGANISM	PRIMARY	ALTERNATIVE	COMMENTS
Blood smear consistent with **P. vivax &/or P. ovale** Ref.: *NEJM 335:800, 1996* CDC: Malaria treatment—(770) 488-7788	**CQ**[2] [1.0 gm (=600 mg base) po, 0.5 gm in 6 hrs, then 0.5 gm daily x2 d] **OR** (1.0 gm po, then 0.5 gm base/kg IV at 12, 24, 36 hrs.) Both regimens total 2.5 gm **+** Primaquine (PQ) 26.3 mg (15 mg base) po daily x14 d. Check for severe G6PD deficiency.	For CQ-resistant P. vivax *(see Comment)*, can try CQ *(CID 23:1171, 1996).* Halofantrine 8 mg/kg x3 d, then repeat at 6 & 12 hrs and at day 7 *(see Table 12B)* PQ 52.6 mg (30 mg base) po daily x28 d. Parenteral rx: CQ 10 mg base/kg IV over 8 hrs, then 15 mg base/kg IV over 24 hrs	CQ-resistant P. vivax reported from Oceania and South America *(CID 23:1171, 1996).* Pregnancy: CQ safe all trimesters. No PQ in pregnancy or to newborns—risk of hemolysis. Peds rx doses: For CQ 10 mg/kg of **base** per kg po, then 5 mg base/kg at 12, 24, 36 hrs. For PQ use 0.25 mg **base/kg** x14 d.
Blood smear consistent with **P. falciparum** or **P. malariae** Only exposure is Central America or Middle East (see Comment)	CQ as for CQ-sensitive P. vivax. Don't need PQ.		Assumes P. falciparum CQ-sensitive, i.e., acquired in Central America (north of Panama Canal), Haiti, or parts of Middle East
Blood smear shows **P. falciparum** assumed **CQ-resistant PO therapy possible.** Ref.: *NEJM 335:800, 1996*	[Quinine sulfate (QS) 300 mg (=250 mg base). Give 600 mg po 3x/d] + (doxycycline 100 mg po bid)—both x7 d. Peds: QS + Fansidar x1 dose on last day of QS in footnote[3]	Atovaquone/proguanil 250/100 mg tab: 4 tabs po, single dose, x3 d. Peds dose in footnote[1]. *(JID 179:1587, 1999; AJTMH 60:533, 1999; JTM 6:518, 1999)*	**Other rx alternatives:** (1) MQ[2]: Give 15 mg base/kg po x1, then 2nd dose of 10 mg base/kg 8–24 hrs later. Max. single dose is 1250 mg. Peds: dose same as for adult. (2) Artemether[4] 4 mg/kg po daily x3 d. (3) Halofantrine 500 mg po q6h x3 d. Repeat regimen in 1 wk. + MQ. **Pregnancy:** Quinine OK; avoid MQ 1st trimester. Can sub clinda 900 mg po tid for doxy. No doxycycline.
Blood smear consistent with **P. falciparum. Pt too ill for initial po therapy.** Ref.: *NEJM 335:800, 1996).* CDC: Malaria info—(770) 488-7788	In U.S.: Quinidine gluconate [10 mg/kg IV over 1 hr, then 0.02 mg/kg/min. (monitor EKG) x72 hrs] **OR** [15 mg/kg IV over 4 hrs, then 7.5 mg/kg IV over 4 hrs q8h x72 hrs] **OR** until patient can take po meds.	Outside U.S.: Quinine dihydrochloride[NS 20] mg/kg IV over 4 hrs, then 10 mg/kg IV q8h x72 hrs **OR** Artemether[4] 4 mg/kg IM, then 2 mg/kg IM, q8h[3]. For both, switch to po regimen when possible to finish 7 days of rx.	Severe falciparum malaria. May be manifest as cerebral malaria, renal failure, or ARDS. **Monitor parasitemia!** If rx effective, expect ≥75% ↓ parasite count after 48 hrs of rx. If parasitemia exceeds 15%, consider exchange transfusion *(CID 26:853, 1998).* **NOTE:** Steroids are harmful in cerebral malaria.

[1] **Peds prophylaxis dosages: Mefloquine** dose by **weight** in kg: 5–9 = 1/8 adult dose; 10–19 = ½ adult dose; 20–30 = ½ adult dose; 31–45 = ¾ adult dose; >45 = adult dose. **Atovaquone/proguanil** by **weight** in kg, single daily dose: 11–20 kg 62.5/25 mg; 21–30 kg 125/50 mg; 31–40 kg 187.5/75 mg; >40 kg 250/100 mg. **Doxycycline**, ages >8–12 yrs.: 2 mg/kg/d up to 100 mg.

[2] **CQ** = chloroquine phosphate; **QS** = quinine sulfate; **MQ** = mefloquine; **PQ** = primaquine

[3] **Pediatric treatment dosage:** QS 25 mg/kg/d po div. q8h x3 d. + a single po dose of Fansidar (pyrimethamine sulfadoxine) given on last day of quinine. Fansidar single dose by age (yr.) of pt: <1 = ¼ tab; 1–3 = ½ tab; 4–8 yrs = 1 tab; 9–14 = 2 tabs; >14 = 3 tabs. Artemether peds dose = 3.2 mg/kg IM, then 1.6 mg/kg IM/d x4 d. Atovaquone/proguanil single daily dose by weight: 11–20 kg 250/100 mg; 21–30 kg 500/200 mg; 31–40 kg 750/300 mg; >40 kg 1 gm/400 mg; all x3 days.

[4] For artemether, contact CDC Drug Service, (770) 488-7788.

NOTE: All dosage recommendations are for adults (unless otherwise indicated) and assume normal renal function. See page 98 for abbreviations.

TABLE 12 (4)

INFECTING ORGANISM	SUGGESTED REGIMENS — PRIMARY	ALTERNATIVE	COMMENTS
PROTOZOA—EXTRAINTESTINAL *(continued)*			
Microsporidia—systemic—*see page 88*			
Pneumocystis carinii Pneumonia (PCP)			
Not acutely ill, able to take po meds. PaO₂ >70 mmHg	(Dapsone 100 mg po qd + trimethoprim 5 mg/kg po tid x21 d.) OR (TMP/SMX-DS, 2 tabs po q8h x21 d.)	[Clindamycin 300-450 mg po q6h + primaquine 15 mg base po qd x21 d.] OR Atovaquone suspension 750 mg po bid with food x21 d.	DAP/TMP, TMP/SMX, clinda/prima regimens equally effective. Rash/fever 10% with DAP/TMP, 19% with TMP/SMX, 21% with clinda/prima. Ref., clinda/prima vs TMP/SMX: *CID* 27:524, 1998. Dapsone ref.: *CID* 27:191, 1998. **After 21 days, chronic suppression in AIDS pts (see below)**.
	NOTE: Concomitant use of corticosteroids usually reserved for sicker pts with PaO₂ <70 (see below)		**Trimetrexate another alternative (See SANFORD GUIDE TO HIV/AIDS THERAPY).**
Acutely ill, po rx not possible. PaO₂ <70 mmHg	[Prednisone 15-30 min. before TMP/SMX—start with 40 mg po bid x5 d., then 40 mg qd x5 d., then 20 mg po qd x11 d.] + [TMP/SMX (15 mg of TMP component/kg/d) IV div. q6-8h x21 d.]	Prednisone as in primary rx PLUS [(Clinda 600 mg IV q8h) + (primaquine 15 mg base po qd)] x21 d. OR Pentamidine 4 mg/kg/d IV x21 d.	**After 21 days, chronic suppression in AIDS pts (see below).** PCP can occur in absence of HIV infection and steroids (*CID* 25:215 & 219, 1997).
	Can substitute IV prednisolone (reduce dose 25%) for po prednisone		
Primary prophylaxis and post-treatment suppression Ref.: *AAC* 42:995, 1998; *MMWR* 48:RR-10, 1999	(TMP/SMX-DS, 1 tab po qd or 3x/wk) OR (dapsone 100 mg po qd) OR (TMP/SMX-SS, 1 tab po qd). DC when CD4 >200 x3 mos. Rare resistance to TMP/SMX: *Ln* 351:1631, 1998	(Pentamidine 300 mg in 6 ml sterile water by aerosol q4 wks) OR (dapsone 200 mg po + pyrimethamine 75 mg po + folinic acid 25 mg po—all once a week) or atovaquone 1500 mg po qd with food.	TMP/SMX-DS regimen provides cross-protection vs toxo and other bacterial infections. Dapsone + pyrimethamine protects vs toxo. Atovaquone suspension 1500 mg once daily as effective as daily dapsone (*NEJM* 339:1889, 1998) & inhaled pentamidine (*JID* 180:369, 1999).
Toxoplasma gondii (Reference: Remington and McLeod in INFECTIOUS DISEASES, Gorbach et al., Eds., 2nd Ed., 1997, pp 1620-40)			
Immunologically normal patients *(For pediatric doses, see reference)*			
Acute illness with lymphadenopathy	No specific rx unless severe/persistent symptoms or evidence of vital organ damage		
Acquired via transfusion (lab accident)	Treat as for active chorioretinitis.		
Active chorioretinitis; meningitis; lowered resistance due to steroids or cytotoxic drugs	[Pyrimethamine (pyri) 50-100 mg po bid on 1st day, then 25 mg qd] + [sulfadiazine (see footnote¹) 1-1.5 gm po qid] + [leucovorin (folinic acid) 10 mg po or more/day]—see *Comment*. Treat 1-2 wks beyond resolution of signs/symptoms; continue leucovorin 1 wk after stopping pyri.		For congenital toxo, toxo meningitis in adults, and chorioretinitis, add prednisone 1 mg/kg/d in 2 div. doses until CSF protein conc. falls or vision-threatening inflammation has subsided. Adjust folinic acid dose by following CBC results.
Pregnancy—1st 18 weeks of gestation, or to term if fetus not infected	Spiramycin [From FDA, call (301) 827-2335] 1.0 gm po q8h. NOTE: Use caution in interpretation of commercial tests for toxoplasma IgM antibody; obtain consultation and/or obtain FDA Advisory—call (301) 594-3060.		For fetal infection after week 17 or late maternal infection—*see text reference above for details.*

¹ Sulfonamides for toxo. Sulfadiazine now commercially available. Sulfisoxazole much less effective.
NOTE: All dosage recommendations are for adults (unless otherwise indicated) and assume normal renal function. *See page 98 for abbreviations.*

TABLE 12 (5)

INFECTING ORGANISM	SUGGESTED REGIMENS		COMMENTS
	PRIMARY	ALTERNATIVE	
PROTOZOA—EXTRAINTESTINAL/Toxoplasma gondii *(continued)*			
Acquired immunodeficiency syndrome (AIDS)			
Cerebral toxoplasmosis Ref.: See *Remington & McLeod ref., above*	[Pyrimethamine (pyri) 200 mg x1 po, then 75–100 mg/d po] + (sulfadiazine 1–1.5 gm po q6h) + (folinic acid 10–15 mg/d po) x3–6 wks and then suppressive rx (see below) OR TMP/SMX 10/50 mg/kg/d po or IV div. q12h x30 d. *(AAC 42:1346, 1998)*	[Pyri + folinic acid (as in primary regimen)] + 1 of the following: (1) Clinda 600 mg po/IV q6h or (2) clarithro 1.0 gm po bid or (3) azithro 1.2–1.5 gm po qd or (4) dapsone 100 mg po qd. Treat 3–6 wks, then suppression.	Use alternative regimen for pts with severe sulfa allergy. If multiple ring-enhancing brain lesions (CT or MRI), >85% of pts respond to 7–10 days of empiric rx; if no response, suggest brain biopsy. IgG toxo antibody positive in approx. 84% *(NEJM 327:1643, 1992).*
Primary prophylaxis, AIDS pts—IgG toxo antibody + CD4 count <100/µl	(TMP/SMX-DS, 1 tab po qd) or (TMP/SMX-SS, 1 tab po qd)	[(Dapsone 50 mg po qd) + (pyri 50 mg po q week) + (folinic acid 25 mg po q week)] OR atovaquone 1500 mg po qd	Prophylaxis for pneumocystis also effective vs toxo. Ref.: *MMWR 48:RR-10, 1999*
Suppression after rx of cerebral toxo	(Sulfadiazine 500–1000 mg 4x(d) + (pyri 25–75 mg po qd) + (folinic acid 10–25 mg po qd)	[(Clinda 300–450 mg po q6–8h) + (pyri 25–75 mg po qd)] + (folinic acid 10–25 mg po qd)] OR atovaquone 750 mg po q6–12h	(Pyri + sulfa) prevents PCP and toxo; (clinda + pyri) prevents toxo only.
Trichomonas vaginalis	See *Vaginitis, Table 1, page 18*		
Trypanosomiasis			
T. brucei gambiense or T. brucei rhodesiense: African sleeping sickness			
Early infection with normal CSF	Suramin[PDS] test dose of 0.2 gm IV, then 20 mg/kg, up to max. of 1.0 gm, IV on days 1, 3, 7, 14 & 21. Children: 20 mg/kg on same schedule.	Pentamidine isethionate 4 mg/kg IM qod x10 doses) or (eflornithine 100 mg/kg q6h IV x14 d. and then 75 mg/kg po for 21–30 d. for gambiense but not rhodesiense)	Peds. dose of eflornithine: 100 mg/kg IV x2 wks, then 75 mg/kg po q6h x4 wks.
Late infection with CNS symptoms and abnormal CSF	Melarsoprol[PDS] 2–3.6 mg/kg/d IV x3 doses, repeat after 1 week and again after 10–21 days (active vs rhodesiense) See *Peds dose in Table 12B, page 96.*	In debilitated pts, can start with suramin 0.2 gm/d IV x2 d., then start melarsoprol. Prednisolone 1 mg/kg/d po may ↓ post-rx encephalopathy (see Comment).	CSF abnormal if ≥5 cells/µl or ↑ protein concentration. Melarsoprol-induced encephalopathy in 10% of pts. NOTE: T. brucei rhodesiense are resistant to nifurtimox and eflornithine.
T. brucei gambiense **relapse** post-rx with melarsoprol	Eflornithine 100 mg/kg q6h IV x14 d., then 75 mg/kg po for 21–30 d.		
T. brucei gambiense prophylaxis	Pentamidine isethionate 3 mg/kg IM q 6 months	Not for casual visitor.	Risk to tourists low. Not effective for T. brucei rhodesiense.
T. cruzi Chagas disease or acute American trypanosomiasis Heart disease ref.: *NEJM 325:763, 1991*	Nifurtimox[PDS] 8–10 mg/kg/d po div. 4x/d. after meals x120 d. Ages 11–16 yrs: 12.5–15 mg/kg/d div. qid po x90 d. Children <11 yrs: 15–20 mg/kg/d div. qid po x90 d.	Benznidazole[NUS] 7.5 mg/kg/d po div. 2x/d x60 d. *(Ln 348:1407, 1996).* NOTE: Avoid tetracycline and steroids.	Treatment of no benefit in chronic late disease. Nifurtimox reported 70–95% effective. Immunosuppression for heart transplant can reactivate chronic Chagas disease.
NEMATODES—INTESTINAL (Roundworms) Ref.: *Int Dis Clin Pract (IDCP) 5:473, 1996*			
Angiostrongylus cantonensis	Mebendazole 100 mg po bid x5 d.	Thiabendazole 22 mg/kg po bid x3 d.	Causes eosinophilic meningitis.
Angiostrongylus costaricensis	Thiabendazole 25 mg/kg po tid x3 d. Give max. dose of 3.0 gm/day.		Can cause inflammatory mass that mimics appendicitis.

[1] **PDS** = available from Parasitic Drug Service of CDC

NOTE: All dosage recommendations are for adults (unless otherwise indicated) and assume normal renal function. *See page 98 for abbreviations.*

TABLE 12 (6)

INFECTING ORGANISM	SUGGESTED REGIMENS		COMMENTS
	PRIMARY	ALTERNATIVE	
NEMATODES—INTESTINAL (Roundworms) *(continued)*			
Ascaris lumbricoides **(ascariasis)**	Albendazole 400 mg po x1 dose or mebendazole 100 mg po bid x3 d.	Pyrantel pamoate 11 mg/kg po x1 dose (max. dose 1.0 gm)	For intestinal or biliary obstruction, use piperazine citrate 75 mg/kg to max. dose of 3.5 gm once daily x2 d. NO concomitant chlorpromazine with piperazine *(Table 21, page 131)*, as seizures can occur.
	If GI obstruction, use piperazine—dosage in Comments		
Capillaria philippinensis (capillariasis)	Mebendazole 200 mg po bid x20 d.	Albendazole 200 mg po bid x10 d.	
Enterobius vermicularis **(pinworm)**	Albendazole 400 mg po x1, repeat in 2 wks OR mebendazole 100 mg po x1, repeat in 2 wks	Pyrantel pamoate 11 mg/kg to max. dose of 1.0 gm) po x1 dose; repeat every 2 wks x2.	*Side-effects in Table 12B, pages 97, 98.*
Hookworm (Necator americanus and Ancylostoma duodenale)	Albendazole 400 mg po x1 or mebendazole 100 mg po bid x3 d.	Pyrantel pamoate 11 mg/kg (to max. dose of 1.0 gm) po daily x3 d.	NOTE: Ivermectin not effective. Eosinophilia may be present but eggs detectable in stool.
Strongyloides stercoralis **(strongyloidiasis)**	Ivermectin 200 µg/kg/d x2 d OR albendazole 400 mg po qd x3 d.	Thiabendazole 25 mg/kg po bid (max. 3 gm/d) x2 d. (7–10 d. for hyperinfection syndrome)	Case report of ivermectin failure in pt with hypogamma-globulinemia *(Am J Med Sci 311:178, 1996)*.
Trichostrongylus orientalis	Albendazole 400 mg po x1 dose	Pyrantel pamoate 11 mg/kg (max. 1.0 gm) po x1	
Trichuris trichiura **(whipworm)**	Albendazole 400 mg po x1 dose	Mebendazole 100 mg po bid x3 d.	May need repeat rx if heavily infected.
NEMATODES—EXTRAINTESTINAL (Roundworms)			
Anisakis simplex **(anisakiasis)**	Physical removal: endoscope or surgery	Mebendazole 200 mg po bid x3 d.	Anisakiasis acquired by eating raw fish: herring, salmon, mackerel, cod, squid. Similar illness due to Pseudoterranova species acquired from cod, halibut, red snapper.
Ancylostoma braziliense: causes **cutaneous larva migrans**	Ivermectin 150 µg/kg po x1 dose	Albendazole 200 mg po bid x3 d.	Also called "creeping eruption"
Dracunculus medinensis: **Guinea worm**	Surgical removal of pre-emergent worm	Metronidazole 250 mg po tid x10 d used by some to ↓ inflammatory response and facilitate removal. Immersion in warm water promotes worm emergence from skin.	
Filariasis			
Lymphatic **(Elephantiasis):** Wuchereria bancrofti or Brugia malayi or B. timori	Ivermectin 100–440 µg/kg x1 dose OR Report of rx of children with both ivermectin 200–400 µg/kg and albendazole 400 mg, one dose of each (*Ln 350:480, 1997*)	Diethylcarbamazine[1] (DEC) over 21 days: Days 1 & 2, 50 mg tid; day 3, 100 mg tid; days 4–21, 2 mg/kg tid. (See Comment)	All drugs clear microfilariae but not adult worms.
Cutaneous			
Loiasis: Loa loa, eyeworm disease[2]	Diethylcarbamazine (DEC)[1]—dose as for Wuchereria; albendazole 200 mg po bid x21d. reported effective.		DEC 300 mg/wk po effective prophylaxis
Onchocerca volvulus[2] (onchocerci-asis) (*Ln 351:1341, 1998*)	Ivermectin 150 µg/kg po x1 dose; repeat q6 months to suppress dermal and ocular micro-filariae. If eye involved, start prednisone 1 mg/kg/d po several days before ivermectin.		Ivermectin ↓ number of microfilariae in skin and impairs female worm fertility; does not kill adult worms (nothing does). Ivermectin OK in pregnancy.
Body cavity			
Mansonella perstans (dipetalonemiasis)	Mebendazole 100 mg po x30 d.	Usually no or vague allergic symptoms + eosinophilia. Ivermectin has no activity against this species.	

[1] Diethylcarbamazine available from Wyeth-Ayerst (610) 971-5509
[2] Occasional serious reactions reported in pts with both loiasis and onchocerciasis given ivermectin (*Ln 350:18, 1997*)
NOTE: All dosage recommendations are for adults (unless otherwise indicated) and assume normal renal function. *See page 98 for abbreviations.*

TABLE 12 (7)

INFECTING ORGANISM	SUGGESTED REGIMENS		COMMENTS
	PRIMARY	ALTERNATIVE	
NEMATODES—EXTRAINTESTINAL (Roundworms)/Filariasis/Cutaneous/Body cavity (continued)			
Mansonella streptocerca	Diethylcarbamazine[1], as above for Wuchereria OR ivermectin 150 μg/kg x1		Chronic pruritic hypopigmented lesions that may be confused with leprosy. Can be asymptomatic.
Mansonella ozzardi	Ivermectin 150 μg/kg x1 dose may be effective		Usually asymptomatic. Articular pain, pruritus, lymphadenopathy reported.
Dirofilariasis: Heartworms			
D. immitis, dog heartworm	No effective drugs; surgical removal only option		Can lodge in pulmonary artery → coin lesion. Eosinophilia rare.
D. tenius (raccoon), D. ursi (bear), D. repens (dogs, cats).	No effective drugs		Worms migrate to conjunctivae, subcutaneous tissue, scrotum, breasts, extremities
Gnathostoma spingerum: eosinophilic myeloencephalitis	Surgical removal + albendazole 400 mg po qd	or bid x21 d.	Can manifest as painful subcutaneous mass with eosinophilia
Toxocariasis	**Direct rx at relief of symptoms as infection self-limited, e.g., steroids & antihistamines; use of anthelminthics controversial.**		
Visceral larval migrans	Diethylcarbamazine[1] 2 mg/kg po tid x10 d.	(Albendazole 400 mg po bid) or (mebendazole 100–200 mg po bid) x5 days	Severe lung, heart or CNS disease may warrant steroids. Differential dx of larval migrans syndromes: Toxocara canis and catis, Ancylostoma spp., Gnathostoma spp., Spirometra spp.
Ocular larval migrans	First 4 wks of illness: (Oral prednisone 30–60 mg po qd + subtenon triamcinolone 40 mg weekly) x2 weeks		No added benefit of antihelminthic drugs. Rx of little effect after 4 wks.
Trichinella spiralis (**trichinosis**)—muscle infection	Albendazole 400 mg po bid x14 d.	Mebendazole 5 mg/kg po bid x10-13 d.	Use albendazole/mebendazole with caution during pregnancy.
	Concomitant prednisone 40–60 mg qd		
TREMATODES (Flukes)			
Clonorchis sinensis (liver fluke)	Praziquantel 25 mg/kg po tid x1 day or albendazole 10 mg/kg/d. po x7 d.		Same dose in children
Fasciola buski (intestinal fluke)	Praziquantel 25 mg/kg po tid x1 day		Same dose in children
Fasciola hepatica (sheep liver fluke)	Bithionol[PDS]: Adults and children: 30–40 mg/kg (max. dose 2 gm/d) qod x10–15 doses		Triclabendazole experimental drug: 10 mg/kg po x1 dose
Heterophyes heterophyes (intestinal fluke); Metagonimus yokogawai (intestinal fluke); Opisthorchis viverrini (liver fluke)	Praziquantel 25 mg/kg po tid x1 day		Same dose in children
Paragonimus westermani (lung fluke)	Praziquantel 25 mg/kg po tid x2 days		Same dose in children
Schistosoma haematobium; GU bilharziasis	Praziquantel 20 mg/kg po bid x1 day (2 doses)		Same dose in children. Alternative: metrifonate 10 mg/kg/dose po q2 wks for 3 doses.
Schistosoma intercalatum	Praziquantel 20 mg/kg po bid x1 day (2 doses)		Same dose in children
Schistosoma japonicum; Oriental schisto	Praziquantel 20 mg/kg po tid x1 day (3 doses)		Same dose in children
Schistosoma mansoni (intestinal bilharziasis) Possible praziquantel resistance (JID 176:304, 1997)	Praziquantel 20 mg/kg po bid x1 day (2 doses)	Oxamniquine. Single dose of 15 mg/kg po once; in North and East Africa 20 mg/kg po daily x3 d.	Same dose for children. For neurological manifestations: CID 18:354, 1994
Schistosoma mekongi	Praziquantel 20 mg/kg po tid x1 day (3 doses)		Same dose for children

[1] Diethylcarbamazine available from Wyeth-Ayerst (610) 971-5509
[2] **PDS** = Available from Parasitic Drug Service of CDC
NOTE: All dosage recommendations are for adults (unless otherwise indicated) and assume normal renal function. *See page 98 for abbreviations.*

TABLE 12 (8)

INFECTING ORGANISM	SUGGESTED REGIMENS		COMMENTS
	PRIMARY	ALTERNATIVE	
TREMATODES (Flukes) *(continued)*			
Toxemic schisto: Katayama fever			Massive infection with either S. japonicum or S. mansoni
CESTODES (Tapeworms)			
Echinococcus granulosus (hydatid disease) Rx renders cyst content non-infectious in 80–90% and cyst disappearance in 30% of pts. (Refs.: *NEJM* 337:881, 1997; *IDCP* 6:159, 1997)	Combine percutaneous drainage with 3 cycles of po albendazole: >60 kg: 400 mg po bid with meals x28 days; <60 kg: 15 mg/kg/d div. bid with meals (max. daily dose 800 mg) x28 days. 74% response with 25% relapse. Can re-treat (*CID* 29:304 & 310, 1999).	Praziquantel 25 mg/kg po q4h with food x3 doses Another option: cyst puncture with ultrasound, content aspiration, injection 95% ethanol or hypertonic saline, re-aspirate & concomitant chemotherapy (*Acta Trop* 64:95, 1997). NOTE: If cyst spillage secondary to trauma or surgery, need praziquantel and then several cycles of albendazole to prevent implantation of secondary cysts.	
	28-day cycle, then 14 days no drug. Repeat for 3 cycles.		
Echinococcus multilocularis (alveolar cyst disease)	Albendazole efficacy not clearly demonstrated, can try in dosages used for hydatid disease. Wide surgical resection; technique evolving (*Radiology* 198:259, 1996).		
Intestinal tapeworms			
Diphyllobothrium latum (fish), Dipylidium caninum (dog), Taenia saginata (beef), and Taenia solium (pork)	Praziquantel 5–10 mg/kg po x1 dose for children and adults	Praziquantel 10 mg/kg po x1 dose for children and adults	
Hymenolepis diminuta (rats) and H. nana (humans)	Praziquantel 25 mg/kg po x1 dose for children and adults		
Cerebral (neuro) cysticercosis Larval stage of T. solium—*see Comment* Management refs.: *IDCP* 6:358, 1997; *EIN* 3:403, 1997; *CID* 24:157, 1997	Praziquantel 50 mg/kg/d po in 3 div. doses x15 d. One refractory pt. treated with praziquantel 100 mg/kg/d + ASA 325 mg/d, cimetidine 800 mg/d, + dexamethasone x21 d. (*WJM* 170:112, 1999)	Albendazole x8–30 d. by weight: >60 kg, 400 mg po bid with meals; <60 kg, 15 mg/kg/d po div. bid with meals (max. daily dose 800 mg)	Dexamethasone ± seizure meds may be needed to control rx-induced inflammation from cyst death. In children, albendazole rx leads to faster resolution of CT lesions and lower risk of late seizures: *PJID* 17:696, 1998.
Sparganosis (Spirometra mansonoides) Larval cysts: source—frogs/snakes	Surgical resection or ethanol injection of subcutaneous masses (*NEJM* 330:1887, 1994).		
ECTOPARASITES			
Pediculus humanus corporis (body lice)	Treat the clothing. Organism lives in, deposits eggs in seams of clothing. Discard clothing; if not possible, treat clothing with 1% malathion powder or 10% DDT powder.		Body louse leaves clothing only for blood meal. Nits in clothing viable for 1 month. Ref.: *Med Lett* 38:6, 1997.
P. humanus var. capitis (**head louse**, nits)	**Permethrin,** 5% prescription strength (ELIMITE) or 1% non-prescription (Nix). Wash hair, apply lotion for 10 min., then rinse off, comb; 2nd treatment 7–10 days after 1st to kill newly hatched lice (all products). **Lindane (Kwell)** 1%, less effective (use only if failed other therapy). Seizures can occur from coverage of broad areas or ingestion. For head lice treatment failures, anecdotal reports of success with ivermectin 200 µg/kg single dose po. Another option (not in neonates/infants): Malathion 0.5% lotion (Ovide). Apply for 8–12 hrs.; comb for nits after washing hair.		Benefit of residual permethrin on hair reduced by shampoos or vinegar. No residual effect with lindane or pyrethrin products. Nit removal important adjunct. Use nit comb ± enzymatic egg remover (CLEAR is one example).
Phthirus pubis (crabs)			Treat sex partners if body or pubic lice. Cost: Permethrin 60 gm $9.20; lindane 60 ml $6.35–16.40; malathion $31.25; ivermectin $9.97.

NOTE: All dosage recommendations are for adults (unless otherwise indicated) and assume normal renal function. See *page 98 for abbreviations.*

TABLE 12 (9)

INFECTING ORGANISM	SUGGESTED REGIMENS		COMMENTS
	PRIMARY	ALTERNATIVE	

ECTOPARASITES *(continued)*

Sarcoptes scabiei **(scabies)** (mites) *(CID 27:646, 1998)*

INFECTING ORGANISM	PRIMARY / ALTERNATIVE	COMMENTS
Immunocompetent patients	Primary: Permethrin 5% cream (ELIMITE). Apply entire skin from chin to toes. Leave on 8–10 hrs. Repeat in 1 week. Safe for children >2 mos. old. Do not use in pregnancy *(see Comment)*. Alternative: Lindane 1% lotion. Apply as for permethrin OR ivermectin 200 μg/kg po x1 *(NEJM 333:26, 1995)*.	Trim fingernails. Reapply to hands after handwashing. Pruritus may persist ≥2 wks after mites gone. Do not use lindane in pregnancy or in young children—absorbed through skin; can use 6–10% precipitated sulfur in petrolatum daily x3 days. Repeated lindane application associated with seizures in children.
AIDS patients, CD4 <150/mm³ **(Norwegian scabies**—see Comments*)	For Norwegian scabies: Permethrin as above on day 1, then repeat x several weeks. Or in petrolatum daily on days 2–7, then repeat x several weeks. Ivermectin 200 μg/kg po x1 reported effective.	Norwegian scabies in AIDS pts: Extensive, crusted. Can mimic psoriasis. Not pruritic. ELIMITE: 60 gm $18.10; lindane 60 ml $2.60–10.50. **Highly contagious—isolate!**

TABLE 12B: DOSAGE, PRICE, AND SELECTED ADVERSE EFFECTS OF ANTIPARASITIC DRUGS

NOTE: Drugs available from CDC Parasitic Drug Service indicated by "PDS". Call (404) 639-3670 (or -3356).

Doses vary with indication. For convenience, drugs divided by type of parasite; some drugs used for multiple types of parasites, e.g., albendazole.

COMMENT: Cost data represent average wholesale prices as listed in Oct. 1997 Medi-Span Hospital Formulary Pricing Guide.

CLASS, AGENT, GENERIC NAME (TRADE NAME)	USUAL ADULT DOSAGE (Cost)	ADVERSE REACTIONS/COMMENTS
Antiprotozoan Drugs		
Intestinal Parasites		
Albendazole (Albenza)	Doses vary with indication, 200–400 mg bid po 200 mg tab $1.10	Teratogenic. Pregnancy Cat. C; give after negative pregnancy test. Abdominal pain, nausea/vomiting, alopecia, ↑ serum transaminase. Rare leukopenia.
Dehydroemetine *(PDS)**	1.5 mg/kg/d to max. of 90 mg IM	Local pain, ECG changes, cardiac arrhythmias, precordial pain, paresthesias, weakness, peripheral neuropathy. GI: nausea/vomiting, diarrhea. Avoid strenuous exercise for 4 wks after rx.
Diloxanide furoate *(PDS)*	500 mg po tid	GI: flatulence, abdominal distention, nausea/vomiting. Pruritus, urticaria.
Furazolidone (Furoxone)	Peds: 6 mg/kg/d div. qid. Not for infants <1 mo. old. Liquid: 60 ml $16.06; 100 mg tab $2.67	Only liquid antigiardiasis drug in U.S. Disulfiram-like reaction with alcohol. Occasional side-effects: Fever, urticaria, ↓ BP, arthralgia, nausea/vomiting, headache. Hemolysis if G6PD deficient. May turn urine brown.
Iodoquinol [was diiodohydroxyquin]NUS	Adults: 650 mg po tid; children: 40 mg/kg/d div. tid.	Rarely causes nausea, abdominal cramps, rash, acne. Contraindicated if iodine intolerance.
Metronidazole/Omidazole NUS (Tiberal)/Tinidazole NUS (Fasigyn)	Side-effects similar for all. *See metronidazole in Table 9A, page 62, & 10B, page 68*	*See metronidazole in Table 9A, page 62, & 10B, page 68*
Paromomycin (Humatin) Aminosidine in U.K.	Up to 750 mg qid. 250 mg caps $2.62	Drug is aminoglycoside similar to neomycin; if absorbed due to concomitant inflammatory bowel disease can result in oto/nephrotoxicity. Doses >3 gm assoc. with nausea, abdominal cramps, diarrhea.
Quinacrine NUS (Atabrine, Mepacrine)	100 mg tid. No longer available in U.S.	Contraindicated for pts with history of psychosis of psoriasis. Yellow staining of skin. Dizziness, headache, vomiting, toxic psychosis (1.5%), hemolytic anemia, leucopenia, thrombocytopenia, urticaria, rash, fever, minor disulfiram-like reactions.

* All doses for adults with normal renal function unless pediatric dose given. **PDS** = Available from Parasitic Drug Service of CDC. *See page 98 for other abbreviations.*

TABLE 12B (2)

CLASS, AGENT, GENERIC NAME (TRADE NAME)	USUAL ADULT DOSAGE (Cost)	ADVERSE REACTIONS/COMMENTS
Antiprotozoan Drugs (continued)		
Extraintestinal Parasites		
Antimony compounds[NUS] Stibogluconate sodium (Pentostam, Tricostam)—PDS Meglumine antimonate (Glucaratime, Glucontim— French tradenames	Solution containing 30–34% pentavalent antimony	Cough/vomiting if IV infusion too fast. Arthralgia 50%. Others: myalgia, bradycardia, cramps/diarrhea, pruritus/rash, renal toxicity, ↑ amylase. **NOTE: EKG abnormalities occur. Combination rx with, or sequential rx with, ampho B may trigger fatal arrhythmias (Ln 351:1928, 1998).**
Artemether[NUS] (Artenam)	Adults: 4 mg/kg IM, then 2 mg/kg IM q8h. Children: 3.2 mg/kg IM, then 1.6 mg/kg IM qd.	Drug fever, abdominal pain, diarrhea, primary heart block. Refs.: NEJM 335:69 & 76, 1996.
Atovaquone (Mepron)	Suspension: 1 tsp (750 mg) po bid 750 mg/5 ml. Cost: 210 ml $613.00	No. pts stopping rx due to side-effects was 9%; rash 22%, GI 20%, headache 16%, insomnia 19%, fever 14%
Atovaquone and proguanil (Malarone)	Prophylaxis: 250 mg + 100 mg qd Treatment: 1000 mg + 400 mg once daily x3 days Tabs: Either 250/100 mg or 62.5/25 mg. Peds dosage: Table 12, page 89, footnote 1	Adverse effects in rx trials: Adults—abd. pain 17%, N/V 12%, headache 10%, dizziness 5%. Rx stopped in 1%. Asymptomatic mild ↑ in ALT/AST. Children—cough, headache, anorexia, vomiting, abd. pain. See drug interactions, Table 21. Safe in G6PD-deficient pts. Can crush tabs for children.
Benznidazole[NUS] (Rochagan, Radinyl)	7.5 mg/kg/d po	Photosensitivity in 50% of pts. GI: abdominal pain, nausea/vomiting/ anorexia. CNS: disorientation, insomnia, twitching/seizures, paresthesias, polyneuritis
Chloroquine phosphate (Aralen)	Dose varies—see Malaria prophylaxis and rx. 500 mg tabs $4.33; IM 250 mg ampule $17.06	Minor: anorexia/nausea/vomiting, headache, dizziness, blurred vision, pruritus in dark-skinned pts. Major: protracted rx in rheumatoid arthritis can lead to retinopathy. Can exacerbate psoriasis. Can block response to rabies vaccine.
Dapsone Ref.: CID 27:191, 1998	100 mg po qd 100 mg tabs $0.20	Usually tolerated by pts with rash after TMP/SMX. Adverse effects: nausea/vomiting, rash, oral lesions (CID 18:630, 1994). Methemoglobinemia (usually asymptomatic); if >10–15%, stop drug. Hemolytic anemia if G6PD deficient. Sulfone syndrome: fever, rash, hemolytic anemia, atypical lymphocytes, and liver injury (West J Med 156:303, 1992).
Eflornithine[NUS] (Ornidyl)	Approved in U.S. for trypanosome infections but not marketed. Contact Hoechst Marion Roussel, (800) 552-3656.	Diarrhea in ½ pts, vomiting, abdominal pain, anemia/leucopenia in ½ pts, seizures, alopecia, jaundice, ↓ hearing
Halofantrine (Halfan)	Adults: 500 mg po q6h x3 doses Children: 8 mg/kg po q6h x3 doses 250 mg tab $9.88	Poor oral bioavailability ↑ with fatty meal. Causes delay in A-V conduction; do not use if long QT interval or pt taking drugs known to ↑ QT interval (e.g., quinine/quinidine, astemizole, chloroquine, antidepressants, neuroleptic drugs). Other side-effects: nausea, abdominal pain, diarrhea.
Mefloquine (Lariam)	One 250 mg tab/week for malaria prophylaxis; for rx, 1250 mg x1 or 750 mg & then 500 mg in 6–8 hrs. 250 mg tab $8.21	Side-effects in roughly 3%. Minor: headache, irritability, insomnia, weakness, diarrhea. Debatable frequency of severe neuropsychiatric reactions; one study (JID 173:1506, 1996) reports 1:13,000; retrospective survey reports 0.7% (BMJ 313:525, 1996); no effect on performance of airplane pilots (AJTMH 56:235, 1997). Rare: Prolonged QT interval and toxic epidermal necrolysis (Ln 349:101, 1997). Not used for self-rx due to neuropsychiatric side-effects.
Melarsoprol (PDS) (Mel B, Arsobal) (Manufactured in France)	See Trypanosomiasis for adult dose. Peds dose: 0.36 mg/kg IV, then gradual ↑ to 3.6 mg/kg q1–5 days for total of 9–10 doses.	Post-rx encephalopathy (10%) with 15–40% mortality overall; risk of death 2° to rx 4–8%. Prednisolone 1 mg/kg/d po may ↓ encephalopathy. Other: Heart damage, albuminuria, abdominal pain, vomiting, peripheral neuropathy, Herxheimer-like reaction, pruritus.
Nifurtimox (PDS) (Manufactured in Germany by Bayer)	8–10 mg/kg/d po div. 4x/day	Side-effects in 40–70% of pts. GI: abdominal pain, nausea/vomiting. CNS: polyneuritis (⅓), disorientation, insomnia, twitching, seizures. Skin rash. Hemolysis with G6PD deficiency.

* All doses for adults with normal renal function unless pediatric dose given. **PDS** = Available from Parasitic Drug Service of CDC. See page 98 for other abbreviations.

CLASS, AGENT, GENERIC NAME (TRADE NAME)	USUAL ADULT DOSAGE (Cost)		ADVERSE REACTIONS/COMMENTS
Antiprotozoan Drugs/Extraintestinal Parasites *(continued)*			
Pentamidine (NebuPent)	300 mg via aerosol q month. Also used IM. 300 mg $98.75 + admin. costs		Hypotension, hypocalcemia, hypoglycemia followed by hyperglycemia, pancreatitis. Neutropenia (15%), thrombocytopenia. Nephrotoxicity. Others: nausea/vomiting, ↑ liver tests, rash.
Primaquine phosphate	26.3 mg (=15 mg base)		In G6PD def. pts, can cause hemolytic anemia with hemoglobinuria. Methemoglobinemia. Nausea/abdominal pain if pt. fasting.
Pyrimethamine (Daraprim, Malodie) Also combined with sulfadoxine as **Fansidar**	100 mg po, then 25 mg qd. 25 mg $0.43. Cost of folinic acid (leuco-vorin) 10 mg $5.75	Major problem is hematologic: megaloblastic anemia, ↓ WBC, ↓ platelets. Can give 5 mg folinic acid/day to ↓ bone marrow depression and not interfere with antitoxoplasmosis effect. If high-dose pyrimethamine, ↑ folinic acid to 10–50 mg/d. Pyrimethamine + sulfadiazine can cause mental changes due to carnitine deficiency *(AJM 95:112, 1993)*. Other: Rash, vomiting, diarrhea, xerostomia	
Quinidine gluconate	Loading dose of 10 mg (equivalent to 6.2 mg of quinidine base)/kg IV over 1–2 hrs, and then constant infusion of 0.02 mg of quinidine gluconate/kg/minute.		Adverse reactions of quinidine/quinine similar: (1) IV bolus injection can cause fatal hypotension, (2) hyperinsulinemic hypoglycemia, esp. in pregnancy, (3) ↓ rate of infusion of IV quinidine if QT interval ↑ >25% of baseline, (4) reduce dose 30–50% after day 3 due to ↓ renal clearance and ↓ vol. of distribution.
Quinine sulfate (300 mg salt = 250 mg base)	325 and 650 mg tabs. No IV prep. in U.S. Oral rx of chloroquine-resistant falciparum malaria: 650 mg po tid x3d., then tetracycline 250 mg po qid x7 d. 325 mg $0.16		Cinchonism; tinnitus, headache, nausea, abdominal pain, blurred vision. Rarely: blood dyscrasias, drug fever, asthma, hypoglycemia.
Spiramycin[1] (Rovamycine) *(JAC 42:572, 1998)*	Up to 3–4 gm/d		GI and allergic reactions have occurred. Not available in U.S.
Sulfadiazine	1.0–1.5 gm po q6h 500 mg $0.34		*See Table 9B, page 69, for sulfonamide side-effects*
Sulfadoxine and pyrimethamine combination (Fansidar)	Contains 500 mg of sulfadoxine and 25 mg of pyrimethamine One tab $3.45		Very long mean half-life of both drugs: Sulfadoxine 169 hrs, pyrimethamine 111 hrs allows weekly dosage. Fatalities reported due to Stevens-Johnson syndrome and toxic epidermal necrolysis. Renal excretion—use with caution in pts with renal impairment.
DRUGS USED TO TREAT NEMATODES, TREMATODES, AND CESTODES			
Bithionol (Manufactured in Japan)	Adults & children: 30–40 mg/kg (to max. of 2 gm/d) po qod x10–15 doses		Photosensitivity, skin reactions, urticaria, GI upset
Diethylcarbamazine[2] (Hetrazan)	Used to treat filariasis. Licensed (Lederle) but not available in U.S.		Headache, dizziness, nausea, fever. Host may experience inflammatory reaction to death of adult worms: fever, urticaria, asthma, GI upset (Mazzotti reaction).
Ivermectin (Stromectol)	Strongyloidiasis dose: 200 µg/kg x1 dose po Onchocerciasis: 150 µg/kg po x1 Scabies: 200 µg/kg po x1 6 mg tabs $7.98		Mild side-effects: fever, pruritus, rash. In rx of onchocerciasis, can see tender lymphadenopathy, headache, bone/joint pain. Can cause Mazzotti reaction *(see above)*.
Mebendazole (Vermox)	Doses vary with indication. 100 mg tab $5.68		Rarely causes abdominal pain, nausea, diarrhea. Contraindicated in pregnancy and children <2 yrs old.
Oxamniquine (Vansil)[NUS]	For S. mansoni. Some experts suggest 40–60 mg/kg over 2–3 days in all of Africa.		Rarely: dizziness, drowsiness, neuropsychiatric symptoms, GI upset. EKG/EEG changes. Orange/red urine.

[1] Available from FDA: (301) 443-5680
[2] Available from Wyeth-Ayerst, (610) 971-5509
* All doses for adults with normal renal function unless pediatric dose given. **PDS** = Available from Parasitic Drug Service of CDC. *See page 98 for other abbreviations.*

97

TABLE 12B (4)

CLASS, AGENT, GENERIC NAME (TRADE NAME)	USUAL ADULT DOSAGE (Cost)	ADVERSE REACTIONS/COMMENTS
DRUGS USED TO TREAT NEMATODES, TREMATODES, AND CESTODES (continued)		
Praziquantel (Biltricide)	Doses vary with parasite; see Table 12A. 600 mg $11.90	Mild: dizziness/drowsiness. Only contraindication is ocular cysticercosis.
Pyrantel pamoate (over-the-counter as Reese's Pinworm Medicine)	Oral suspension. Dose for all ages: 11 mg/kg (to max. of 1 gm) x1 dose	Rare GI upset, headache, dizziness, rash
Suramin (Germanin) (Can obtain via PDS)	For early trypanosomiasis. Drug powder mixed to 10% solution with 5 ml water and used within 30 minutes.	Does not cross blood-brain barrier; no effect on CNS infection. Side-effects: vomiting, pruritus, urticaria, fever, paresthesias, albuminuria (discontinue drug if casts appear). Do not use if renal/liver disease present. Deaths from vascular collapse reported.
Thiabendazole (Mintezol)	Take after meals. Dose varies with parasite; see Table 12A. 500 mg $1.08	Nausea/vomiting, headache, dizziness. Rarely: liver damage, ↓ BP, angioneurotic edema, Stevens-Johnson syndrome. May ↓ mental alertness.

Abbreviations: Clinda = clindamycin; **CQ** = chloroquine phosphate; **MQ** = mefloquine; **NUS** = not available in the U.S.; **PQ** = primaquine; **Pyri** = pyrimethamine; **QS** = quinine sulfate; **TMP/SMX** = trimethoprim/sulfamethoxazole

* All doses for adults with normal renal function unless pediatric dose given. PDS = Available from Parasitic Drug Service of CDC.

TABLE 13A: METHODS FOR PENICILLIN DESENSITIZATION

Perform in ICU setting. Discontinue all β-adrenergic antagonists. Have IV line, ECG and spirometer (Curr Clin Topics Inf Dis 13:131; 1993). Once desensitized, rx must not lapse or risk of allergic reactions ↑. A history of Stevens-Johnson syndrome, exfoliative dermatitis, erythroderma are nearly absolute contraindications to desensitization (use only as an approach to IgE sensitivity).

Oral Route: If oral prep available and pt has functional GI tract, oral route is preferred. 1/3 pts will develop transient reaction during desensitization or treatment, usually mild.

Step *	1	2	3	4	5	6	7	8	9	10	11	12	13	14
Drug (mg/ml)	0.5	0.5	0.5	0.5	0.5	0.5	0.5	5.0	5.0	5.0	50	50	50	50
Amount (ml)	0.1	0.2	0.4	0.8	1.6	3.2	6.4	1.2	2.4	4.8	1.0	2.0	4.0	8.0

* Interval between doses: 15 min. After Step 14, observe for 30 minutes, then 1.0 gm IV

Parenteral Route:

Step **	1	2	3	4	5	6	7	8	9	10	11	12	13	14	15	16	17
Drug (mg/ml)	0.1	0.1	0.1	0.1	1.0	1.0	1.0	10	10	10	100	100	100	100	1000	1000	1000
Amount (ml)	0.1	0.2	0.4	0.8	0.16	0.32	0.64	0.12	0.24	0.48	0.1	0.2	0.4	0.8	0.16	0.32	0.64

** Interval between doses: 15 min. After Step 17, observe for 30 minutes, then 1.0 gm IV

[Adapted from Sullivan, TJ, in Allergy: Principles and Practice, Middleton, E., et al. Eds. C.V. Mosby, 1993, p. 1726, with permission]

TABLE 13B: RAPID ORAL TMP/SMX DESENSITIZATION*

Hour	Dose TMP/SMX (mg)	Comment
0	0.004/0.02	Perform in hospital or clinic. Use oral suspension [40mg TMP/200 mg SMX/5 ml (tsp)]. Take 6 oz water after each dose. Corticosteroids, antihistamines NOT used. Refs.: CID 20:849, 1995; AIDS 5:311, 1991
1	0.04/0.2	
2	0.4/2	
3	4/20	
4	40/200	
5	160/800	

TABLE 14: ANTIVIRAL THERAPY (Non-HIV)
(See NEJM 340:1255, 1999)

VIRUS/DISEASE	DRUG/DOSAGE	SIDE EFFECTS/COMMENTS
Enterovirus—Meningitis: most common cause of aseptic meningitis in U.S. (CID 27:896, 1998)	No rx currently recommended; however, pleconaril (VP 63849), 200–400 mg po tid x7 d (Inv). [For compassionate use (for chronic enteroviral meningoencephalitis in pts with immunodeficiency, neonatal sepsis syndrome, myocarditis, enterovirus infection complicating bone marrow transplant or vaccine-associated paralytic polio), call Virophama (610) 651-0200]	Reduced symptoms of aseptic meningitis caused by enteroviruses by approx. 50% in a placebo-controlled trial in 39 adults (ICAAC Abst., 1997; Antiviral Research 38:1, 1998).
Hemorrhagic Fever Virus Infections		
Congo-Crimean HF	Ribavirin po 4 gm qd x4 d, then 2.4 gm qd x6 d (see Comment)	Ln 346:472, 1995. (For oral drug, contact Virazole, ICN Pharmaceuticals, Costa Mesa, CA, USA)
Ebola/Marburg HF	No data to date on antiviral therapy	
With pulmonary syndrome: Hantavirus pulmonary syndrome, "sin nombre virus"	No benefit from ribavirin has been demonstrated to date (controlled trial in progress). Refs: JID 173:1297, 1996; Emerg Inf Dis 3:95, 1997.	Acute onset of fever, headache, myalgias, non-productive cough, thrombocytopenia and non-cardiogenic pulmonary edema with respiratory insufficiency following exposure to rodents. Serological studies available through CDC (Ln 347:739, 1996). Inhaled nitric oxide associated with improved pulmonary function in single case (PIDJ 17:749, 1998).
With renal syndrome: Lassa, Venezuelan, Korean, HF, Sabia, Argentinian HF, Junin, Machupo	Ribavirin IV 2.0 gm loading dose, then 1.0 gm q6h x4 days, then 0.5 gm q8h x6 days. (See Comment: Congo-Crimean HF.)	Toxicity low, hemolysis reported but recovery when treatment stopped. No significant changes in WBC, platelets, hepatic or renal function. Effective in Lassa and in 2 cases of Bolivian HF (CID 24:718, 1997). No data on others. Venezuelan HF may look like dengue (CID 26:308, 1998).
Dengue and dengue hemorrhagic fever (DHF) Aedes aegypti major vector (JID 176:313, 1997)	No data on antiviral rx. Appropriate fluid replacement with careful hemodynamic monitoring critical (Ln 352:971, 1998).	Resurgence in Southeast Asia, Central and South America and Caribbean. No vaccine; best prevention is to limit mosquito contact (AnIM 128:931, 1998 gives specifics).
Yellow fever	No data on antiviral rx	Reemergence across Africa and South America (200,000 cases/yr). Vaccination effective and should be used (JAMA 276:1157, 1996).
Hepatitis Viral Infections		
Hepatitis A (Ln 351:1643, 1998)	No therapy recommended. If within 2 wks of exposure, gamma globulin 0.02 ml/kg IM injection x1 is protective.	For vaccine recommendations, see Table 20 (MMWR 45, Dec. 27, 1996). 40% of pts with chronic Hep C who developed superinfection with Hep A developed fulminant hepatic failure in 1 study (NEJM 338:286, 1998).
Hepatitis B		
Acute	No therapy recommended	
Chronic (NEJM 336:347, 1997; 337:1733, 1997)	**interferon alfa** available as alfa-2a (Roferon-A), alfa-2b (Intron-A) & interferon alfa-n3 (Alferon N). Dosages: 5 million units daily or 10 million units tiw sc x4–6 mos. 33% will respond (AnIM 126:805, 1997).	53/103 treated >5 yrs responded with loss of HBe antigen 33% reduction in HBe antigen overall (NEJM 336:347, 1997). Survival 95% in responders vs <50% in non-responders (NEJM 334:1422, 1996). Toxicity was not a limiting factor in this trial.
Consider treatment in pts with **persistent elevation of aminotransferase;** detectable levels of HBsAg, HBeAg and HBV DNA in serum; hepatitis on liver bx; & compensated liver disease	Lamivudine (Epivir-HBV) 100 mg qd. Safety & efficacy of rx beyond 1 yr not established & optimal duration of rx not known —see Comment. Formulation & dsage of lamivudine in Epivir-HBV are not appropriate for pts dually infected with HBV & HIV; the higher dosage indicated for HIV rx should be used as part of an appropriate combination regimen.	↑ fibrosis, ↓ ALT, ↓ HBV DNA & ↑ HBeAg seroconversion compared with placebo with little toxicity over 1 year (NEJM 339:61, 1998; 341:1256, 1999). With 3 yrs of rx, up to 65% HBeAg pos. pts lost HBeAg & gained HBeAb (Hpt 30:420A, 1999). Hepatitis may flare when lamivudine stopped. YMDD variant HBV has occurred during rx in up to 32% over 1 yr (NEJM 341:1256, 1999) & ~50% over 3 yrs (J Hpt 30:59, 1999). Long-term clinical significance of YMDD variant HBV is unknown.

NOTE: All dosage recommendations are for adults (unless otherwise indicated) and assume normal renal function.

TABLE 14 (2)

VIRUS/DISEASE	DRUG/DOSAGE	SIDE EFFECTS/COMMENTS
Hepatitis Viral Infections/Hepatitis B *(continued)*		
Prevention Re-infection after transplantation for hepatitis B-induced cirrhosis *(See Table 15A, page 114 for post-exposure prophylaxis recommendations)*	Lamivudine 100 mg qd. Start at least 4 wks pre-transplant and continue for at least 12 months post-transplant *(Hpt 30:222A, 1999; Tpt 62:1456, 1996; Ln 348:1212, 1996).*	Based on 3 uncontrolled studies, data suggest that lamivudine may reduce the rate of HBV reinfection post-transplant. Most pts were clinically stable at 1 yr. Post-transplant recurrence of HBV was observed in some pts & YMDD variant HBV was detected in some cases *(Hpt 30:222A, 1999; Tpt 62:1456, 1996; Ln 348:1212, 1996).* Long-term clinical significance of YMDD variant HBV is ?.
Hepatitis C (up to 3% of world infected) **Chronic** (acute infection usually asymptomatic) 6 genotypes (1 is most common in U.S., 72%, & least responsive to rx) **Rx recommended for persistent elevations AST, HCV RNA+, & findings of fibrosis & moderate inflammation by liver bx** *(MMWR 47:RR-19, 1998).* Consultant care network available for rx questions: 1-800-640-2144.	**Ribavirin + Interferon alfa-2B** Weight ≤75 kg 400 mg a.m. & 3 mIU sc 3x/wk 600 mg p.m., po >75 kg 600 mg po, bid 3 mIU sc 3x/wk Duration: **48 wks genotype 1** (28% sustained response), **24 wks other genotypes** (66% sustained response). Toxicity ↑ with 48 wks vs 24 wks (21% rx for 48 wks discontinued rx secondary to side-effects).	Obtain baseline CBC and at wks 2 & 4 of rx *(see Table 14B, page 107)* In 912 pts with Hep C the combination of interferon alfa-2b + ribavirin was more successful in obtaining sustained virologic response (undetectable serum HCV RNA level 24 wks after 28 or 48 wks of rx) than alfa-2b alone: 31% vs 6% after 6 mos. rx and 38% vs 13% as initial rx *(NEJM 339:1485, 1998).* In 345 pts who relapsed after alfa-2b alone, 82% of combination rx vs 47% of alfa-2b alone responded but only 49% vs 5% of responders had sustained suppression 6 mos. later *(NEJM 339:1493, 1998).* Lack of early virological response did not predict sustained response in rx-naive (50% with sustained response after initial rx with combination did not clear HCV RNA until after wk 12 or 24 of rx). Renal disease present in 50% may respond to rx which correlates with disappearance of HCV-RNA *(AJM 106:347, 1999).* Occult HBV infection might account for lack of response to rx in some pts *(NEJM 341:22, 1999).* Rx associated with reduction of hepatocellular carcinoma *(AnIM 131:174, 1999).*
Prevention **Risk factors:** (1) contaminated blood via transfusion (0.001%/ unit in U.S.); (2) injection drug use (in IVDU, prevalence of Hep C 79%); (3) occupation exposure—risk of infection from needlestick from HCV+ source is 1.8%; highest from hollow-bore needles; (4) sexual activity risk low but ♂→♀ > ♀→♂. **Perinatal transmission:** infants born to HCV + mothers have 5–6% risk of infection (when co-infection of HCV + HIV, risk is 14%)		
Herpes Viral Infections (see review: *CID 26:541, 1998)*		
Cytomegalovirus (CMV) **Normal host**	No rx indicated for acute mononucleosis-like syndrome and not established for congenital CMV *(see Comment)*	A study of newborns with symptomatic congenital CMV infection suggests 8 and 12 mg/kg/d of IV ganciclovir has limited efficacy but ↓ platelets and ↓ PMNs common *(JID 175: 1080, 1997).*
Immunocompromised host	Treatment of AIDS patients with highly active antiretroviral therapy (HAART) is effective in suppressing CMV viremia; 16/16 pts became CMV-negative by PCR without specific CMV therapy and none developed retinitis *(AIDS 13:1203, 1999).* See *MMWR 47(RR-19), Oct. 16, 1998.*	
Colitis/esophagitis	**Ganciclovir** as with retinitis except induction period extended for 3–6 wks. No agreement on use of maintenance *(AnIM 158:957, 1998).* Responses less predictable than for retinitis *(AJM 98:109, 1995).* Foscarnet 90 mg/kg q12h effective in 9/10 pts *(AAC 41:1226, 1997).*	
CMV of the nervous system: Encephalitis & ventriculitis	**Ganciclovir**, as *with retinitis.* Consider combination of ganciclovir and foscarnet as suppressive therapy	Treatment not defined, but disease develops while taking ganciclovir as suppressive therapy
Lumbosacral poly-radiculopathy	**Ganciclovir**, as *with retinitis.* Consider combination of ganciclovir and foscarnet if prior CMV rx used.	About 50% will respond *(CID 20:747, 1995).* survival ↑ (5.4 wks to 14.6 wks) *(CID 27:345, 1998).*
Mononeuritis multiplex	Not defined	Due to vasculitis and may not be responsive to antiviral rx *(ArNeurol 29:139, 1991).*
CMV pneumonia—seen predominantly in transplants (esp. bone marrow), rare in HIV	**Ganciclovir** 2.5 mg/kg q8h IV x20 days + IVIG 500 mg/kg qod x10 doses, then ganciclovir 5 mg/kg/d 3–5 x/week for 20 doses + IVIG 500 mg/kg 2x/week x8 more doses *(AnIM 109:777, 1988)*	11/16 pts showed initial improvement with either ganciclovir or foscarnet but disease eventually progressed despite maintenance *(CID 23:76, 1996).* For preventive therapy, *see Table 15, page 116.*

NOTE: All dosage recommendations are for adults (unless otherwise indicated) and assume normal renal function.

TABLE 14 (3)

VIRUS/DISEASE	DRUG/DOSAGE	SIDE EFFECTS/COMMENTS
Herpes Viral Infections/Cytomegalovirus/Immunocompromised host *(continued)*		

Retinitis (most common in AIDS)
 	
19/30 pts (63%) with inactive CMV retinitis who responded to HAART (↑ of ≥60 CD4 cells/ml) developed immune recovery vitreitis (vision ↓ & floaters with posterior segment inflammation— vitreitis, papillitis & macular changes) an average of 43 wks after rx started *(JID 179:697, 1999).*
 	
See *Guidelines of International Panel: AnIM 158: 957, 1998.*
	Induction therapy, primary:
	Ganciclovir (GCV) 5.0 mg/kg IV (at constant rate over 1 hr) q12h x14–21 days
	OR
	Foscarnet (FOS) 90 mg/kg (adjusted for renal function) IV at constant rate (requires infusion pump) over minimum of 1 hr q12h x14–21 days
	OR
	Combination of **intraocular ganciclovir (GCV) implant** (delivers 1–2 μg/hr x6–7 mos.) + (either concomitant IV GCV as above or oral GCV 1.0 gm tid)
	
	Induction therapy, alternative:
	Cidofovir 5 mg/kg IV q week x2 wks with probenecid (2 gm po 3 hrs before cidofovir dose, 1 gm 2 hrs immediately after dose, and 1 gm 8 hrs after dose) and 1 liter of normal saline IV 1 hr before cidofovir infusion *(AnIM 126:257 & 264, 1997)*.
	
	For pts who fail monotherapy with GCV or FOS, consider combination rx with both: (1) GCV 5 mg/kg q12h IV and (2) FOS as either 60 mg/kg q8h or 90 mg/kg q12h
	
	Suppression (maintenance therapy):
	May be indefinite but with immune reconstitution (response to HAART) most authorities now **discontinuing** suppression *(CID 28:534, 1999; JAMA 282:1633, 1999)*.
	Primary:
	GCV 5 mg/kg IV qd or 6 mg/kg IV qd 5 days/week
	OR
	FOS 90–120 mg/kg/day IV with hydration and dose adjusted for renal function (NOTE: oral and IV hydration found equally effective: 1700 ml/day, *Abst 298 from 4th CRV, 1997*)
	Alternative:
	Combination of GCV intraocular implant q6 mos. + oral GCV as under induction therapy
	OR
	Cidofovir 5 mg/kg IV q2 wks + probenecid and hydration (as above under induction rx)
		Comprehensive reviews of many important clinical issues: *J AIDS & HR 14(Suppl. 1), 1997* and *Arch Ophthal 114:863, 1996.* Corticosteroid rx ↓ inflammatory reaction of immune recovery vitreitis without reactivation of CMV retinitis *(5th CRV, Abst. 751).*
		  Differential dx: HIV retinopathy, herpes simplex retinitis *(Arch Ophthal 114:834, 1996)*, varicella-zoster retinitis (rare, hard to diagnose).
		  Cannot use GCV ocular implant alone as approx. 50% risk of CMV retinitis other eye at 6 mos. and 31% risk visceral disease *(Arch Ophthal 12:153, 1994)*. Risk ↓ with systemic rx *(CID 24:620, 1997; NEJM 337:83, 1997)*.
		  Watch for retinal detachments; 50–60% within 1 yr of dx of retinitis.
		  Equal efficacy of IV GCV and FOS. FOS rx takes more time to administer due to saline hydration. GCV avoids nephrotoxicity of FOS; FOS avoids bone marrow suppression of GCV.
		
		Potential emergence of resistant CMV. 27.5% pts treated 9 months developed CMV isolates resistant to GCV *(JID 177:770, 1998)*, hence may be reason for clinical failure. Treatment options: reinduction with same drug IV, switch to 2nd drug, or add (combine) with local rx. Local rx includes GCV implants or experimental intravitreal rx: (1) GCV 2x/wk or q wk *(CID 23:76, 1996)*; (2) FOS q wk or less often *(Am J Ophth 114:742, 1992)*; (3) cidofovir 20 μg q6 wks *(AnIM 125:98, 1996)*.

EBV—Mononucleosis See *JAMA 281:454, 1999*	No treatment. Corticosteroids for tonsillar obstruction of airway or CNS complications.	Acyclovir and prednisolone inhibited oropharyngeal EBV replication but did not affect duration of symptoms *(JID 174:324, 1996)*.
HHV-6—[implicated as cause of roseola (exanthem subitem) in childhood. Fever & rash documented in transplant pts but association with pneumonitis & prolonged bone marrow suppression questionable *(JID 179:311, 1999)*. In 1 series, 5 BMT pts with encephalitic picture had HHV-6 isolated from CSF *(CID 28:563, 1999)*.	No rx. Foscarnet active in vitro. 3/4 BMT pts with CNS symptoms & HHV-6 DNA in CSF responded to foscarnet (60 mg/kg IV 3x/d).	Role of rx or prophylaxis currently uncertain. Dx depends on separating latent virus from active infection. The rapid shell vial assay, serum PCR assay or immunohistochemical stain for viral proteins may be of value *(AnIM 124:1065, 1996)*. Rx with acyclovir or IVIG did not lower HHV-6 DNA levels in BMT pts *(JID 179:311, 1999)*.
HHV-7—a ubiquitous virus (probably >85% of the population is infected). Appears to infect CD4 lymphocytes via CD4 receptor, is probably transmitted via saliva and its role in human disease has not been clearly elucidated (some cases of exanthem subitem and other febrile illnesses of childhood have been associated with HHV-7).	No antiviral treatment currently recommended. Effective anti-HIV rx may help.	No rx. *(Ln 349:558, 1997; AnIM 127:48, 1997)*.
HHV-8 (probable agent of Kaposi's sarcoma and body cavity lymphoma)—may cause interstitial pneumonia *(NEJM 335:351, 1996)*. Isolated from nasal secretions and saliva *(JID 177:213, 1998)*.	Localized lesions; radiotherapy, laser surgery or intralesional chemotherapy. Systemic: chemotherapy. Anecdotal report of remission in 5 pts given foscarnet 80 mg/kg/d *(Scand J Inf Dis 26: 749, 1994)*. Also, less KS in pts given foscarnet for CMV and associated with ↓ KS in retrospective analysis *(Sci 267:1078, 1995)*. One report implicates HHV-8's association with multiple myeloma *(Science 276:851, 1997)*, another with Castleman's disease *(CID 28:678, 1999)*.	

NOTE: All dosage recommendations are for adults (unless otherwise indicated) and assume normal renal function.

TABLE 14 (4)

VIRUS/DISEASE	DRUG/DOSAGE	SIDE EFFECTS/COMMENTS
Herpes simplex (Types 1 & 2)		
Bell's palsy (May also be caused by H. zoster, Lyme disease)	No rx or [Acyclovir (400 mg po 5x/d for 10 days)] with or without [prednisone po (30 mg bid or 1 mg/kg daily dose given bid x5 d, then taper to 5 mg bid dc after total of 10 days)]	HSV-1 genomes were detected in 11/14 pts in facial nerves by PCR (AnIM 124:27, 1996). In one study, 99 pts with symptoms <3 days had better recovery and less neural degeneration when rx with acyclovir + prednisone compared to prednisone alone (Ann Oto/Rhino/Laryngol 105: 371, 1996).
Encephalitis (Excellent reviews: CID 23:219, 1996; 25:89, 1997))	**Acyclovir** IV 10 mg/kg IV (infuse over 1 hr) q8h x14–21 days	HSV-1 is most common cause of sporadic encephalitis. Survival and recovery from neurological sequelae are related to mental status at time of initiation of rx. **Early dx and rx imperative.** Mortality rate reduced from >70% to 19% with acyclovir rx. PCR analysis of CSF for HSV-1 DNA is 100% specific and 75–98% sensitive. CSF IgG Ab usually appears late (>1st week). Dose: Up to 20 mg/kg q8h in children <12 yrs.
Genital, immunocompetent		
Primary See excellent review: CID 28(Suppl.1):S4, 1999	**Acyclovir** (Zovirax or generic) 400 mg po tid x10 days (FDA-approved dosage is 200 mg 5x/d po x10 days) (Cost: NB 200 mg $1.14; 400 mg $2.21; G 200 mg $0.34) OR **Valacyclovir** (Valtrex) 1000 mg po bid x10 days (Cost: 1.0 gm $3.31) OR **Famciclovir** (Famvir) 250 mg po tid x5–10 days (not FDA-approved for this indication) (Cost: 250 mg $3.18)	Increases rate of healing but does not prevent recurrences. Metabolized to penciclovir, which is active component. Side effects and activity similar to acyclovir. Found to be equal to acyclovir (200 mg 5x/d) tid (ICAAC Abst. H8, 1995). An ester of acyclovir which is well absorbed, bioavailability 3–5x greater than acyclovir. Found to be equal to acyclovir (Sex Trans Dis 24:481, 1997).
Recurrent	Acyclovir 400 mg po tid x5 days or famciclovir 125 mg po bid x3–5 days or valacyclovir 500 mg po bid x5 days	All effective with few differences. Choice can be made on basis of cost & convenience (Arch IM 156:1729, 1996; JAMA 276:44, 1996; Genitourin Med 73:110, 1997). 3 days rx = 5 d. for vala.
Chronic suppression	Acyclovir 400 mg po bid [cost/yr $1387 (JAMA 280:928, 1998)], famciclovir 250 mg po bid ($2321), valacyclovir 250 mg po bid or 500 mg po qd ($1055) or 1000 mg po qd ($1329) [some use if >10 recurrences/yr, others fewer (JID 778:603, 1998)]. Decision to rx arbitrary.	All suppress subclinical HSV-2 shedding between episodes and ↓ symptomatic recurrences (AnIM 124:8, 1996; JCI 99:1092, 1997; JAMA 280:887, 1998). Drug resistance unlikely to develop with ↑ use (Nature Med 4:673, 1998). Since in a large natural hx study 2/3 of pts demonstrated ↓ in recurrences between yrs 1 & 5 (approx. median 6 to 3 episodes/yr), daily suppressive rx should be reassessed periodically and after 3–5 yrs episodic rx may become more practical (AnIM 131:14, 1999).
Gingivostomatitis, primary (children)	Acyclovir 15 mg/kg po 5x/d x7 d. [Efficacy demonstrated in randomized double-blind placebo-controlled trial (BMJ 315:1800, 1992]	
Kerato-conjunctivitis and recurrent epithelial keratitis	Trifluridine (Viroptic), 1 drop 1% solution q2h (max. 9 drops/d.) for max. of 21 days (see Table 1, page 9)	In controlled trials, response % > idoxuridine. Suppressive rx with acyclovir (400 mg bid) reduced recurrences of ocular HSV from 32% to 19% over 12-month period (NEJM 339:300, 1998).
Mucocutaneous		
Oral labial, "fever blisters"		
Normal host	Rx usually not indicated; however, some use (1) penciclovir 1% cream applied q2h while awake for 4 d. or (2) acyclovir topical formulation applied q2h as above (see Comment)	Penciclovir given topically ↓ duration of pain (3.4 vs 4.1 days) (JAMA 277:1374, 1997). Some pts with severe blisters associated with other infections (e.g., pneumococcal sepsis) may benefit from acyclovir 400 mg po tid x5 days (reduces viral shedding and ↓ healing time). Oral famciclovir ↓ maximal lesion size and days to healing in a dose-dependent fashion (125, 250, or 500 mg 3x/d. for 5 d.) when started 48 hrs after experimental ultraviolet radiation-induced herpes labialis. The 500 mg dosage ↓ healing time from 6 to 4 days mean (p < 0.01) (JID 179:303, 1999).
Herpes Whitlow	See Table 7, page 79	

NOTE: All dosage recommendations are for adults (unless otherwise indicated) and assume normal renal function.

TABLE 14 (5)

VIRUS/DISEASE	DRUG/DOSAGE	SIDE EFFECTS/COMMENTS
Herpes Viral Infections/Herpes simplex (Types 1 & 2)/Oral labial, "fever blisters" *(continued)*		
Immunocompromised (includes pts with AIDS)	**Acyclovir** 5.0 mg/kg IV (infused over 1 hr) q8h x7 d. (250 mg/M²) or 400 mg po bid x14–21 d. *(see Comment if suspect acyclovir-resistant).* or Famciclovir 500 mg po bid x7 d. *(not FDA-approved for this indication)* or Valacyclovir 1 gm po 3x/d. x7 d. *(not FDA-approved for this indication)*	Acyclovir-resistant HSV occurs, esp. in large ulcers. Most will respond to **IV foscarnet**, but recur after drug discontinued [median 6 weeks *(NEJM 325:551, 1991)*]. Topical 1% ophthalmic trifluridine q8h gave modest response *(J Acq Immunodef Syn & Human Retrovir 12:147, 1996).* Cidofovir gel effective in 50% of pts (30% healed) with acyclovir-unresponsive ulcers *(JID 176:892, 1997).* Suppressive rx with famciclovir (500 mg po bid) reduced viral shedding and clinical recurrences (total days with lesions 18% vs 5%) in HIV-infected pts *(AnIM 128:21, 1998),* similar to findings with acyclovir. IV penciclovir *(investigational)* (5 mg/kg q12h) was equivalent to IV acyclovir q8h *(AAC 43:1192, 1999).*
Perinatal (genital in pregnancy at delivery)		In 25% HSV reactivated in last month of pregnancy. Infant exposure during vaginal delivery: primary lesion 50% risk, if recurrent lesion 4%. 50% mortality in infected neonates. If visible genital lesion, deliver by **C-section,** regardless of duration of membrane rupture. If no lesions or symptoms, vaginal delivery. Routine HSV cultures no longer recommended. Preliminary trials suggest acyclovir may be useful in dose of 10 mg/kg (20 mg/kg if premature) q8h x10–21 days IV *(PIDJ 14:827, 1995; NEJM 337:509, 1997).*
Herpes simiae—Monkey bite (Herpes B virus)	**Acyclovir** 12 mg/kg IV q8h or ganciclovir 5 mg/kg IV q12h until symptoms improve or resolve, then acyclovir 800 mg po 5x/d for prolonged duration. (Prompt rx may limit infection to 1° site.)	*CID 20:421, 1995.* Fatal human cases of myelitis and hemorrhagic encephalitis have been reported following bites, scratches, or eye inoculation of saliva from monkeys. Initial sx include fever, headache, myalgias and diffuse adenopathy, incubation period of 2–14 days.
Herpes zoster/Varicella—CDC Recommendations for Prevention: Since <5% of cases of varicella but >50% of varicella-related deaths occur in adults >20 yrs of age, the CDC recommends a more aggressive approach in this age group: **1st, varicella-zoster immune globulin** (VZIG) is recommended for post-exposure prophylaxis in susceptible persons at greater risk for complications (immunocompromised adults such as HIV, malignancies and steroid rx) as soon as possible after exposure (<96 hrs). If varicella develops, initiate rx quickly (<24 hrs of rash) with **acyclovir** as below. **2nd,** susceptible adults should be vaccinated. Check antibody in adults with negative or uncertain hx of varicella (10–30% will be Ab-neg.) and vaccinate those who are Ab-neg. **3rd,** susceptible children should receive vaccination. Recommended routinely before age 12–18 mos. but OK at any age *(MMWR 4:410, 19 May 1997).* Varicella is the leading cause of vaccine-preventable deaths in children in the U.S. *(MMWR 47:365, 1998).*		
Varicella		
Normal host (chickenpox)		
Child (2–12 years)	Rx not recommended by AAP. Oral acyclovir for healthy persons at ↑ risk for moderate to severe varicella, i.e., >12 yrs of age; chronic cutaneous or pulmonary diseases; chronic salicylate rx (↑ risk of Reye syndrome). Use **acyclovir 20 mg/kg** po qid x5 days (start within 24 hrs of rash).	Modest response to acyclovir. Slowed development or ↓ number of new lesions. Analgesic requirements decreased *(J Ped 116:633, 1990; NEJM 325:1539, 1991).* Oral dose of acyclovir in children should not exceed 80 mg/kg/d or 3200 mg/d *(1997 Red Book, Am Acad Ped).*
Adolescents, young adults	**Acyclovir** 800 mg po 5x/d x5–7 days (start within 24 hrs of rash). Valacyclovir 1000 mg po 3x/d. x5 d. or famciclovir 500 mg po 3x/d. also probably effective but not FDA-approved for this indication and data lacking *(AnIM 130:922, 1999).*	↓ duration of fever, time to healing, and symptoms *(AnIM 117:358, 1992).*
Pneumonia or pregnancy in 3rd trimester	**Acyclovir** 800 mg po 5x/d or 10 mg/kg IV q8h x5 days. Risks and benefits to fetus and mother still unknown. Many experts recommend rx, especially in 3rd trimester.	Varicella pneumonia severe in pregnancy (41% mortality. *ObGyn 25:734, 1965)* and acyclovir → incidence and severity. If varicella-susceptible mother exposed, then respiratory symptoms develop within 10 days after exposure, start acyclovir *(CCTID 13:123, 1993).* Acyclovir is pregnancy category B; no evidence of ↑ birth defects *(MMWR 42:806, 1993).*
Immunocompromised host	**Acyclovir** 10–12 mg/kg IV (infused over 1 hr) q8h x7 days (500 mg/M²)	Continuous infusion of high-dose acyclovir (2 mg/kg/hr) was used successfully in 1 pt with severe hemorrhagic varicella *(NEJM 336:732, 1997).*

NOTE: All dosage recommendations are for adults (unless otherwise indicated) and assume normal renal function.

TABLE 14 (6)

VIRUS/DISEASE	DRUG/DOSAGE	SIDE EFFECTS/COMMENTS
Herpes Viral Infections (continued)		
Herpes zoster		
Normal host (See *IDCP 4:293, 1995* for excellent review) [NOTE: Trials showing benefit of rx: only pts treated within 3 days of onset of rash] (For rx of post-herpetic neuralgia, see *NEJM 335:32, 1996; ArIM 157:1166, 1997; JID 178:581, 1998; Ln 353:1636, 1999*).	**Valacyclovir** (Valtrex) 1000 mg po tid x7 days or	Valacyclovir ↓ post-herpetic neuralgia more rapidly than acyclovir in pts >50 yrs of age: median duration of zoster-associated pain was 38 days with valacyclovir and 51 days on acyclovir (*AAC 39:1546, 1995*). toxicity of both drugs similar.
	Famciclovir (Famvir) 500 mg po q8h x7 days or	Time to healing more rapid. Reduced post-herpetic neuralgia (PHN) vs placebo in pts >50 yrs of age: duration of PHN with famciclovir 63 days, placebo 163 days. Famciclovir similar to acyclovir in reduction of acute pain and PHN (*Int J Antimicrob Agents 4:241, 1994; AnIM 123:89, 1995*).
	Acyclovir 800 mg po 5x/d x7–10 days [Prednisone po 30 mg bid days 1–7, 15 mg bid days 8–14 and 7.5 mg bid days 15–21 also recommended by some authorities in pts >50 yrs of age (*NEJM 335:32, 1996*)] and especially when pt has large number of lesions (>21 and/or severe pain at presentation (*JID 179:9, 1999*).	A meta-analysis of 4 placebo-controlled trials (691 pts) demonstrated that acyclovir accelerated by approx. 2-fold pain resolution at all measures employed and reduced post-herpetic neuralgia at 3 & 6 mos (*CID 22:341, 1996*). Prednisone added to acyclovir improved quality of life measurements (↓ acute pain, sleep, and return to normal activity) (*AnIM 125:376, 1996*). In post-herpetic neuralgia, antidepressant (amitriptyline, desipramine) ↓ pain (*Ann Neurol 35:550, 1994*).
Immunocompromised host		
Not severe	**Acyclovir** 800 mg po 5x/d x7 days (famciclovir and valacyclovir not FDA-approved for this indication)	If progression, switch to IV
Severe: >1 dermatome, trigeminal nerve or disseminated	Acyclovir 10–12 mg/kg IV (infusion over 1 hr) q8h x7–14 days. In older pts, ↓ to 7.5 mg/kg. If nephrotoxicity and pt improving, ↓ to 5.0 mg/kg q8h.	Rx must be begun within 72 hrs. Acyclovir-resistant VZV occurs in HIV + pts previously treated with acyclovir. **Foscarnet** (40 mg/kg IV q8h for 14–26 days) successful in 4/5 pts but 2 relapsed in 7 and 14 days (*AnIM 115:19, 1991*).
Influenza (A & B) (*JID 178:53, 1998; Ln 354:1277, 1999*)	If fever, cough, myalgia; known community influenza activity; and 1st 48 hrs of illness, consider:	Pts with COPD or asthma, potential risk of bronchospasm with zanamivir. If using inhaled bronchodilator, use before dose of zanamivir. Both zanamivir & oseltamivir are neuraminidase inhibitors effective against influenza A & B and are equally effective as amantadine & rimantadine against influenza A, all reduce duration of symptoms by approx. 50% (1.5–3 days) if given within 30–36 hrs after onset of symptoms (*Med Lett 41:91, 1999; JAMA 282:1240, 1999*).
Suspect or proven acute disease	**For influenza A & B: zanamivir** 2 inhalations (2x5 mg) bid x5 d. 2 doses on day 1 if at least 2 hrs apart (*JID 180:254, 1999*) or **Oseltamivir** 75 mg po bid x5 d. For efficacy, start within 48 hrs of onset of symptoms	**For influenza A only: Rimantadine or amantadine: age 1–9 yrs, 5 mg/kg/d to max. of 75 mg po bid: 10–65 yrs, 100 mg po bid: >65 yrs, 100 mg po qd (adjust for ↓ renal function)**
Prevention (*MMWR 48:RR-4, 1999*)	Annual immunization	If high-risk non-immunized pt during influenza disease activity, give vaccine & then either Zanamivir (see Comment) or rimantadine x4 wks. Zanamivir dose: 2 inhalations 1x/day; oseltamivir 75 mg qd	Neither oseltamivir nor zanamivir FDA-approved for prevention but reported efficacious in clinical trials (*JAMA 282:31 & 75, 1999; NEJM 341:1336 & 1387, 1999*).
Measles		
Children	No therapy or vitamin A 200,000 u po x2 days	Vitamin A ↓ severity of measles in one study (*NEJM 323:160, 1990*), not in others.
Adults	No rx or ribavirin IV (!) 20–35 mg/kg/d x7 days	↓ severity of illness in adults (*CID 20:454, 1994*).

NOTE: All dosage recommendations are for adults (unless otherwise indicated) and assume normal renal function.

TABLE 14 (7)

VIRUS/DISEASE	DRUG/DOSAGE	SIDE EFFECTS/COMMENTS
Papillomaviruses		
Anogenital Warts: Condyloma acuminatum [*See CID 28(Suppl.1):S37, 1999*] [NOTE: Results of Pap smear should be available prior to rx; **avoid rx in pregnant women**] *NOTE: Recurrences common after all treatments*	*See CID 27:796, 1998, for consensus statement:* [**Podofilox** (Condylox) 2x daily application with cotton swab for 3 days followed by 4 days without rx; repeat cycle 4-6x as necessary] or [25% **podophyllin** in tincture of benzoin (Podocon-25): apply once weekly for up to 6 wks, wash after 1-4 hrs.] If no regression after 4 weekly applications, use alternate rx. Interferon alfa-2b (Intron a); alfa-n3 (Alferon N): 1 million units (0.1 ml) into lesion 3x/week x3 weeks Cryotherapy or electrosurgery	Podofilox: Local reactions—pain, burning, inflammation in 50%. No systemic effects. Efficacy in penile warts 74% vs placebo 8%. Recurrences 55% vs 100% with placebo. (Podocon-25 15 ml $32.40, Condylox 3.5 ml $56.64.) Warts recur in ⅓ with either agent within 1st month after rx. Painful; dilute to 10 million units/1.0 ml. Other concentrations are hypertonic *(CID 28:S537, 1999)*. Use when other rx fails, esp. in AIDS.
	Imiquimod (5% cream). Apply 3x/week prior to sleep; remove 6-10 hrs later when awake. Continue until cleared or max. of 16 wks.	When applied 3x/wk overnight for up to 16 wks or until warts completely cured, produced clearance rates of 52% vs 14% for controls *(AAC 42:789, 1998)*. Cost of 1-4 wks rx: $108-432. Imiquimod: Local reactions—mild erythema 60%, erosion 30% *[AJM 102(5A):34, 1997]*.
Parvo B19 Virus Uncomplicated or self-limited acute arthritis. May be chronic in children.	No treatment recommended	Bone marrow shows selective erythrocyte maturation arrest with giant pronormoblasts. IgM antibody available for diagnosis: Specialty Labs, Santa Monica, CA. Parvo B19 also associated with respiratory distress syndrome *(CID 27:900, 1998)* and myocarditis/myocardiopathy *(CID 28:1343, 1999)*.
Acute profound anemia: in utero, in hemolytic anemia, in HIV.	IVIG 0.4 gm/kg IV qd x5 d in immune def. states with severe anemia has been reported	IVIG contains anti-parvo B19 antibody. In pts with pre-existing hemolytic anemia, parvo B19-induced bone marrow arrest can result in sudden severe anemia. *See Am J Hematol 61:16, 1999 for new suggestions on management.*
Papovavirus/Polyoma Virus **Progressive multifocal leuco-encephalopathy** (PML)(JC virus) Usually in pts with advanced HIV disease	*See SANFORD GUIDE TO HIV/AIDS THERAPY.* HAART ↑ survival (545 d. vs 60 d., p < 0.001) and either improved (50%) or stabilized (50%) neurological deficits in 12 pts *(AIDS 12:2467, 1999)*. Others less optimistic *(CID 28:1152, 1999)*.	Cytarabine of no value in controlled trial *(NEJM 338:1345, 1998)*. Camptothecin, a human topoisomerase I inhibitor, was administered to a single pt with slowing of progression *(Ln 349:1366, 1997)*.
Respiratory Syncytial Virus Major cause of morbidity in neonates/infants *(JID 180:41, 1999)*. ↑ recognition in adults: 2–9% of pts >65 yrs of age with pneumonia requiring hospitalization are due to RSV *(JID 179:25, 1999)*.	Rapid dx by antigen detection on nasopharyngeal wash. **No rx controversial!** or ribavirin (Virazole) rx 1.1 gm/d. by aerosol. **Use controversial!** Consider use in pts at high risk for complications (congenital heart disease, cystic fibrosis, premature infants, immunodeficiencies) or severely ill (PO₂ <65 mmHg)—can't make recommendation.	Ribavirin reported to ↓ fever and other symptoms and signs. However, in a retrospective case controlled study of children on mechanical ventilators for severe RSV & in a prospective placebo-controlled trial of otherwise normal children, **ribavirin had no beneficial effect** and was associated with prolonged time on the ventilator *(J Ped 128:422, 1996; AJRCCM 160:829, 1999)*. Drug complications include anemia, rash & conjunctivitis. (6 gm vial $319.85). *See Table 14B, page 108 for use of RSV immunoglobulin to prevent RSV in infants and children.*
Prevention (1) Children <24 mos. old with bronchopulmonary dysplasia (BPD) requiring supplemental O₂ (2) Perhaps premature infants (<32 wks gestation) and <6 mos. old at start of RSV season	**Read important footnote[1]** **RSV immune globulin intravenous** (RSV-IGIV) 750 mg/kg IV once monthly Nov.-through April (for northern hemisphere) 1st year of life for prematures. Perhaps up to 60 months of age for pts with BPD OR **Palivizumab** 15 mg/kg IM q month Nov.-April as above.	RSV-IVIG very expensive—estimated cost per infusion $1,175. See consensus opinion for details: *Ped Inf Dis J 15:1059, 1996. See Ln 354:847, 1999 for updated review.* Palivizumab reduced hospitalization rates for RSV in 1500 premature infants & children with chronic lung disease from 10.6% to 4.8% *(Pediatrics 102:531, 1998)*.

[1] Dilute to 20 mg/ml, deliver as small particle aerosol by O₂ mask over 12-18 hours/day for at least 3, no more than 7 days. Use with extreme caution in patients requiring mechanical ventilation (crystals precipitate with valve failure, avoidable with frequent cleaning). **Ribavirin is teratogenic in animals,** contraindicated in pregnancy. Potential inhalation exposure of pregnant health care workers is at or above permissible limits *(PIDJ 12:2, 1993)*.

NOTE: All dosage recommendations are for adults (unless otherwise indicated) and assume normal renal function.

TABLE 14 (8)

VIRUS/DISEASE	DRUG/DOSAGE	SIDE EFFECTS/COMMENTS
Rhinovirus (Colds)	No antiviral rx indicated. Symptomatic rx (studied): • ipratropium bromide nasal spray (2/nostril tid q4d) • clemastine fumarate (1.34 mg tab) 1 tab po bid q4d	Ipratropium nasal spray reduced rhinorrhea and sneezing vs placebo (AnIM 125:89, 1996). Clemastine (an antihistamine) reduced sneezing, rhinorrhea and nasal secretions but was associated with dry nose, mouth and throat in 6–19% (CID 22:656, 1996). Zinc gluconate lozenges (1 lozenge q2h when awake for duration of symptoms) also reduced symptoms vs placebo (AnIM 125:81, 1996). Products vary in Zn ion availability; see JAC 40:483, 1997.
Transfusion Transmitted Virus (TTV)	None—not proven to be associated with human disease but common in U.S. volunteer blood donors (10%) and IV drug abusers (17%) (JID 179:1242, 1999).	

TABLE 14B: ANTIVIRAL DRUGS (Other Than Retroviral)

DRUG NAME(S) GENERIC (TRADE)	DOSAGE/ROUTE/COST*	COMMENTS/ADVERSE EFFECTS
CMV (See SANFORD GUIDE TO HIV/AIDS THERAPY)		
Cidofovir (Vistide)	5 mg/kg IV qweek x2, then q2 weeks. (375 mg $727) Properly timed IV prehydration with normal saline and oral probenecid **must be used with each cidofovir infusion** (see pkg insert for details). Renal function (serum creatinine and urine protein) must be monitored prior to each dose (see pkg insert for details).	**Adverse effects: Nephrotoxicity:** dose-dependent proximal tubular injury (Fanconi-like syndrome): proteinuria, glycosuria, bicarbonaturia, phosphaturia, polyuria (nephrogenic diabetic insipidus now reported. Ln 350:413, 1997.) ↑ creatinine. Concomitant saline prehydration, probenecid, extended dosing intervals allowed use. Other toxicities: nausea 48%, fever 31%, alopecia 16%, myalgia 16%, probenecid hypersensitivity 16%, neutropenia 29%. No effect on hematocrit, platelets, LFTs. 25% of pts dc IV cidofovir due to toxicity. **Comment:** Recommended dosage, frequency or infusion rate of cidofovir must not be exceeded. Dose must be reduced or discontinued if changes in renal function occur during rx. For ↑ of 0.3–0.4 mg/dl in serum creatinine, cidofovir dose must be ↓ from 5 to 3 mg/kg; discontinue cidofovir if ↑ to 0.5 mg/dl above baseline or 3+ proteinuria develops (for 2+ proteinuria, observe pts carefully and consider discontinuation).
Cidofovir gel (Forvade)		Available for topical rx of acyclovir-resistant mucocutaneous HSV in AIDS pts through "expanded access" from Gilead, 1-800-GILEAD5.
Fomivirsen (Vitravene)	330 µg by direct intravitreal injection q2 wks x2, then q month	This is an antisense drug approved for local treatment of CMV retinitis in AIDS pts who are intolerant of, have a contraindication to or are unresponsive to other treatments for CMV. It inhibits production of proteins responsible for regulation of viral gene expression essential for virulence. Toxicity includes ocular inflammation (uveitis), iritis and vitreitis, ↑ intraocular pressure, abnormal vision, anterior chamber inflammation and cataracts. Do not give if pt had received IV or intravitreal cidofovir (Vistide) within last 2–4 wks; may exaggerate ocular inflammation (Priority Pharmacy 3, #8, Oct. 30, 1998).
Foscarnet (Foscavir)	60 mg/kg q8h IV (6 gm $3.27)	**Adverse effects: Major clinical toxicity is renal impairment (⅓ of patients)**— ↑ creatinine, proteinuria, nephrogenic diabetes insipidus. ↓ Ca++, ↓ Ca++, ↓ Mg++. Toxicity ↑ with other nephrotoxic drugs [amphotericin B, aminoglycosides or pentamidine (especially severe ↓ Ca++)]. Adequate hydration may ↓ toxicity. Other: headache, mild (100%); fatigue (100%); nausea (80%), fever (25%). CNS: seizures. Hematol.: ↓ WBC, ↓ Hgb. Hepatic: liver function tests ↑. Neuropathy. Penile ulcers.
Ganciclovir (Cytovene)	IV: 5 mg/kg q12h x14 days (induction) 5 mg/kg IV qd or 6 mg/kg 5x/wk (suspension) (500 mg IV $34.80)	**Adverse effects:** Granulocytopenia 25%, thrombocytopenia 25%, thrombocytopenia 21%, anemia 6% Fever 48%, GI 50%: nausea, vomiting, diarrhea, abdominal pain 19%, rash 10%. Retinal detachment 11% (relationship to ganciclovir ?). Confusion, headache, psychiatric disturbances and seizures. Neutropenia may respond to granulocyte colony stimulating factor (G-CSF or GM-CSF). Severe myelosuppression may be ↑ with coadministration of zidovudine or azathioprine. **Comment:** Drug should be reconstituted immediately before use and unused portion discarded. Reconstituted solution should not be refrigerated.
	Oral: 1.0 gm tid with food (fatty meal) (250 mg cap $3.90)	**Adverse effects:** Hematologic less frequent than with IV. Granulocytopenia 18%, anemia 12%, thrombocytopenia 6%. GI, skin same as with IV. Retinal detachment 8%.
	Intraocular implant (~$4000/device + cost of surgery)	**Adverse effects:** Late retinal detachment (7/30 eyes). Does not prevent CMV retinitis in good eye or visceral dissemination. **Comment:** Replacement every 6 months recommended.

NOTE: All dosage recommendations are for adults (unless otherwise indicated) and assume normal renal function.
* From Oct. 1998 Hospital Formulary Pricing Guide. Price is average wholesale price (AWP). NB = name brand, G = generic, DC = discontinue

TABLE 14B(2)

DRUG NAME(S) GENERIC (TRADE)	DOSAGE/ROUTE/COST*	COMMENTS/ADVERSE EFFECTS
Herpesvirus (non-CMV)		
Acyclovir (Zovirax or generic)	Zovirax: 200 mg po tab $1.14 400 mg po tab $2.22 800 mg po tab $4.31 500 mg IV $59.51 G: 200 mg po tab $0.34	**po:** Generally well-tolerated with occ. diarrhea, vertigo, fatigue, arthralgia. Less frequent rash, fatigue, insomnia, fever, menstrual abnormalities, acne, sore throat, muscle cramps, lymphadenopathy. CNS (1%): lethargy, tremors, confusion, hallucinations, delirium, seizures, coma *(CID 21:435, 1995)*. Renal (5%): ↑ creatinine, hematuria. With high doses may crystalize in renal tubules → **IV:** Phlebitis, caustic with vesicular lesions with IV infiltration, CNS (1%): obstructive uropathy (rapid infusion, dehydration, renal insufficiency and ↑ dose ↑ risk). Hepatic: ↑ ALT, AST. Uncommon: neutropenia *(CID 20: 1557, 1995)*, rash, diaphoresis, hypotension, headache, nausea.
Famciclovir (Famvir)	250 mg po cap $3.18 500 mg po cap $6.39	Metabolized to penciclovir. Side-effects similar to acyclovir, included headache, nausea, diarrhea, and dizziness but incidence did not differ from placebo *(JAMA 276:47, 1996)*. May be taken without regard to meals.
Penciclovir (Denavir)	Topical 1% cream: apply to area of recurrence of herpes labialis with start of sx then q2h x4 d.	Adverse effects: Well tolerated.
Trifluridine (Viroptic)	1 drop 1% solution q2h (max. 9 drops/d.) for max. of 21 d. (7.5 ml 1% solution $66.66)	Mild burning (5%), palpebral edema (3%), punctate keratopathy, stromal edema
Valacyclovir (Valtrex)	500 mg cap $2.82	An ester of acyclovir that is well-absorbed, bioavailability 3–5x greater than acyclovir. Side-effects similar to acyclovir. Thrombotic thrombocytopenic purpura/hemolytic uremic syndrome reported in pts with advanced HIV disease and transplant recipients participating in clinical trials of valacyclovir at doses of 8 gm/day, no reports at approved doses.
Hepatitis		
Interferon alfa is available as alfa-2a (Roferon-A), alfa-2b (Intron-A)	3 million units: Roferon $33.94, Intron $33.92; Infergen 9 µg $37.00	**Adverse effects (IV dosage):** Flu-like syndrome is common, esp. during 1st week of rx: fever 98%, fatigue 89%, myalgia 73%, headache 71%. GI: anorexia 46%, diarrhea 29%. CNS: dizziness 21%. Rash 18%, later profound fatigue & psychiatric symptoms (depression, anxiety, emotional lability and agitation), alopecia, ↑ TSH, autoimmune thyroid disorders with hypo- or hyperthyroidism. Hematol.: ↓ WBC 49%, ↓ Hgb 27%, ↓ platelets 35%. Acute reversible hearing loss and/or tinnitus in up to ⅓ *(Ln 343:1134, 1994)*. Side-effects ↑ with ↑ doses and dose reduction necessary in up to 46% receiving chronic rx for HSV.
Lamivudine (3TC) (Epivir & Epivir-HBV)	Side-effects: See Table 14D, page 111. NOTE: Available as 150 mg for HIV and 100 mg for hepatitis B.	
Ribavirin-Interferon alfa-2b combination (Rebetron)	Ribavirin (Rebetol) 200 mg capsules, adult dose: 400 mg am + 600 mg pm (<75 kg body weight) or 600 mg bid (>75 kg body weight) + Interferon (Intron A), adult dose: 3 m,u (1 vial) tiw subcutaneous. Rebetron cost with 1000 mg/d. ribavirin is $7,819 for 24-wk supply (according to wholesale price in Drugs Topics Red Book Update, May 1999).	Side-effects common with flu-like symptoms (>50%), see *interferon alfa above*. Hemolytic anemia common (mean reduction in Hgb 3 gm/dl) but usually responds to ↓ ribavirin dosage (see package insert). Severe psychiatric effects, esp. depression, most common (23–36%) reason for discontinuation of rx. Suicidal behavior reported. Hyper- and hypothyroidism, alopecia (30%) and pulmonary disease reported *(Mayo Clin Proc 74:367, 1999)*. **Since ribavirin is teratogenic, drug must not be used during pregnancy or within 6 months of pregnancy.** Dose changes:<table><tr><td></td><td>Ribavirin</td><td>Interferon</td></tr><tr><td>Hgb: <10</td><td>↓ to 200 mg a.m., 400 mg p.m.</td><td>No change</td></tr><tr><td><8.5</td><td>DC</td><td>DC</td></tr><tr><td>WBC <1500</td><td>No change</td><td>↓ to 1.5 mIU sc 3x/wk</td></tr><tr><td><1000</td><td>DC</td><td>DC</td></tr><tr><td>Abs. PMNs <750</td><td>No change</td><td>↓ to 1.5 mIU sc 3x/wk</td></tr><tr><td><500</td><td>DC</td><td>DC</td></tr><tr><td>Platelets: <50,000</td><td>No change</td><td>↓ to 1.5 mIU sc 3x/wk</td></tr><tr><td><25,000</td><td>DC</td><td>DC</td></tr></table>Response of immune complex renal disease: *AJM 106:347, 1999*.

NOTE: All dosage recommendations are for adults (unless otherwise indicated) and assume normal renal function.
* From Oct. 1998 Hospital Formulary Pricing Guide. Price is average wholesale price (AWP). NB = name brand, G = generic, DC = discontinue

TABLE 14B(3)

DRUG NAME(S) GENERIC (TRADE)	DOSAGE/ROUTE/COST*	COMMENTS/ADVERSE EFFECTS
Influenza A **Amantadine (Symmetrel, Intuition) or Rimantadine (Flumadine HCI)**	Amantadine and rimantadine doses are the same (rimantadine approved only for prophylaxis in children, not treatment). Adult dose: 100 mg bid. Amantadine 100 mg of syrup $1.81 Rimantadine 100 mg tab $1.61	**Side-effects/toxicity:** CNS (nervousness, anxiety, difficulty concentrating, and lightheadedness). Symptoms occurred in 6% on rimantadine vs 14% on amantadine. They usually ↓ after 1st week and disappear when drug dc. GI (nausea, anorexia). Some serious side-effects—delirium, hallucinations, and seizures—are associated with high plasma drug levels resulting from renal insufficiency, esp. in older pts, those with prior seizure disorders, or psychiatric disorders. In pts with impaired renal function, dosage of both drugs should be reduced (amantadine: creatinine clearance <50 ml/min, rimantadine: CrCl <10 ml/min); *see package inserts and Table 17, pages 124 & 125*. Both drugs teratogenic in animals and contraindicated during pregnancy *(Med Lett 39:72, 1997)*.
Influenza A and B—For both drugs, initiate within 48 hrs of symptom onset		
Zanamivir (Relenza) For pts ≥12 yrs of age	2 inhalations (2 x 5 mg) bid x5 d—initiate within 48 hrs of symptoms. Powder is inhaled using specially designed breath-activated device. Each medication-containing blister contains 5 mg of zanamivir. $44.40 for 5 days rx	Active by inhalation against neuraminidase of both influenza A and B and inhibits release of virus from epithelial cells of respiratory tract. Approx. 4–17% of inhaled dose absorbed into plasma. Excreted by kidney but with low absorption, dose reduction not necessary in renal impairment. Minimal side-effects: <3% cough, sinusitis, diarrhea, nausea and vomiting.
Oseltamivir (Tamiflu)	75 mg po bid x5 d. Cost: 10 capsules $53.00	Well absorbed from GI tract as ethyl ester of active compound GS 4071. Bioavailability after activation by gut & liver 80%. T½ 6–10 hrs; excreted unchanged by kidney. Adverse effects in 15% include nausea, vomiting, headache. Nausea ↓ with food.
Respiratory Syncytial Virus (RSV) and other		
Palivizumab (Synagis) *(See Med Lett 41:1, 1999)* Used only for prevention of RSV infection in high-risk children *(Ped 102:1211, 1998)*	15 mg/kg IM q month 100 mg vial (for 1 injection) $1,216.58	A monoclonal antibody directed against the F glycoprotein on surface of virus; side-effects are nominal, occ. ↑ ALT *(JID 176:1215, 1997)*.
Ribavirin (Virazole) Aerosol	1.1 gm/day (6 gm vial for inhalation $1319.85)	**Ribavirin side-effects:** Anemia, rash, conjunctivitis: Read package insert. Avoid procedures that lead to drug precipitation in ventilator tubing with subsequent dysfunction. Significant teratogenicity in animals. Pregnant health care workers should avoid direct care of pts receiving aerosolized ribavirin.
RSV-IV immunoglobulin (RespiGam) (RSV-IVIG)	750 mg/kg IV q month (50 ml) $661.53	RespiGam side-effects rare: fatal anaphylaxis, pruritus, rash, wheezing, fever, joint pain.
Warts *(See CID 28:S37, 1999)*		
Interferon alfa-2b or alpha-n3	1 million units (0.1 ml) into lesion	**Side-effects:** Have to use vials containing 10 million units/1.0 ml. Cost: 0.1 ml $10.50
Podofilox (Condylox)	3.5 ml for topical application, $62.30	**Side-effects:** Local reactions—pain, burning, inflammation in 50%. No systemic effects.
Imiquimod (Aldara)	Cream applied 3x/week to maximum of 16 weeks. 250 mg packets $9 each	Mild erythema, erosions, itching and burning

NOTE: All dosage recommendations are for adults (unless otherwise indicated) and assume normal renal function.
* From Oct. 1998 Hospital Formulary Pricing Guide. Price is average wholesale price (AWP). **NB** = name brand. **G** = generic. **DC** = discontinue

TABLE 14C: ANTIRETROVIRAL THERAPY IN ADULTS 1999-2000

1. **When should antiretroviral treatment be started?**
The **most important factor in answering this question is to find out if the patient is ready to comply with the difficult regimens** since lack of compliance guarantees failure of the treatment and facilitates the emergence of resistant subpopulations of virus making it much more difficult to treat the patient later *(AnIM 129:503, 1998; JAMA 280:567, 1998)*. It also creates the potential for spread of resistant viruses to others. Studies indicate that about ⅓ of patients are totally adherent, ⅓ partially adherent and ⅓ almost totally nonadherent to prescribed rx. 2 important factors affect adherence: (1) the number of pills and (2), ease of administration of the regimen, qd better than bid, which is better than tid; mixing bid with tid medications with food and without food makes total adherence nearly impossible. Every effort should be made to come to an agreement or contract with the patient as to what he/she is capable or willing to comply with prior to initiating rx. Frequent follow-up with advice & encouragement to the patient is important to help maintain compliance and to detect non-compliance. 1998 recommendations from 2 major panels are available and are remarkably similar: International AIDS Society *(JAMA 280:78, 1998)* and Kaiser Family Foundation *(AnIM 128:1079, 1998)*. Another in 1999: *Journal of the International Assn of Physicians in AIDS Care 5:Suppl. 1, 1999.* Summary below:

TABLE 14C (2)

Situation 1: CD4 count <500/mm³ or Viral burden >5000-10,000 copies/ml	Situation 2: CD4 count <500/mm³ Viral burden: >50-<5000 copies/ml (any detectable virus)	Situation 3: CD4 count >500/mm³ Viral burden >50-<5,000 copies/ml	Situation 4: CD4 count >500/mm³ Viral burden undetectable.
Comment: Treatment indicated	Comment: Recommendations vary. Authors favor rx if pt compliant and committed.	Comment: Recommendations vary, Authors favor rx if pt compliant and committed.	Comment: Retest periodically. No rx

2. Available drugs: categories, names, and dosages (Summary in Medical Letter 39:111, 1997; Deeks & Volberding in Medical Management of AIDS, Sande & Volberding, Eds., 6th Ed., 1999)

There are currently 12 FDA-approved drugs available in the United States for use against HIV:

The **nucleoside reverse-transcriptase inhibitors (NRTI)**, which include:

Group A drugs:
  Zidovudine (ZDV)—Retrovir   Standard dosage:
  Stavudine (d4T)—Zerit   300 mg bid or 200 mg tid
     40 mg bid for >60 kg, 30 mg bid for <60 kg

Group B drugs:
  Didanosine (ddl)—Videx
    200 mg bid (empty stomach) for >60 kg, 125 mg bid for <60 kg. A single daily dose of 400 mg po hs is commonly used.

  Zalcitabine (ddC)— HIVID   0.75 mg tid
  Lamivudine (3TC)—Epivir   150 mg bid

Also:
  Abacavir—Ziagen   300 mg bid. Recently approved (12/98), can be used in combination with all other NRTIs.

  ZDV/3TC (Combivir)   One combination tab bid

The **non-nucleoside reverse-transcriptase inhibitors (NNRT)**, which include:
  Nevirapine—Viramune   200 mg bid x2 weeks, then 200 mg bid
  Delavirdine—Rescriptor   400 mg tid
  Efavirenz—Sustiva   600 mg qd hs (at bedtime)

The **protease inhibitors (PI)**, which include:
  Saquinavir—Invirase   600 mg q8h with meals
  Saquinavir—Fortovase   1200 mg q8h with meals
  Indinavir—Crixivan   800 mg q8h, empty stomach or with light meal **[1200 mg bid is less effective and NOT recommended]**
  Ritonavir—Norvir   300 mg q12h with food, then dose escalate over 2 wks to 600 mg bid
  Nelfinavir—Viracept   750 mg q8h with food [1250 mg bid looks promising (5th CRV, Abst. 373)]
  Ritonavir/saquinavir   Each drug taken 400 mg bid
  Indinavir/ritonavir   Each 400 mg bid [also produces serum levels similar to each drug alone at tid—promising (ICAAC Abst. A-57, 1997)]
  Amprenavir—Agenerase   1200 mg po bid (softgel capsules) with or without food; high-fat meal should be avoided. Oral solution available. (Approved 4/99)

When using 2 NRTIs together, it is recommended that an A drug be combined with a B drug, not an A with an A or a B with a B drug to prevent additive toxicities and possible antagonism of action. **Most recommend initiating triple combinations:** combine 2 NRTIs (A+B) with either a PI or an NNRTI. Addition of the PI (Indinavir) improved results of both clinical & virologic parameters in antiretroviral naive & experienced patients (NEJM 337:725 & 734, 1997). Significant drug-drug interactions occur with PIs (esp. with ritonavir). Drug tolerance and the ability of the patient to balance food intake and convenience (quality of life issues) are major considerations. Virologic failure after 1 yr in 50% of pts (S. Deeks, ICAAC 1997). Factors: previous rx, late-stage disease, poor compliance, and drug toxicity. The role of abacavir in initial therapy has not been determined.

3. Summary of Suggested Treatment of HIV Infection (see text for details)

CLINICAL CIRCUMSTANCE	PREFERRED	ALTERNATIVE	NOT GENERALLY RECOMMENDED	NOT RECOMMENDED
Normal CD4 T-lymphocyte count: no quantifiable virus in plasma with ultrasensitive test	No treatment. Repeat plasma viral burden every 6 months.			

Quantifiable virus in plasma (most authorities use viral titers of >5000 to 10,000 copies/ml of plasma as an indicator to initiate antiretroviral rx); **CD4 count normal or decreased; treatment-naive patient**	Combine 1 drug from protease inhibitor (PI) list with 2-drug regimen from list of **nucleoside reverse transcriptase inhibitors (NRTI)**:
	PIs NRTIs
	Indinavir ZDV + 3TC (potent)
	Nelfinavir d4T + ddl (potent)
	Ritonavir ZDV + ddl
	Amprenavir ZDV + ddC
	(Saquinavir-SGC* ± ritonavir) d4T + 3TC (potent)
		Combine 2 NRTIs from list in Preferred Rx box with 1 of the following list of **non-nucleoside reverse transcriptase inhibitors (NNRTIs)**:
		Efavirenz (most potent)
		or
		Nevirapine
		or
		Triple NRTI: ZDV + 3TC + abacavir
			2 NRTIs	1. All monotherapies
				2. Certain combinations of NRTIs:
				  d4T + ZDV
				  ddC + ddl
				  ddC + d4T
				  ddC + 3TC

* See next page for footnotes and abbreviations

TABLE 14C (3)

CLINICAL CIRCUMSTANCE	PREFERRED	ALTERNATIVE	NOT GENERALLY RECOMMENDED	NOT RECOMMENDED
Failure of initial therapy	Options: 1. As for treatment-naive, but switch to a different PI and a different combination of NRTIs. 2. Double PI rx (ritonavir + saquinavir-SGC*) ± NNRTI 3. Efavirenz + a different combination of NRTIs 4. Double PI + 2 different NRTIs	Options: 1. Different PI + d4T + ddl + hydroxyurea 2. Substitute an investigational drug as part of new combination rx. Drugs available on compassionate use basis by category.		Change of only 1 or 2 drugs of 3-drug regimen
Acute retroviral syndrome	ZDV + 3TC + PI x2 years minimum (or other similar rx)	Hope is to ↓ viral setpoint and slow progression of disease (data still pending)		
Needlestick injury	See Table 15			
Pregnancy	See Table 15			

Abbreviations: NRTI = nucleoside reverse transcriptase inhibitor; **NNRTI** = non-nucleoside reverse transcriptase inhibitor; **PI** = protease inhibitor; **ZDV** = zidovudine; **3TC** = lamivudine; **d4T** = stavudine; **ddl** = didanosine; **A & B** refer to Group A & B drugs *(see page 109)*; **SGC** = softgel capsules; **5th CRV** = 5th Conference on Retroviruses & Opportunistic Infections, 1998

4. How should patients be monitored?
Most authorities recommend measurements of viral load after 1 month, then every 3–4 months, and more frequently if non-compliance is suspected, CD4 counts drop, or clinical symptoms appear or progress. It is also recommended that viral load be quantified every time adjustments in drugs or dosages are made, at 2–4 weeks, and again at 8–12 weeks, in order to document drug effect.

TABLE 14D: ANTIRETROVIRAL DRUGS AND SIDE-EFFECTS

DRUG NAME(S) GENERIC (TRADE)	DOSAGE/ROUTE/COST*	COMMENTS/ADVERSE EFFECTS
Antiretroviral Drugs. *For detailed pharmacology: Chap. by Flexner & Hendrix in AIDS, Ed. DeVita, 1997*		
Nucleoside Reverse Transcriptase Inhibitors (NRTI) (FDA-approved): All have potential for severe steatosis, hepatomegaly and lactic acidosis (rare)		
Abacavir (Ziagen)	300 mg tabs Dose: 300 mg bid with no food or water restrictions (300 mg $5.00 or **$300/month**)	Approved based on data of abacavir + ZDV + 3TC. **Adverse effects:** Headache, nausea/vomiting, malaise, & diarrhea most common. Most serious is hypersensitivity reaction in 3–5%: malaise, fever, GI upset, rash, resolves in 2 days: **do not rechallenge—may be life-threatening.**
Didanosine (ddl) (Dideoxyinosine) (Videx) *See Comment for hydroxyurea*	≥60 kg body weight Tablets 200 mg q12h on empty stomach Powder 250 mg q12h on empty stomach <60 kg body weight Tablets 125 mg q12h on empty stomach Powder 167 mg q12h on empty stomach

Chewable tablets (25, 50, 100, 150 mg) must be chewed or crushed thoroughly before swallowing. Buffered powder for oral solution (100, 167, 250 mg packets) to be dissolved in 4 oz water is available. New tablet formulations are 35% smaller & softer (easier to chew) than original tablets. (100 mg tablet $1.80, 250 mg powder $4.53) (Approx. **$216/month** for 400 mg/d) | **Adverse effects: Pancreatitis** 6% (0.35% fatal), ↑ amylase 10%. ↑ amylase can be of salivary origin esp. with xerostomia. No intervention necessary unless symptomatic. In pts with history of pancreatitis 8/27 (30%) developed pancreatitis, avoid or use with caution in alcoholics. Hyperglycemia, occasional diabetes mellitus. **Peripheral neuropathy** 20%, 12% required dose reduction. Hepatic: ↑ SGOT 13%, fatal liver failure in 0.2%, hypertriglyceridemia. **Other:** GI—**diarrhea** 28%, abdominal pain 10% nausea 6%, skin—rash 9%. CNS—headache 7%, fever 12%. Lab: anemia (<8.0 gm, 2%), leucopenia (<2,000, 16%), thrombocytopenia (<50,000, 2%), ↑ uric acid 2%. Pregnancy—use only if clearly needed. Approved for children. Drugs on Na+ restriction, buffered tablets each contain 265 mg Na+. **Note:** Drugs whose absorption requires gastric acidity and can be blocked by buffers in ddl, e.g. indinavir, dapsone, ketoconazole, fluoroquinolones, should be given 2 hours apart from ddl. **Hydroxyurea** (500 mg bid) has been shown to ↑ available concentration of nucleoside analogs, particularly ddl, and ↑ antiretroviral activity. In a Swiss HIV Cohort Study, d4T, ddl & hydroxyurea achieved a log 4.5 reduction in viral RNA and 54% (39/72) were undetectable at 12 wks vs 28% with d4T and ddl alone. May blunt CD4 cell response and ↑ risk of pancreatitis and peripheral neuropathy. The drug is inexpensive and no cross-resistance has been found. We await further trials. |

NOTE: All dosage recommendations are for adults (unless otherwise indicated) and assume normal renal function.
* From 1999 Red Book Update (8/99), Medical Economics Co. Price is average wholesale price (AWP). **NB** = name brand. **G** = generic

TABLE 14D (2)

DRUG NAME(S) GENERIC (TRADE)	DOSAGE/ROUTE/COST*	COMMENTS/ADVERSE EFFECTS
Nucleoside Reverse Transcriptase Inhibitors (NRT) *(continued)*		
Lamivudine (3TC) (Epivir or Epivir-HBV)	For HIV (Epivir): 150 kg po bid in combination with ZDV (200 mg bid or 300 mg/day). Also, oral solution of 10 mg/ml. (150 mg tab $4.33) (Approx. **$260/month**). **NOTE: Combination tablets available** (150 mg 3TC + 300 mg ZDV) = Combivir $9.40 ea. (**$564/mo.**). Dose: 1 Combivir bid po. For Hepatitis B (Epivir-HBV): 100 mg po qd. 100 tab = $4.33	**Adverse effects: Well tolerated.** Side-effects reported for combination ZDV + 3TC, most due to ZDV. 13/276 pts on the combination developed precipitous ↓ in hemoglobin. (>50%) (*CID 27:908, 1998*). Fatigue & headache 35%, malaise 27%, nasal symptoms 20%, fever 10%. GI: nausea 33%, diarrhea 18%, nausea/vomiting 12%, anorexia 10%, abdominal pain 9%. Neurol.: neuropathy 12%, dizziness 10%, insomnia 11%, depression 9%, anemia 3%. In **pediatric trials: pancreatitis** 15%, Lab: leucopenia 7%, anemia 3%. In **pediatric trials: pancreatitis** 15%. In hepatitis B trials with 100 mg daily rx: ear, nose & throat infections 25%, malaise & fatigue 24%, & headache 21%. Hepatitis may flare when lamivudine stopped.
Stavudine, d4T (Zerit)	≥60 kg: 40 mg bid po (40 mg tab $4.56) <60 kg: 30 mg bid po (30 mg tab $4.40) (Approx. **$274/month** for 40 mg bid). Oral solution available.	**Adverse effects: Peripheral neuropathy** (15–20%). GI: nausea/vomiting, abdominal pain, diarrhea, pancreatitis 1% with 6 deaths attributed to d4T. CNS: sleep disorders, mania. Skin: rash. Hepatic: ↑ AST, ALT.
Zalcitabine **(Dideoxycytidine),** **ddC** (HIVID)	0.75 mg po q8h. Higher doses too toxic. (0.75 mg tablet $2.42) (Approx. **$218/month** for 0.75 mg q8h)	**Adverse effects:** Major clinical toxicity is **peripheral neuropathy** (22–35%) (numbness and paresthesias → severe continuous pain, slowly reversible when ddC discontinued, ↑ with diabetes mellitus). Other: GI—**oral ulcers** 13%, dysphagia 3%, abdominal pain 3%, skin—**rash** 8%. CNS—headache 9%, myalgia 5%. Lab: Anemia (<7.5 gm) 5%, leucopenia (<1500, 9%). Fertile women should not receive ddC unless on effective contraception. Safety in children <13 yrs not established. Irreversible ototoxicity has been reported (*Int J STD & AIDS 8:201, 1997*).
Zidovudine (ZDV), formerly azido- thymidine (AZT) (Retrovir) *See lamivudine for Combivir cost*	300 mg po bid 100 mg tab (po) $1.69, 300 mg tab (po) $5.06 200 mg IV $18.24 50 mg/tsp, 240 ml $40.50 (Approx. **$304/month** for 600 mg/d) **NOTE: Combination tablets of ZDV (300 mg) + 3TC (150 mg) available. Dose: 1 tab bid**	**Adverse effects:** Most are dose-dependent. On 600 mg/d: Major clinical toxicity: **hematologic:** anemia (<8 gm, 1%), granulocytopenia (<750, 1.8%). **Macrocytosis expected with all dosage regimens.** Anemia may respond to epoetin alfa if endogenous serum erythropoietin levels are ≤500 mU/ml. Other: GI—**nausea 50%**, xerostomia, hypertriglyceridemia, anorexia 20%, vomiting 17%. CNS—**headache** 62%, **malaise** 53% (headache, malaise at initiation of rx less frequent if dose 200 mg qd for 5–7 days, then 400 mg q12h for 5–7 days, then 200 mg q8h); pigmentation of nails, **[myopathy** (creatine kinase ↑ 2 months before clinical signs, biopsies show abnormal giant mitochondria, strength returns ~8 weeks after ZDV discontinued, *Quart J Med 86:5, 1993*]. **Asthenia and insomnia common complaints.**
Non-Nucleoside Reverse Transcriptase Inhibitors (NNRT)		
Delavirdine (Rescriptor)	400 mg po tid (mix 4 100 mg tablets in 3 oz. of water to produce slurry). (100 mg $0.67). (Approx. **$233/month**)	Adverse events of moderate or severe intensity reported in ≥2% of pts but **skin rash has occurred in 18% attributed to the drug;** can continue or restart drug in most cases. Other side-effects include headache, nausea, vomiting, diarrhea and ↑ in liver enzymes in <5% of pts. See *drug-drug interactions, Table 21*. Cross-resistant HIV strains develop with nevirapine.
Efavirenz (Sustiva)	600 mg. Three 200 mg capsules with or without food usually at bedtime to minimize CNS side effects. 200 mg $4.38 (approx. **$394/month**)	**Adverse effects: CNS side effects** including dizziness, insomnia, somnolence, impaired concentration and abnormal dreaming in 52%. Symptoms improve over 1st month. Discontinuation rate 2.6%. **Rash** in 28% of pts in clinical trials (treatment-related in 18%) leading to discontinuation in 1.7%. Rash improves with antihistamines. **Drug interactions:** See *Table 21.* **Pregnancy Category C.**
Nevirapine (Viramune)	200 mg daily for 2 wks, followed by full dose of 200 mg 2x/day (may lower risk of rash). (200 mg $4.65) (**$279/month**)	**Adverse effects: Rash in 37% enrolled in trials;** grade 3 rash in 5.6%, 6.7% stopped nevirapine because of rash. Stevens-Johnson reported (*Lancet 351:567, 1998*). Rash resolves in 50% of pts within 2 wks of stopping rx and in 80% by 1 month. **Severe rash or any rash with constitutional symptoms: drug should be stopped and pts should NOT be rechallenged** (*Ln 351: 1133, 1998*). Fever, nausea and headache can occur. ↑ gamma glutamyl transpeptidase (GGT) in 10% of 252 vs 2% of controls. Nevirapine has good CSF penetration.
Protease Inhibitors: Recommend use only in combination with 2 NRTI (A+B) drugs (see *NEJM 338:1281, 1998*)	**Comment:** There are 15 case reports of **spontaneous bleeding** episodes in HIV+ pts with hemophilia being treated with protease inhibitors. There is no proven causal relationship; however, FDA & manufacturers recommend monitoring hemophiliac pts for spontaneous bleeding whenever protease inhibitors are used. All PIs may be associated with **hyperglycemia and/or hyperlipidemia.** 6/105 pts given PIs developed symptomatic **diabetes mellitus** (*ICAAC Abst. LB-8, 1997*). 13/24 PI-rx pts had abnormal glucose tolerance tests & 17/24 had evidence of peripheral insulin resistance (*AIDS 12: F167, 1998*). Central obesity (*Ln 351:871, 1998*), gynecomastia, and **"buffalo hump"** [fatty distributions [median time after initiation of PI rx 22 wks (4–61 wks)], as well as symmetrical fat wasting of face, limbs, and upper trunk (**peripheral lipodystrophy**) [median time after PI rx 10 months] reported with all PIs (*CID 27:65 & 68, 1998; AIDS 12:F37 & 51, 1998*). The mechanism of glucose and lipid abnormalities is unknown but PIs have molecular similarities to 2 human proteins that regulate lipid metabolism (*Ln 351:1881, 1998*). PIs also enhance adipogenesis in cell culture (*Ln 352:1032, 1998*).	

NOTE: All dosage recommendations are for adults (unless otherwise indicated) and assume normal renal function.
* From 1999 Red Book Update (8/99), Medical Economics Co. Price is average wholesale price (AWP). **NB** = name brand, **G** = generic

TABLE 14D (3)

DRUG NAME(S) GENERIC (TRADE)	DOSAGE/ROUTE/COST*	COMMENTS/ADVERSE EFFECTS
Protease Inhibitors *(continued)*		
Amprenavir (Agenerase)	1200 mg po bid (soft-gel capsules) as 8 150 mg caps bid. Oral solution available. 150 mg $1.26 **($604/ month)**	**Adverse effects: Skin rash in 28% of pts.** Most maculopapular of mild-moderate intensity, some with pruritus; severe or life-threatening rash, including Stevens-Johnson syndrome, in 1% of pts (4% of amprenavir recipients who developed rash). Rash onset 7–73 days, median 10 days. When amprenavir dc for mild rash, reintroduction of drug generally did not result in rash recurrence. DC drug for severe life-threatening rash & for moderate rash accompanied by systemic symptoms. **GI events common:** nausea 38–73%, vomiting 19–20%, diarrhea 33–56%. **Paresthesias** in up to 30% & **depression** or mood disorders in 4–15%. **Many drug-drug interactions—see Table 21.**
Indinavir sulfate (Crixivan)	800 mg po tid (capsules). Rx: Two 400 mg caps po tid with 12 oz. liquid, without food. (400 mg cap $2.57) [Approx. **$464/month** + NRTI drug(s)]. Also avail. as 200 & 333 mg tabs.	**Adverse effects: Kidney stones** due to indinavir crystals in collecting system (2–3% on 2.4 gm/d but higher in "hot climates" *(AIDS 14:296, 1997; 12/174 (6.9%) developed nephrolithiasis within 4 mos. of starting indinavir; 5/8 who continued rx had a 2nd episode (ICAAC Abst. 183, 1997). Rapid onset crystalluria also reported in HIV-neg. persons (CID 27:917, 1998). Prevent (minimize) by good hydration (≥48 oz. water/ day) (AAC 42:332, 1998).* **↑ indirect bilirubin 10–15% (≥2.5 mg/dl) due to a drug-induced Gilbert's syndrome (of no clinical significance),** but severe hepatitis reported in 3 cases *(Ln 349:924, 1997)* **GI:** nausea 12%, vomiting 4%, diarrhea 5%. Anemia/neutropenia ~5% *(Abst 287, 3rd CRV, 1996).* Headache 6%. Hyperglycemia has been reported in 77/1000 pts 1–7 months after initiation of rx *(Ln 350:713, 1997).* Rarely severe allergic reactions with repeated exposure *(CID 26:523, 1998).* 10 pts receiving indinavir had ↑ from 95 to 142 mg/dl cholesterol from 145 to 172 mg/dl and triglycerides ↑ *(IDSA Abst. 233, 1997).* **Drug interactions: see Table 21.**
Nelfinavir (Viracept)	750 mg po tid with food (250 mg $2.16) (Approx. **$582/mo.**) Oral powder: 50 mg/gm (144 gm $59.45) In combination with d4T and 3TC, nelfinavir 1250 mg **bid** as effective as 750 mg **tid** in ↓ viral load (2–2.5 log) and ↑ CD4 (120 cells/mm³) with 16-wk follow-up *(5th CRV, Abst. 373).*	**Adverse effects: GI: Mild to moderate diarrhea in 14–52%,** but may be better tolerated than other approved PIs. Toxicity profile similar to other PIs. Potential for bid dosing. Well absorbed with food. Resistance develops slowly and resistant strains have remained susceptible to other PIs. However, because of potential HIV cross-resistance between nelfinavir and other PIs, it is unknown what effect nelfinavir rx will have on the activity of coadministered or subsequently administered PIs. **Drug-drug interactions: see Table 21.**
Ritonavir (RTV) (Norvir)	600 mg po bid with food (capsules). Capsules must be kept in refrigerator. [Rx: start with 3 100 mg caps po with chocolate milk (or Ensure® or Advera®) bid day 1; 4 caps bid day 2, 3; 5 caps bid day 5; then 6 caps bid po qd.] (100 mg cap $1.85) [Approx. **$668/month** + NRTI drug(s)] Take with food.	**Adverse effects:** Common (85–100% but only 12% withdrawals). More than any other anti-HIV drug. See *Table 21 and review package insert.* **GI:** bitter aftertaste (↓ by taking with chocolate milk, Ensure®, Advera®), nausea 23%, ↓ by initial dose escalation (titration) regimen; vomiting 13%; diarrhea 13%; **circumoral paresthesias 5–6%;** ↑ γGTT, ↑ **triglycerides;** ↑ **LFTs/CPK/uric acid.** 1 case of acute hepatic failure *(AnIM 129:670, 1998);* other: lightheadedness 9–14%. **Many important drug-drug interactions: see Table 21.**
Saquinavir (SQV) (Invirase) (Fortovase for softgel tab)	600 mg po tid (capsules). Rx: Three 200 mg caps po tid with food—high fat preferred. Soft capsules preferred. (Hard capsule 200 mg $2.24; softgel 200 mg $1.15) Invirase—hard capsules 600 mg po tid with meals **($604/month)** Fortovase—soft capsules 1200 mg po tid with meals **($623/month)**	Oral bioavailability hard caps ~ 4%, take with food. **Soft gelatin capsule formulation shows ↑ absorption to 10–13%.** **Adverse effects:** Overall 37%—mostly mild, <5% moderate. GI: diarrhea, abdominal discomfort, nausea; headache *(Ln 345:952, 1995).*

NOTE: All dosage recommendations are for adults (unless otherwise indicated) and assume normal renal function.
** From 1999 Red Book Update (8/99). Medical Economics Co. Price is average wholesale price (AWP). **NB** = name brand. **G** = generic*

TABLE 15A

PREVENTION OF INFECTION WITH CHEMOTHERAPY

CLASS OF ETIOLOGIC AGENT/DISEASE/CONDITION	PROPHYLAXIS: AGENT/DOSE/ROUTE/DURATION	COMMENTS
Group B streptococcal disease, neonatal: Vaginal colonization with group B strep. Assoc. with ↑ neonatal sepsis & maternal peripartum and postpartum infectious complications (*JID 179:1410, 1999; Ln 353:51, 1999*)		
Pregnant women—intrapartum antimicrobial prophylaxis—**2** approaches to management [CDC Guidelines, *MMWR 45(RR-7):1, 1996*—some question this strategy (*IDCP 7:188, 1998; PID 17:973, 1998*)]: **1. Prenatal screening cultures**—from vagina & rectum, by swab, at 35–37 wks gestation. Use transport media (Amies); survive at room temp. up to 96 hr. **2. Risk factor approach**—Rx if any of the following are present: (a) previously delivered infant with invasive GBS infection; (b) GBS bacteriuria during this pregnancy; (c) delivery at <37 wks gestation; (d) duration of ruptured membranes ≥18 hrs; (e) intrapartum temp. ≥100.4°F (≥38.0°C)	If culture positive or risk factors dictate prophylaxis: Rx mother during labor with pen G 5 MU IV (load) then 2.5 MU IV q4h until delivery. Alternate rx: Ampicillin 2 gm IV (load) then give 1 gm IV q4h until delivery. Pen-allergic: Clindamycin 900 mg IV q8h until delivery or erythromycin 500 mg IV q6h until delivery.	
Neonate delivered from mother who received prophylaxis	Careful observation of signs & symptoms (*see MMWR 45:RR-7, 1996 for specifics*)	
Preterm, premature rupture of the membranes in Group B strep-negative women (*JAMA 278:989, 1997*)	[IV ampicillin 2 gm q6h + IV erythromycin 250 mg q8h) for 48 hrs followed by po amoxicillin 250 mg q8h + po erythromycin base 333 mg q8h x5 d. Effective in ↓ infant morbidity.	Antibiotic rx reduced respiratory distress syndrome (50.6% to 40.8%, p = 0.03), necrotizing enterocolitis (5.8% to 2.3%, p = 0.03) and prolonged pregnancy (2.9 to 6.1 days, p < 0.001) vs placebo.
Meningitis prevention:		
Hemophilus influenzae type b Household and/or day care contact: residing with index case or ≥4 hrs. Day care contact: same day care as index case for 5–7 days before onset	Rifampin 20 mg/kg po (not to exceed 600 mg) qd x4 doses	**Household:** If there is one unvaccinated contact ≤4 yrs in the household, rifampin recommended for all household contacts except pregnant women. **Child Care Facilities:** With 1 case, if attended by unvaccinated children ≤2 yrs, consider prophylaxis + vaccinate susceptibles. If all contacts >2 yrs: no prophylaxis. If ≥2 cases in 60 days and unvaccinated children attend, prophylaxis recommended for children and personnel (*Am Acad Ped Red Book 1997, page 222*).
Neisseria meningitidis exposure (close contact) Ref.: *MMWR 46(RR-5):1–21, 1997*	Rifampin 600 mg q12h x4 doses, po. (Children 10 mg/kg po q12h x4 doses)] or [ciprofloxacin (adults) 500 mg po single dose) or [ceftriaxone 250 mg IM x1 dose (child <15 yrs, 125 mg IM x1)] Spiramycin 500 mg q6h x5 d, po. Children 10 mg/kg po q6h x5 d	N. meningitidis spread by respiratory droplets, not aerosols, hence close contact required. ↑ risk if close contact for at least 4 hrs during week before illness onset (e.g., housemates, day care contacts, cellmates) or exposure to pt's nasopharyngeal secretions (e.g., via kissing, mouth-to-mouth resuscitation, intubation, nasotracheal suctioning). Azithro 500 mg x1 as effective as RIF 600 mg bid x2 d. (*PIDJ 17:816, 1998*). Primary prophylactic regimen in many European countries.
Neutropenic patients, afebrile, e.g., post-chemotherapy See *CID 25:551, 1997; CID 27:235, 1998*	IDSA guidelines for afebrile neutropenic pts: **Routine prophylaxis should be avoided** even though TMP/SMX 2 double strength tablets po bid or FQ (norfloxacin 400 mg po bid, ofloxacin 400 mg po bid, or ciprofloxacin 500 mg po bid) have been shown to reduce febrile episodes. No reduction in mortality and	TMP/SMX (>30 studies) reduces infection rates (vs placebo) with fewer adverse effects (*JID 161:381, 1990*). In a meta-analysis of 19 randomized studies, **quinolone** use reduced Gm-neg. bacteremia (OR = 0.09) but not Gm+ bacteremia (OR = 1.05). Addition of penicillin, vancomycin, macrolide or rifampin reduced Gm+ bacteremia (OR = 0.46) but had no impact on fever-related morbidity (OR = 0.83) or infection-related mortality (OR = 0.74) (*CID 23:795, 1996; AnIM 125:183, 1996*). Oral fluconazole and itraconazole shown to reduce fungal infections but use remains controversial (*CID 28:331, 1999; CID 28:250, 1999*). Use of selective bowel decontamination did not reduce overall infection rate follow-

TABLE 15A (2)

Management of Exposure to Blood, Vaginal/Penile Secretions With Risk of Transmission of Hepatitis B/C and/or HIV (Needlestick Injury) *(Adapted from CDC recommendations: MMWR 47:R-7, 1998; also see JAMA 281:931, 1999)*

General steps in management:

1. Wash clean wounds/flush mucous membranes immediately (use of caustic agents or squeezing the wound is discouraged; data lacking regarding antiseptics).
2. Assess risk by doing the following: (a) Characterize exposure; (b) Determine/evaluate source of exposure by medical history, risk behavior, & testing for hepatitis B/C, HIV; (c) Evaluate and test exposed individual for hepatitis B/C & HIV

Hepatitis B Exposure

Exposed Person		Exposure Source	
	HBs Ag+	HBs Ag –	Status Unknown
Unvaccinated	Give HBIG 5 ml IM & initiate HB vaccine	Initiate HB vaccine	If possible, do HBs Ag on source person
Vaccinated (antibody status unknown)	Do anti-HBs on exposed person	No rx necessary	Do anti-HBs on exposed person
	If titer ≥10 IU/ml, no rx		If titer <10 IU/ml, give 1 dose HB vaccine + HBIG
	If titer <10 IU/ml, HBIG + 1 dose HB vaccine		If titer ≥10 IU/ml, no rx

Hepatitis C Exposure

Determine antibody to hepatitis C for both exposed person and, if possible, exposure source. **No recommended prophylaxis;** immune serum globulin not effective.

HIV: Occupational exposure management *(for sexual exposure to HIV, see below)*

- The decision to initiate post-exposure prophylaxis (PEP) for HIV is a clinical judgment that should be made in concert with the exposed healthcare worker (HCW). It is based on:
    1. Likelihood of the source patient having HIV infection: ↑ with history of high-risk activity—injection drug use, sexual activity with known HIV+ person, unprotected sex with multiple partners (either hetero- or homosexual), receipt of blood products 1978–1985. ↑ with clinical signs suggestive of advanced HIV (unexplained wasting, night sweats, thrush, seborrheic dermatitis, etc.). Remember, the vast majority of persons are **not** infected with HIV (0.5% of women in larger U.S. cities) and likelihood of infection **extremely rare** if not in above risk groups.
    2. Type of exposure (approx. 1 in 300–400 needlesticks from infected source will transmit HIV.
    3. Limited data regarding efficacy of PEP (PEP with ZDV alone reduced transmission by 90% in 1 retrospective case-controlled study—*NEJM 337:1485, 1997*).
    4. Side-effects of PEP drugs.

- If source person is **known positive for HIV** or **likely to be infected** and **status of exposure warrants PEP**, antiretroviral drugs should be started **immediately.** If ELISA for HIV is negative, drugs can be stopped. The HCW should be re-tested at 3–4 weeks, 3 & 6 months whether PEP is used or not (the vast majority of seroconversions will occur by 3 months; delayed conversions after 6 months are exceedingly rare). Tests for HIV RNA should not be used for dx of HIV infection because of false-positives (esp. at low titers) & these tests are only approved for established HIV infection [a possible exception is if pt develops signs of acute HIV (mononucleosis-like) syndrome within the 1st 4–6 wks of exposure when antibody tests might still be negative.]

- PEP for HIV is usually given for **4 weeks** and monitoring of side-effects recommended: baseline complete blood count, renal and hepatic panel to be repeated at **2 weeks.** 50–75% of HCW on PEP demonstrate mild side-effects (nausea, diarrhea, myalgias, headache, etc.) but in up to ⅓ severe enough to discontinue PEP. Consultation with infectious diseases/HIV specialist valuable when questions regarding PEP arise.

TABLE 15A (3)

3 Steps to HIV Post-Exposure Prophylaxis (PEP) After Occupational Exposure:

Step 1: Determine the exposure code (EC)

Is source material blood, bloody fluid, semen/vaginal fluid or other normally sterile fluid or tissue?

→ Yes

→ No → No PEP

What type of exposure occurred?

Mucous membrane or skin integrity compromised (e.g., dermatitis, open wound) → Volume

Percutaneous exposure → Severity

Intact skin → No PEP

Volume:
- Small: Few drops → EC1
- Large: Major splash and/or long duration → EC2

Severity:
- Less severe: Solid needle, scratch → EC2
- More severe: Large-bore hollow needle, deep puncture, visible blood, needle used in vein of source (risk 1:300/400) → EC3

Step 2: Determine the HIV Status Code (HIV SC)

What is the HIV status of the exposure source?

HIV negative → No PEP

HIV positive

Status unknown → HIV SC unknown

Source unknown → HIV SC unknown

HIV positive:
- Low titer exposure: asymptomatic & high CD4 count → HIV SC 1
- High titer exposure: advanced AIDS, prin. HIV high viral load or low CD4 count → HIV SC 2

Step 3: Determine Post-Exposure Prophylaxis (PEP) Recommendation

EC	HIV SC	PEP
1	1	May not be warranted
1	2	Consider basic regimen—see footnote[1]
2	1	Recommend basic regimen—see footnote[1]
2	2	Recommend expanded regimen—see footnote[1]
3	1 or 2	Recommend expanded regimen—see footnote[1]
	Unknown	If exposure setting suggests risks of HIV exposure & EC in 2 or 3, consider basic regimen.

Post-Exposure Prophylaxis: Management Following Sexual Exposure *(Adapted from MMWR 47:RR-17, 1998; also see NEJM 336:1097, 1997)*
Since the probability of transmission of HIV via sexual contact may approach that of a needlestick, it is reasonable to consider PEP in persons who have had a sexual encounter with an HIV+ person. Currently there are no data on effectiveness of PEP in this setting. The same assessment as suggested above for occupational exposure might be followed in an attempt to determine relative risk. It has been estimated that transmission of HIV following an episode of receptive penile-anal sexual exposure 0.1–0.3%, for receptive vaginal exposure 0.1–0.2%, and unknown for receptive oral intercourse (although less risky than others).

PEP should not be used for low-risk exposure (potentially infected body fluids on intact skin) or for persons who seek care too late for anticipated effect (>72 hrs after exposure). Consideration might be given for PEP when risk is high; PEP can be initiated promptly, and adherence is likely. It is prudent to weigh relative low per-act probability of transmission with reported exposure against uncertain effectiveness, potential toxicities, and cost (approx. $600–1000/course).
Management and drug selection as above. Patient should also be screened for other sexually transmitted diseases.

[1] Treat for 4 weeks: Monitor for drug side-effects q2 weeks
Basic regimen: **Zidovudine 300 mg with lamivudine 150 mg po bid**
Expanded regimen: **Basic regimen + either (indinavir 800 mg po q8h) or (nelfinavir 750 mg po q8h)**

TABLE 15A (4)

CLASS OF ETIOLOGIC AGENT/DISEASE/CONDITION	PROPHYLAXIS: AGENT/DOSE/ROUTE/DURATION	COMMENTS
V transmission from mother to neonate (vertical transmission) If mother not breastfed if possible since risk of transmission is 7% at 11 months & 10.3% at 23 months in a study in Malawi (JAMA 282: 744, 1999).	**Standard for developed countries with prenatal care: Zidovudine** (ZDV) 300 mg bid po starting last ½ of pregnancy, then IV 2 mg/kg loading dose then 1 mg/kg/hr during labor & then 2 mg/kg po q6h for baby beginning 8–12 hrs after birth for 6 weeks. (Cost: $200/mother-baby pair) If mother already receiving antiretroviral rx, consult with HIV/ID specialist.	This is ACTG 076 trial which reduced infection in neonate to **8.3% vs 25.5%** in placebo. Minimal side-effects & no evidence of fetal abnormalities in neonates attributed to drug. None of the mothers breastfed (NEJM 331:1173, 1994).
	For infants born to HIV-infected mother who received no antiretroviral rx during or before delivery: Zidovudine 2 mg/kg po q6h to baby beginning 8–12 hrs after birth for 6 wks.	Observational study of 900 births showed ZDV rx to infant reduced transmission from 30% to 10% (NEJM 339:1409, 1998).
	Suggested regimen for less-developed countries: Nevirapine 200 mg po to mother at onset of labor & a single 2 mg/kg dose to baby within 72 hrs of birth (not FDA-approved indication). (Cost: $4.00/mother-baby pair)	Nevirapine rx reduced HIV transmission to neonate to **8.2%** at birth, **11.9%** by 6–8 wks & **13.1%** by **14–16 wks** compared to ZDV rx given at onset of labor & to baby bid for 1 wk: birth 10.4%, 6–8 wks 21.3%, **14–16 wks 25.1%, 98% of mothers breastfed**. No evidence for drug-associated fetal abnormalities, but follow-up short (Ln 354:795, 1999).
Post-splenectomy bacteremia. Likely agents: Pneumococci, meningococci, H. influenzae type b (also at ↑ risk of fatal malaria, severe babesiosis) (immunization important, see Comments)	Penicillin V: Children—Age: <5 yrs 125 mg po bid, >5 yrs 250 mg po bid; Adults: 250 mg po bid. (Alternatives: Amoxicillin, TMP/SMX) NOTE: Repeat pneumococcal vaccine every 6 years	Daily antimicrobial prophylaxis effective with sickle-cell disease, but should be considered for asplenic children <5 yrs. Also recommended in children and adolescents for 3 yrs post splenectomy. **Adjunct measures for all ages: meningococcal A & C, pneumococcal and Hib vaccines before elective splenectomy.** Some authorities prescribe AM/CL for self-administration with onset of any fever for all ages.
Sexual Exposure		
Sexual assault victim (likely agents and risks, see NEJM 322:713, 1990)	(Ceftriaxone 125 mg IM) + (doxycycline 100 mg bid po x7 d.) + (metronidazole 2 gm po single dose) (NEJM 332: 234, 1995)	Perform bimanual pelvic exam. Examine wet mount for motile sperm. T. vaginalis. Culture for gonococci, chlamydia (if available), syphilis & HIV antibody test. Pregnancy test. Follow-up exam at 2 wks. Repeat STS & serology for HIV at 12 weeks (MMWR 42(RR-14), 1993).
Sexual contacts, likely agents: N. gonorrhoeae, C. trachomatis	[(Ceftriaxone 125 mg IM) + (doxycycline 100 mg bid, po x7 d)] or [(cefixime 400 mg po) + (azithromycin 1.0 gm po), each as single dose]	Be sure to check for syphilis since all regimens may not eradicate incubating syphilis (JID 170:689, 1994).
Syphilis exposure		Rx for exposure within 3 months. Make effort to dx syphilis
Sickle-cell disease. Likely agent: S. pneumoniae (see post-splenectomy, above)	3 mos.–5 yrs: Amoxicillin 125 mg po bid >5 yrs: Penicillin V 250 mg po bid	Start prophylaxis before age 4 mos (Am Acad Ped Red Book 1994, p. 375). Children with SCD should receive vaccines: DTP, OPV, MMR, Hep B, Hib, pneumococcus, influenza ± meningococcal. Treat febrile episodes with ceftriaxone (50 mg/kg IV) (NEJM 329:472,1993).
Transplantation		
Bone marrow	Regimens continue to evolve. Current "standard" regimens include drugs active vs bacteria, fungi, pneumocystis, herpes simplex and CMV (see Comment).	Details of specific drugs and timing of administration vary from one transplant center to another. Representative regimen presented in AnIM 123:205, 1995. Similar regimen for solid organ transplants.
Solid organ transplants: liver, kidney, heart, lung	Range of opportunistic infections and variability in prophylaxis protocols is greater than in bone marrow recipients. Many use TMP/SMX 1 single-strength tab po qd for 4–12 mos. post-transplant. Special concern for CMV infections (see Comment)	For extent of infections, see NEJM 338:1741, 1998. For "optimal" CMV prophylaxis, see Transplantation 61:1279, 1996. Hard to define best regimens, as unethical to use placebo control. Ganciclovir better than acyclovir in prevention of CMV (N Ln 346:69, 1995). Valacyclovir also effective (NEJM 340:1462, 1999).
Wegener's granulomatosis	TMP/SMX 800/160 tab po bid	Reduced relapses of pts in remission [18% (TMP/SMX) vs 40% (placebo)] over 24 months (NEJM 335:16, 1996).

TABLE 15B: SURGICAL ANTIBIOTIC PROPHYLAXIS

Surgical Procedures: To be optimally effective, antibiotics must be started in the interval: 2 hrs before time of surgical incision (NEJM 326:281, 1992). For most procedures the number of doses needed for optimal coverage has not been defined. Current practice is to give a single dose (Ln 344:1547, 1999) although FDA-approved product labeling is often for 2 or more doses. If surgical procedure lasts >3 hrs, intraoperative doses should be given at approx. 3-hr intervals. (Note: The dose/route/durations listed below are for the most part those approved in FDA product labeling. For single dose regimens, the dosage & route are the same.) Preventing hypothermia at surgery appears to be important in preventing postoperative infections (NEJM 334:1209, 1996).

TYPE OF SURGERY	PROPHYLAXIS	COMMENTS
Cardiovascular Surgery Antibiotic prophylaxis in cardiovascular surgery has been proven beneficial only in the following procedures: • Reconstruction of abdominal aorta • Procedures on the leg that involve a groin incision • Any vascular procedure that inserts prosthesis/foreign body • Lower extremity amputation for ischemia • Cardiac surgery (Eur J Clin Microbio Inf Dis 13:1033, 1994)	Cefazolin 1.0 gm IV as a single dose or q8h x1-2 d or cefuroxime 1.5 gm IV as a single dose or q12h for total of 6 gm or vancomycin 1.0 gm IV as single dose	Single injection just before surgery probably as effective as multiple doses. Not recommended for cardiac catheterization. For prosthetic heart valves, customary to stop prophylaxis either after removal of retrosternal drainage catheters or just a 2nd dose after coming off bypass. Vancomycin may be preferable in hospitals with ↑ frequency of MRSA but no coverage for Gm-neg. bacilli, therefore would add cefazolin for groin incisions. A meta-analysis of 7 placebo-controlled randomized studies of antimicrobial prophylaxis for implantation of permanent pacemakers, sig. ↓ in incidence of infection (Circ 97:1796, 1998).
Gastric, Biliary and Colonic Surgery **Gastroduodenal/Biliary** Gastroduodenal, includes percutaneous endoscopic gastrostomy (high-risk only; see Comments)	Cefazolin or cefoxitin or cefotetan or ceftizoxime or cefuroxime 1.5 gm IV as a single dose (some give additional doses q12h x2-3 d). Dosage as with C-section, above, except ceftizoxime 1 gm IV, repeat at 12-24 hrs	Gastroduodenal: High-risk is marked obesity, obstruction, ↓ gastric acid or ↓ GI motility. Biliary: Cephalosporins not active vs enterococci yet clinically effective as prophylaxis in biliary surgery. With cholangitis, treat as infection, not prophylaxis: TC/C 3.1 gm q4-6h IV or PIP/TZ 3.375 gm q6h or 4.5 gm q8h IV) or AM/SB 3.0 gm q4-6h IV. Biliary high-risk: age >70, acute cholecystitis, non-functioning gallbladder, obstructive jaundice or common duct stones.
Biliary, includes laparoscopic cholecystectomy (high-risk only, see Comments) Endoscopic retrograde cholangiopancreatography Controversial: No benefit from single dose piperacillin in randomized placebo-controlled trial, AnIM 125:442, 1996 (see Comment)	No rx without obstruction. If obstruction: Ciprofloxacin 500 mg-1 gm po 2 hr prior to procedure Ceftizoxime 1.5 gm IV 1 hr prior to procedure Piperacillin 4 gm IV 1 hr prior to procedure	Most studies show that **achieving adequate drainage** will prevent postprocedural cholangitis or sepsis and no further benefit from prophylactic antibiotics. With inadequate drainage antibiotics may be of value. American Society for GI Endoscopy recommends use for known or suspected biliary obstruction. Oral cipro as effective as cephalosporins in 2 studies & less expensive (CID 23:380, 1996).
Colorectal; includes appendectomy		Elective colorectal prep: Pre-op day: (1) 10:00 am 4 L polyethylene glycol electrolyte solution (Colyte, GoLYTELY) po over 2 hr. (2) Clear liquid diet only. (3) 1:00 pm, 2:00 pm and 10:00 pm, neomycin 1 gm + erythro base 1 gm po. (4) NPO after midnight. There are alternative regimens which have been less well studied. GoLYTELY 1-6 pm, then neomycin 2 gm po + metronidazole 2.0 gm po at 7:00 pm and 11:00 pm. Oral regimen as effective as parenteral; parenteral in addition to oral not required. For emergency colorectal surgery, use parenteral. (CID 15 Suppl. 1:S313, 1992).
Elective surgery	Neomycin + erythromycin po (see Comment for dose)	
Emergency surgery	[Cefazolin 1-2 gm IV + metronidazole 0.5 gm IV (single dose)] or cefoxitin or cefotetan 1-2 gm IV	
Ruptured viscus: See Peritoneum, Table 1, page 33	Cefoxitin 2.0 gm IV, then 1.0 gm IV q8h x ≥5 d. (base on clinical signs) or [clindamycin 600 mg IV q6h + gentamicin 1.5 mg/kg IV q8h) x ≥5 d.	Cefazolin 2.0 gm IV (single dose) or clindamycin 600-900 mg IV (single dose) ± gentamicin 1.5 mg/kg IV
Head and Neck Surgery (Ann Otol Rhinol Laryngol 101 Suppl:16, 1992) Antimicrobial prophylaxis in head & neck surgery appears efficacious only for procedures involving oral/pharyngeal mucosa (i.e., laryngeal or pharyngeal tumor). Uncontaminated head & neck surgery does not require prophylaxis.		
Neurosurgical Procedures Clean, non-implant; e.g., craniotomy	Cefazolin 1.0 gm IV x1. Alternative: vanco 1.0 gm IV x1	Reference: Ln 344:1547, 1994
Clean, contaminated (cross sinuses, or naso/oropharynx)	Clindamycin 900 mg IV (single dose)	British recommend amoxicillin/clavulanate 1.2 gm IV or (cefuroxime 1.5 gm IV + metronidazole 0.5 gm IV)
CSF shunt surgery: controversial (Meta-analysis: CID 17:98, 1993)	Vancomycin 10 mg into cerebral ventricles + gentamicin 3 mg into cerebral ventricles (Ln 344:1547, 1994)	Efficacy when infection rate >15%. Alternative: TMP (160 mg) + SMX (800 mg) IV pre-op and q12h x3 doses

TABLE 15B(2)

TYPE OF SURGERY	PROPHYLAXIS	COMMENTS
atric/Gynecologic Surgery		
...ginal or abdominal hysterectomy	Cefazolin 1–2 gm or cefoxitin 1–2 gm or cefotetan 1–2 gm or cefuroxime 1.5 gm all IV 30 min. before surgery. See Comment NOTE.	1 study found cefotetan superior to cefazolin (CID 20:677, 1995). For prolonged procedures, doses can be repeated q4–8h for duration of procedure. NOTE: Also approved is trovafloxacin 200 mg IV/po 1 to 2 hrs pre-op.
Cesarean section for premature rupture of membranes or active labor	Cefazolin, administer IV as soon as umbilical cord clamped.	
Abortion	1st trimester: high-risk only (see Comments) aqueous pen G 2 mu IV or doxycycline 300 mg po. 2nd trimester: Cefazolin 1 gm IV	High-risk: Pts with previous pelvic inflammatory disease, gonorrhea or multiple sexual partners (Drugs 41:19, 1991).
Orthopedic Surgery (Generally pts with prosthetic joints do not require prophylaxis for dental procedures. Individual considerations prevail (J Am Dental Assn 128G:1004, 1997). See Table 1, p. 24		
Hip arthroplasty,[1] spinal fusion	Same as cardiac	"Customarily stopped after "Hemovac" removed.
Total joint replacement (other than hip)	Cefazolin 1–2 gm IV pre-op (± 2nd dose) or vancomycin 1.0 gm IV on call to OR	Post-op: some would give no further rx (Med Lett 39:98, 1997)
Open reduction of closed fracture with internal fixation	Ceftriaxone 2 gm IV or IM x1 dose	8.3% vs 3.6% (for placebo) reduction found in Dutch trauma trial (Lancet 347:1133, 1996).
Urologic Surgery/Procedures		
	Antimicrobials not recommended in pts with sterile urine. Pts with pre-operative bacteriuria should be treated.	Recommended antibiotic to pts with pre-operative bacteriuria: Cefazolin 1 gm IV q8h x1–3 doses perioperatively, followed by oral antibiotics (nitrofurantoin or TMP/SMX) until catheter is removed or for 10 d.
Transrectal prostate biopsy	Ciprofloxacin 500 mg po 12 hrs prior to biopsy and repeated 12 hrs after biopsy (levo, norflox should work)	Cipro reduced bacteremia from 37% (in gentamicin-rx group) to 7% (Urology 38:84, 1991, and review in JAC 39:115, 1997.
Others		
Breast surgery, herniorrhaphy	P Ceph 1,2, dosage as C-section above	
Traumatic (non-bite) wound	Either cefazolin 1.0 gm IV q8h or ceftriaxone 2.0 gm IV q24h x ≥5 d. (base on clinical signs)	

TABLE 15C: ANTIMICROBIAL PROPHYLAXIS FOR THE PREVENTION OF BACTERIAL ENDOCARDITIS IN PATIENTS WITH UNDERLYING CARDIAC CONDITIONS

[These are the recommendations of the American Heart Association (JAMA 277:1794, 1997). However, a recent population-based retrospective case-controlled study brings into serious question whether dental procedures predispose to endocarditis and whether antibiotic prophylaxis is of any value (see AnIM 129:761, 1998)]

ENDOCARDITIS PROPHYLAXIS RECOMMENDED	ENDOCARDITIS PROPHYLAXIS NOT RECOMMENDED
Cardiac conditions associated with endocarditis	
High-risk conditions:[2] Prosthetic valves—both bioprosthetic and homograft Previous bacterial endocarditis Complex cyanotic congenital heart disease (CHD), e.g., single ventricle, transposition, tetralogy of Fallot Surgically constructed systemic pulmonic shunts or conduits **Moderate-risk conditions:** Most other CHD; hypertrophic cardiac myopathy; mitral prolapse with regurgitation	Negligible-risk (same as general population): Atrial septal defect or repaired ASD/VSD, or PDA (beyond 6 months) Previous CABG, mitral prolapse without MI Physiologic, functional, or innocent heart murmurs Previous Kawasaki or rheumatic fever without valve dysfunction Cardiac pacemakers (all) and implanted defibrillators

[1] Gentamicin (12.5 mg/gm of acrylic bone cement) is released for at least 3 weeks. Usefulness not proven.

[2] Some now recommend that prophylaxis prior to dental procedures should **only** be used for **extractions** and **gingival surgery** (including implant replacement) and **only** for patients with **prosthetic cardiac valves** or **previous endocarditis** (AnIM 129:829, 1998). If any of these 4 conditions exist = prophylactic antibiotics according to American Heart Association are recommended.

TABLE 15C(2)

ENDOCARDITIS PROPHYLAXIS RECOMMENDED	ENDOCARDITIS PROPHYLAXIS NOT RECOMMENDED

Dental and other procedures where prophylaxis is considered for patients with moderate- or high-risk cardiac conditions

Dental: Extractions, periodontal procedures[1]	Dental: Filling cavities with local anesthetic
implants, root canal, subgingival antibiotic fibers/strips	Rubber dams, suture removal, orthodontic removal
Initial orthodontic bands (not brackets); intraligamentary local anesthetic	Orthodontic adjustments, dental x-rays
Cleaning of teeth/implants if bleeding anticipated	Shedding of primary teeth
Respiratory: T&A, surgery on respiratory mucosa, rigid bronchoscopy	Respiratory: Intubation, flexible bronchoscopy[2], tympanostomy tube
GI: Sclerotherapy of esophageal varices; dilation of esophageal stricture; ERCP with	Transesophageal cardiac ECHO[2], EGD without biopsy[2]
biliary obstruction	GU: Vaginal hysterectomy[2], vaginal delivery[2], C-section
GU: Biliary tract surgery; surgery on/through intestinal mucosa	If uninfected; Foley catheter, uterine D&C, therapeutic abortion, tubal ligation, insert/remove IUD
Prostate surgery; cystoscopy; urethral dilatation	Other: Cardiac cath, angioplasty, implanted pacemaker, defibrillators, coronary stents
	Skin biopsy, circumcision

Abbreviations: ***CHD*** = cyanotic heart disease, ***T&A*** = tonsillectomy/adenoidectomy, ***ERCP*** = endoscopic retrograde cholangiography, ***ASD/VSD*** = atrial septal defect/ventricular septal defect, ***PDA*** = patent ductus arteriosus, ***EGD*** = esophagogastroduodenostomy, ***D&C*** = dilation and curettage

PROPHYLACTIC REGIMENS FOR DENTAL, ORAL, RESPIRATORY TRACT, OR ESOPHAGEAL PROCEDURES

SITUATION	AGENT	REGIMEN[3]
Standard general prophylaxis	Amoxicillin	Adults: 2.0 gm; children 50 mg/kg orally 1 hr before procedure
Unable to take oral medications	Ampicillin	Adults: 2.0 gm IM or IV; children 50 mg/kg IM or IV within 30 min. before procedure
Allergic to penicillin	Clindamycin OR	Adults: 600 mg; children 20 mg/kg orally 1 hr before procedure
	(Cephalexin[4] or cefadroxil[4]) OR	Adults: 2.0 gm; children 50 mg/kg orally 1 hr before procedure
	Azithromycin or clarithromycin	Adults: 500 mg; children 15 mg/kg orally 1 hr before procedure
Allergic to penicillin and unable to take oral medications	Clindamycin OR	Adults: 600 mg; children 20 mg/kg IV within 30 min. before procedure
	Cefazolin[4]	Adults: 1.0 gm; children 25 mg/kg IM or IV within 30 min. before procedure

PROPHYLACTIC REGIMENS FOR GENITOURINARY/GASTROINTESTINAL (EXCLUDING ESOPHAGEAL) PROCEDURES[5]

SITUATION	AGENT[2]	REGIMEN
High-risk patients	Ampicillin + gentamicin	Adults: ampicillin 2.0 gm IM or IV + gentamicin 1.5 mg/kg (not to exceed 120 mg) within 30 min. of starting the procedure; 6 hr later, ampicillin 1 gm IM/IV or amoxicillin 1 gm orally
		Children: ampicillin 50 mg/kg IM or IV (not to exceed 2.0 gm) + gentamicin 1.5 mg/kg within 30 min. of starting the procedure; 6 hrs later, ampicillin 25 mg/kg IM/IV or amoxicillin 25 mg/kg orally
High-risk patients allergic to ampicillin/amoxicillin	Vancomycin + gentamicin	Adults: vancomycin 1.0 gm IV over 1–2 hrs + gentamicin 1.5 mg/kg IV/IM (not to exceed 120 mg); complete injection/infusion within 30 min. of starting the procedure
		Children: vancomycin 20 mg/kg IV over 1–2 hrs + gentamicin 1.5 mg/kg IV/IM; complete injection/ infusion within 30 min. of starting the procedure
Moderate-risk patients	Amoxicillin or ampicillin	Adults: amoxicillin 2.0 gm orally 1 hr before procedure, or ampicillin 2.0 gm IM/IV within 30 min. of starting the procedure
		Children: amoxicillin 50 mg/kg orally 1 hr before procedure, or ampicillin 50 mg/kg IM/IV within 30 min. of starting the procedure
Moderate-risk patients allergic to ampicillin/ amoxicillin	Vancomycin	Adults: vancomycin 1.0 gm IV over 1–2 hrs; complete infusion within 30 min. of starting the procedure
		Children: vancomycin 20 mg/kg IV over 1–2 hrs; complete infusion within 30 min. of starting the procedure

[1] Some now recommend that prophylaxis prior to dental procedures should **only** be used for **extractions** and **gingival surgery** (including implant replacement) and **only** for patients with **prosthetic cardiac valves** or **previous endocarditis** (*An/M 129:829, 1998*). If any of these 4 conditions exist = prophylactic antibiotics according to American Heart Association are recommended.

[2] Prophylaxis optional for high-risk patients

[3] Total children's dose should not exceed adult dose

[4] Cephalosporins should not be used in individuals with immediate-type hypersensitivity reaction (urticaria, angioedema, or anaphylaxis) to penicillins.

[5] No second dose of vancomycin or gentamicin is recommended.

TABLE 16: PEDIATRIC DOSAGES OF SELECTED ANTIBACTERIAL AGENTS
[Adapted from both: (1) Nelson's Pocket Book of Pediatric Antimicrobial Therapy, 2000-2001, 14th Ed., J Nelson & J. Bradley, eds., Lippincott Williams and Wilkins, and (2) 1997 Red Book, 24th Ed., American Academy of Pediatrics, pages 607-636]

DRUG	BODY WEIGHT <2000 gm		BODY WEIGHT >2000 gm		>28 DAYS OLD
	0–7 days old	8–28 days old	0–7 days old	8–28 days old	
Aminoglycosides, IV or IM					
Amikacin	7.5 q18–24h	7.5 q12h	10 q12h	10 q12h	10 q8h
Gent/tobra	2.5 q18–24h	2.5 q12h	2.5 q12h	2.5 q12h	2.5 q8h
Aztreonam, IV	30 q12h	30 q8h	30 q8h	30 q6h	30 q6h
Cephalosporins					
Cefaclor					20–40 mg div tid
Cefadroxil					30 div bid (max 2 g/d)
Cefazolin	20 q12h	20 q12h	20 q12h	20 q8h	20 q8h
Cefepime					150 div q8h
Cefixime					8 as qd or div bid
Cefotaxime	50 q12h	50 q8h	50 q12h	50 q8h	50 q6h (75 q6h for meningitis)
Cefoxitin			20 q12h		80–160 div q6h
Cefpodoxime					10 div bid (max 400 mg/d)
Cefprozil					15–30 div bid (max 1 g/d)
Ceftazidime	50 q12h	50 q8h	50 q8h	50 q8h	50 q8h
Ceftibuten					4.5 bid
Ceftizoxime					33–66 q8h
Ceftriaxone	50 qd	50 qd	50 qd	75 qd	50–75 qd (meningitis 100)
Cefuroxime IV	50 q12h	50 q8h	50 q12h	50 q8h	50 q8h (80 q8h for meningitis)
po					10–15 bid (max 1 g/d)
Cephalexin					25–50 4x/d (max 4 g/d)
Loracarbef					15–30 div bid (max 0.8 g/d)
Chloramphen. IV					12.5–25 q6h (max 2–4 g/d
Clindamycin IV	5 q12h	5 q8h	5 q8h	5 q6h	7.5 q6h
po					5–6 q8h
Ciprofloxacin po[2]					20–30 div bid (max 1.5 g/d)
Imipenem[3] IV			25 q12h	25 q8h	15–25 q6h (max 2 g/d)
Macrolides					
Erythro IV & po	10 q12h	10 q8h	10 q12h	13 q8h	10 q6h
Azithro po					10–12 day 1, then 5/d[4]
Clarithro po					7.5 q12h (max. 1 g/d)
Meropenem IV					60–120 div q8h (120 for meningitis)
Metro IV & po	7.5 q24h	7.5 q12h	7.5 q12h	15 q12h	7.5 q6h
Penicillins					
Ampicillin	50 q12h	50 q8h	50 q8h	50 q6h	50 q6h
Amp-sulbactam					100–300 div q6h
Amoxicillin po			30 div bid		25–50 div tid
Amox-Clav po					For 875/125 formulation:45 div bid
Cloxacillin					50–100 div 4x/d
Dicloxacillin					12–25 div 4x/d
Mezlocillin	75 q12h	75 q8h	75 q12h	75 q8h	75 q6h
Nafcillin,oxacillin IV	25 q12h	25 q8h	25 q8h	37 q6h	37 q6h
Piperacillin, PIP/tazo IV					100–300 div q4–6h
Ticarcillin,T.clav IV	75 q12h	75 q8h	75 q8h	75 q6h	75 q6h
Penicillin G IV	50,000 u q12h	75,000 u q8h	50,000 u q8h	50,000 q q6h	50,000 q6h
Penicillin V					25–50 div 3–4x/d
Rifampin po			10, single dose	20, single dose	20, single dose (max. 600 mg)
Sulfisoxazole po				120–150	120–150/d div. q4–6h
TMP/SMX po,IV; UTI: 8–12 TMP component div bid; Pneumocystis: 20 TMP component div 4x/d					
Tetracycline po (age 8 or older)					25–50 4x/d
Doxycycline po,IV (age 8 or older)					2–4 div bid
Vancomycin IV					40–60 div q6h

Abbreviations: **Chloramphen** = chloramphenicol; **Clav** = clavulanate; **div** = divided; **Gent/tobra** = gentamicin/tobramycin; **Metro** = metronidazole; **Tazo** = tazobactam; **TMP** = trimethoprim; **TMP/SMX** = trimethoprim/sulfamethoxazole; **UTI** = urinary tract infection

[1] May need higher doses in patients with meningitis
[2] With exception of cystic fibrosis, not approved for use under age 18.
[3] recommended in children with CNS infections due to risk of seizures.
[4] for otitis; for pharyngitis, 12 mg/kg x5 d.

TABLE 17
DOSAGE OF ANTIMICROBIAL DRUGS IN ADULT PATIENTS WITH RENAL IMPAIRMENT

Adapted from DRUG PRESCRIBING IN RENAL FAILURE, 4th Ed. Aronoff et al (Eds.), American College of Physicians, 1999 and Berns et al, Renal Aspects of Antimicrobial Therapy for HIV Infection. In: P. Kenimel & J. Berns, Eds., HIV INFECTION AND THE KIDNEY, Churchill-Livingstone, 1995, pp 195–236.
UNLESS STATED, ADJUSTED DOSES ARE % OF DOSE OF NORMAL RENAL FUNCTION.

Drug adjustments are based on the patient's estimated endogenous creatinine clearance, which can be calculated as:

$$\frac{(140-age)(ideal\ body\ weight\ in\ kg)}{(72)(serum\ creatinine,\ mg/dL)}\ \text{for men (x 0.85 for women)}$$

| Ideal body weight for men: | 50.0 kg + 2.3 kg per inch over 5 feet |
| Ideal body weight for women: | 45.5 kg + 2.3 kg per inch over 5 feet |

NOTE: For the following drugs, **there is no need for adjustment of dosage** in patients with renal impairment: **amphotericin B, amprenavir, azithromycin, ceftriaxone, chloramphenicol, clindamycin, delavirdine, dirithromycin, doxycycline, minocycline, moxifloxacin, nafcillin, pyrimethamine, rifabutin, rifapentine, trovafloxacin**

ANTIMICROBIAL	HALF-LIFE (NORMAL/ESRD) hr	DOSE FOR NORMAL RENAL FUNCTION[5]	METHOD* (see footnote)	ADJUSTMENT FOR RENAL FAILURE Estimated creatinine clearance (CrCl), ml/min			SUPPLEMENT FOR HEMODIALYSIS, CAPD	COMMENTS AND DOSAGE FOR CAVH
				>50–90	10–50	<10		
ANTIBACTERIAL ANTIBIOTICS								
Aminoglycoside Antibiotics:			Traditional multiple daily doses—adjustment for renal disease					
Amikacin	1.4–2.3/17–150	7.5 mg/kg q12h	D&I	60–90% q12h	30–70% q12–18h **Dose for CAVH[1]**	20–30% q24–48h	HEMO: ⅔ normal dose AD[2] CAPD: 15–20 mg lost/L dialysate/day¶ (see Comment)	High flux hemodialysis membranes lead to unpredictable aminoglycoside clearance, measure post-dialysis drug levels for efficacy and toxicity. With CAPD, pharmacokinetics highly variable— check serum levels. ¶Usual method for CAPD: 2 liters of dialysis fluid placed q.id or 8 liters/day (give 8Lx20 mg lost/L = 160 mg of amikacin supplement IV per day). Adjust dosing weight for obesity: [ideal body weight + 0.4(actual body weight – ideal body weight)] (CID 25:112, 1997).
Gentamicin, Tobramycin	2–3/20–60	1.7 mg/kg q8h	D&I	60–90% q8–12h	30–70% q12h **Dose for CAVH[1]**	20–30% q24–48h	HEMO: ⅔ normal dose AD[2] CAPD: 3–4 mg lost/L dialysate/day	
Netilmicin	2–3/35–72	2.0 mg/kg q8h	D&I	50–90% q8–12h	20–60% q12h **Dose for CAVH[1]**	10–20% q24–48h	HEMO: ⅔ normal dose AD[2] CAPD: 3–4 mg lost/L dialysate/day	
Streptomycin	2–3/30–80	15 mg/kg (max. of 1.0 gm) q24h	I	50% q24h	q24–72h **Dose for CAVH[1]**	q72–96h	HEMO: ½ normal dose AD[2] CAPD: 20–40 mg lost/L dialysate/day	

ONCE-DAILY AMINOGLYCOSIDE THERAPY: ADJUSTMENT IN RENAL INSUFFICIENCY (see Table 9C for OD dosing/normal renal function)

Creatinine Clearance (ml/min.)	>80	60–80	40–60	30–40	20–30	10–20	<10
Drug		Dose q24h (mg/kg)			Dose q48h (mg/kg)		
Gentamicin/Tobramycin	5.1	4	3.5	2.5	4	3	2
Amikacin/kanamycin/streptomycin	15	12	7.5	4	7.5	8 q72h	8 q96h
Isepamicin[NUS]	8	8	8	8 q48h	8	2.5	2.0
Netilmicin	6.5	5	4	2	3		

Carbapenem Antibiotics								
Imipenem (see Comment)	½	0.5 gm q6h	D&I	250–500 mg q6–8h	250 mg q6–12h **Dose for CAVH**	125–250 mg q12h	HEMO: 250 mg AD + q12h CAPD: Dose for CrCl <10	↑ potential for seizures if recommended doses exceeded in pts with CrCl <20 ml/min. See package insert, esp. for pts <70 kg
Meropenem	1/6–8	1.0 gm q8h	D&I	1.0 gm q8h	1.0 gm q12h **Dose for CAVH**	0.5 gm q24h	HEMO: Dose AD CAPD: Dose for CrCl <10	

[1] **CAVH** = continuous arteriovenous hemofiltration (NEJM 336:1303, 1997); [2] **AD** = after dialysis; give dose under CrCl <10 ml/min after dialysis. See page 125 for other footnotes and abbreviations.

TABLE 17 (2)

ANTIMICROBIAL	HALF-LIFE (NORMAL/ESRD) hr	DOSE FOR NORMAL RENAL FUNCTION[3]	METHOD* (see footnote)	ADJUSTMENT FOR RENAL FAILURE — Estimated creatinine clearance (CrCl), ml/min >50-90	10-50	<10	SUPPLEMENT FOR HEMODIALYSIS, CAPD	COMMENTS AND DOSAGE FOR CAVH
Cephalosporin Antibiotics: DATA ON SELECTED PARENTERAL CEPHALOSPORINS								
Cefazolin	1.9/40-70	1.0-2.0 gm q8h	I	q8h	q12h **Dose for CAVH**	q24-48h	HEMO: 0.5-1.0 gm AD; CAPD: 0.5 gm q12h	
Cefepime	2.2/18	2.0 gm q12h	I	q12h	q16-24h	q24-48h	HEMO: 1 gm AD; CAPD: 1-2 gm q48h	CAVH not recommended
Cefotaxime, Ceftizoxime	1.7/15-35	2.0 gm q8h	I	q8-12h	q12-24h **Dose for CAVH**	q24h	HEMO: 1 gm AD; CAPD: 0.5-1 gm qd	Active metabolite of cefotaxime in ESRD. Reduce dose further for hepatic and renal failure.
Cefotetan	3.5/13-25	1-2 gm q12h	D	100%	50%	25%	HEMO: 1 gm AD; CAPD: 1 gm qd	CAVH: 750 mg q12h
Cefoxitin	0.8/13-23	2.0 gm q8h	I	q8h	q8-12h **Dose for CAVH**	q24-48h	HEMO: 1 gm AD; CAPD: 1 gm qd	May falsely increase serum creatinine by interference with assay.
Ceftazidime	1.2/13-25	2 gm q8h	I	q8-12h	q24-48h **Dose for CAVH**	q48h	HEMO: 1 gm AD; CAPD: 0.5 gm qd	Volume of distribution increases with infection.
Cefuroxime sodium	1.2/17	0.75-1.5 gm q8h	I	q8h	q8-12h	q24h	HEMO: Dose AD[2]; CAPD: Dose for CrCl <10	For CAVH: 1.5 gm, then 750 mg IV q24h
Fluoroquinolone Antibiotics								
Ciprofloxacin	4/6-9	500-750 mg po (or 400 mg IV) q12h	D	100%	50-75%	50%	HEMO: 250 mg po or 200 mg IV q12h; CAPD: 250 mg po or 200 mg IV q8h	CAVH: 200 mg IV q12h
Gatifloxacin	7-14/36	400 mg po/IV q24h	D	400 mg q24h	200 mg q24h	200 mg q24h	HEMO: 200 mg q24h AD; CAPD: 200 mg q24h	CAVH: As for CrCl 10-50
Levofloxacin	4-8/76	500 mg qd IV, PO	D[1]	100%	50%	25-50%	HEMO/CAPD: Dose for CrCl <10	CAVH: No data
Ofloxacin	7.0/28-37	400 mg po/IV q12h	D&I	100%	50% q12h	50% q24h	HEMO: 100 mg bid; CAPD: Dose for CrCl <10	CAVH: 300 mg/d
Sparfloxacin	15-20/38.5	400 mg day 1, then 200 mg qd	D&I	100%	50-75%	50% q48h	HEMO: Dose for CrCl <10; CAPD/CAVH: No data	
Macrolide Antibiotics								
Clarithromycin	5-7/22	0.5-1.0 gm q12h	D	100%	75%	50-75%	HEMO: Dose AD[2]; CAPD: None	ESRD dosing recommendations based on extrapolation
Erythromycin	1.4/5-6	250-500 mg q6h	D	100%	100%	50-75%	HEMO/CAPD/CAVH: None	Ototoxicity with high doses in ESRD. Vol. of distribution increases in ESRD.

1 Regardless of CrCl, 1st dose is 500 mg, and then adjust dose and interval

2 **AD** = after dialysis; give dose as for CrCl <10 ml/min after dialysis. **CAVH** = continuous arteriovenous hemofiltration. *See page 125 for other footnotes and abbreviations*

TABLE 17 (3)

ANTIMICROBIAL	HALF-LIFE (NORMAL/ESRD) hr	DOSE FOR NORMAL RENAL FUNCTION	METHOD* (see footnote)	ADJUSTMENT FOR RENAL FAILURE Estimated creatinine clearance (CrCl), ml/min			SUPPLEMENT FOR HEMODIALYSIS, CAPD	COMMENTS AND DOSAGE FOR CAVH
				>50-90	10-50	<10		
Miscellaneous Antibacterial Antibiotics								
Metronidazole	6-14/7-21	7.5 mg/kg q6h	D	100%	100% **Dose for CAVH**	50%	HEMO: Dose AD[2] CAPD: Dose for CrCl <10	Hemo clears metronidazole and its metabolites (AAC 29:235, 1986)
Sulfamethoxa-zole	10/20-50	1.0 gm q8h	I	q12h	q18h **Dose for CAVH**	q24h	HEMO: 1 gm AD CAPD: 1 gm qd	
Teicoplanin[NUS]	45/62-230	6 mg/kg/day	I	q24h	q48h **Dose for CAVH**	q72h	HEMO: Dose for CrCl <10 CAPD: Dose for CrCl <10	
Trimethoprim	11/20-49	100-200 mg q12h	I	q12h	q18h	q24h	HEMO: Dose AD CAPD: q24h	CAVH: q18h
Vancomycin[1]	6/200-250	1 gm q12h	D&I	1 gm q12h	1 gm q24-96h	1 gm q4-7 d.	HEMO/CAPD: 1.0 gm q1 wk	CAVH: 500 mg q24-48h. New hemo-dialysis membranes ↑ clear. of vanco; check levels
Penicillins								
Amoxicillin Ampicillin	1.0/5-20 1.0/7-20	250-500 mg q8h 250 mg-2 gm q6h	I I	q8h q6h	q8-12h q6-12h	q24h q12-24h	HEMO: Dose AD[2] CAPD: 250 mg q12h	IV amoxicillin not available in the U.S.
Aztreonam	2.0/6-8	2 gm q8h	D	100%	50-75% **Dose for CAVH**	25%	HEMO: 0.5 gm AD CAPD: Dose for CrCl <10	Technically is a β-lactam antibiotic.
Mezlocillin	1.1/2.6-5.4	1.5-4.0 gm q4-6h	I	q4-6h	q6-8h	q8h	HEMO/CAPD/CAVH: None	1.9 mEq sodium/gm. Reduce dose further for liver and kidney disease.
Penicillin G	0.5/6-20	0.5-4 million U q4h	D	100%	75% **Dose for CAVH**	20-50%	HEMO: Dose AD as for CrCl <10 CAPD: Dose for CrCl <10	1.7 mEq potassium/mU. ↑ potential for seizures. 6 mU/d upper limit dose in ESRD.
Piperacillin	1.0/3.3-5.1	3-4 gm q4-6h	I	q4-6h	q6-8h **Dose for CAVH**	q8h	HEMO: Dose AD as for CrCl <10 CAPD: Dose for CrCl <10	1.9 mEq sodium/gm
Pip (P)/Tazo(T)	1.0 P/1.0 T 3.0 P/4.0 T	3.375 gm q6h	D&I	3.375 gm q6h	2.25 gm q8h	2.25 gm q8h	HEMO: Dose for CrCl <10 + 0.75 gm AD CAPD: Dose for CrCl <10	
Ticarcillin	1.2/13	3 gm q4h	D&I	1-2 gm q4h	1-2 gm q8h **Dose for CAVH**	1-2 gm q12h	HEMO: 3.0 gm AD CAPD: Dose for CrCl <10	5.2 mEq sodium/gm
Ticarcillin/Clavulanate	1.0 (TC)/1.0(CL) 13 (TC)/4.0 (CL)	3.1 gm q4h	D&I	3.1 gm q4h	2.0 gm q4-8h	2.0 gm q12h	HEMO: CrCl <10 + 3.1 gm AD CAPD: 3.1 gm q12h	

[1] Vancomycin serum levels may be overestimated in renal failure if measured by either fluorescence polarization immunoassay or radioimmunoassay; vanco breakdown products interfere. EMIT method OK.

[2] **AD** = after dialysis; give dose as for CrCl <10 ml/min after dialysis. **CAVH** = continuous arteriovenous hemofiltration. *See page 125 for other footnotes and abbreviations*

TABLE 17 (4)

ANTIMICROBIAL	HALF-LIFE (NORMAL/ESRD) hr	DOSE FOR NORMAL RENAL FUNCTION[§]	METHOD* (see footnote)	ADJUSTMENT FOR RENAL FAILURE Estimated creatinine clearance (CrCl), ml/min			SUPPLEMENT FOR HEMODIALYSIS, CAPD	COMMENTS AND DOSAGE FOR CAVH
				>50-90	10-50	<10		
Tetracycline Antibiotics								
Tetracycline	6-10/57-108	250-500 mg qid	I	q8-12h	q12-24h	q24h	HEMO/CAPD/CAVH: None	Avoid in ESRD
ANTIFUNGAL ANTIBIOTICS								
Amphotericin B	24/unchanged	Non-lipid: 0.4-1.0 mg/kg/d; ABCC:[1] 3-6 mg/kg/d; ABLC:[1] 5 mg/kg/d; LAB:[1] 3-5 mg/kg/d	I	q24h	q24h	q24-48h	HEMO: None CAPD: Dose for CrCl <10	Toxicity lessened by saline loading; risk amplified by concomitant cyclosporine A, aminoglycosides, or pentamidine
Fluconazole	37/100	100-400 mg q24h	I	q24h	q24-48h Dose for CAVH	q48-72h	HEMO: 200 mg AD CAPD: Dose for CrCl <10	
Flucytosine	3-6/75-200	37.5 mg/kg q6h	I	q12h	q12-24h Dose for CAVH	q24h	HEMO: Dose AD[2] CAPD: 0.5-1.0 gm q24h	Goal is peak serum level >25 μg/ml and <100 μg/ml
Itraconazole	21/25	100-200 mg q12h	I	q12h	q12h	q12-24h	HEMO/CAPD/CAVH: 100 mg q12-24h	
Terbinafine	36-200/?	250 mg po/day	–	q24h	Use has not been studied. Recommend avoidance of drug.			
ANTIPARASITIC ANTIBIOTICS								
Pentamidine	29/118	4 mg/kg/d	I	q24h	q24-36h	q48h	HEMO/CAPD/CAVH: None	
Quinine	5-16/5-16	650 mg q8h	I	650 mg q8h	650 mg q8-12h Dose for CAVH	650 mg q24h	HEMO: Dose AD[2] CAPD: Dose for CrCl <10	Marked tissue accumulation
ANTITUBERCULOUS ANTIBIOTICS *(Excellent review: Nephron 64:169, 1993)*								
Ethambutol	4/7-15	15-25 mg/kg q24h	I	q24h Dose for CAVH	q24-36h	q48h	HEMO: Dose AD[2] CAPD: Dose for CrCl <10	25 mg/kg 4-6 hr prior to dialysis for usual 3x/week dialysis. Streptomycin recommended in lieu of ethambutol in renal failure.
Ethionamide	2.1/?	250-500 mg q12h	D	100%	100%	50%	HEMO/CAPD/CAVH: None	
Isoniazid	0.7-4/8-17	5 mg/kg/d (max. 300 mg)	D	100%	100%	100%	HEMO: Dose AD[2] CAPD/CAVH: Dose for CrCl <10	
Pyrazinamide	9/26	25 mg/kg q24h (max. dose 2.5 gm qd)	D	25 mg/kg q24h	25 mg/kg q24h	12-25 mg/kg q24h	HEMO: 40 mg/kg 24 hrs prior to each 3x/wk dialysis CAPD: No reduction; CAVH: No data	
Rifampin	1.5-5/1.8-11	600 mg/d	D	600 mg q24h	300-600 mg q24-48h	300-600 mg q48h	HEMO: None CAPD/CAVH: Dose for CrCl <10	Biologically active metabolite
ANTIVIRAL AGENTS								
Acyclovir, IV	2.5/20	5-12.4 mg/kg q8h	D&I	5-12.4 mg/kg q8h	5-12.4 mg/kg q12-24h	2.5 mg/kg q24h	HEMO: Dose AD[2] CAPD: Dose for CrCl <10	Rapid IV infusion can cause renal failure. CAVH: 3.5 mg/kg/d
Amantadine	12/500	100 mg po bid	I	q24-48h	q48-72h	q7d	HEMO/CAPD/CAVH: None	

[1] ABCC = ampho B cholesteryl complex; ABLC = ampho B lipid complex; LAB = liposomal ampho B

[2] AD = after dialysis; give dose as for CrCl <10 ml/min after dialysis. CAVH = continuous arteriovenous hemofiltration. *See page 125 for other footnotes and abbreviations*

TABLE 17 (5)

ANTIMICROBIAL	HALF-LIFE (NORMAL/ESRD) hr	DOSE FOR NORMAL RENAL FUNCTION§	METHOD* (see footnote)	ADJUSTMENT FOR RENAL FAILURE Estimated creatinine clearance (CrCl), ml/min >50-90	10-50	<10	SUPPLEMENT FOR HEMODIALYSIS, CAPD	COMMENTS AND DOSAGE FOR CAVH
ANTIVIRAL AGENTS *(continued)*								
Cidofovir: Complicated dosing—see package insert								
Induction	2.5/unknown	5 mg/kg 1x/wk for 2 wks	—	5 mg/kg 1x/wk	0.5-2 mg/kg 1x/wk	0.5 mg/kg 1x/wk	No data	Major toxicity is renal. No efficacy, safety, or pharmacokinetic data in pts with moderate/severe renal disease.
Maintenance	2.5/unknown	5 mg/kg q2wks	—	5 mg/kg q2wks	0.5-2 mg/kg q2wks	0.5 mg/kg q2wks	No data	
Didanosine tablets	0.6-1.6/4.5	125-200 mg q12h	D	200 mg q12h	200 mg q24h	150 mg q24h	HEMO: Dose AD†; CAPD/CAVH: Dose for CrCl <10	Based on incomplete data. Data are estimates.
Famciclovir	1.6-2.9/10-22	500 mg q8h	D&I	500 mg q8h	500 mg q12-48h	250 mg q48h	HEMO: 250 mg AD; CAPD: No data	CAVH: Dose for CrCl 10-50
Foscarnet (CMV dosage) Dosage adjustment based on est. CrCl (ml/min) div. by pt's kg	Normal half-life (T½) 3 hrs with terminal T½ of 18-88 hrs. T½ very long with ESRD	Induction: 60 mg/kg q8h x2-3 wks IV; Maintenance: 90-120 mg/kg/d IV	*CrCl as ml/min/kg body weight—ONLY FOR FOSCARNET* >1.4 — Induction: 60 q8h; Maintenance: 120 q24h	>1.0-1.4 — Ind: 45 q8h; Maint: 90 q24h	>0.8-1.0 — Ind: 50 q12h; Maint: 65 q24h	>0.6-0.8 — Ind: 40 q12h; Maint: 105 q48h	>0.5-0.6 — Ind: 60 q24h; Maint: 80 q48h. >0.4-0.5 — Ind: 50 q24h; Maint: 65 q48h. <0.4 — Do not use	See package insert for further details
Ganciclovir IV:	2.9/30	Induction 5 mg/kg q12h IV	D&I	5 mg/kg q12h	1.25-2.5 mg/kg q24h	1.25 mg/kg 3x/wk	HEMO: Dose AD†; CAPD: Dose for CrCl <10	
		Maintenance 5 mg/kg q24h IV	D&I	2.5-5.0 mg/kg q24h	0.6-1.25 mg/kg q24h	0.625 mg/kg 3x/week	HEMO: 0.6 mg/kg AD; CAPD: Dose for CrCl <10	
po:		1.0 gm tid po	D&I	0.5-1.0 gm tid	0.5-1.0 gm qd	0.5 gm 3x/week	HEMO: 0.5 gm AD	
Indinavir/nelfinavir/nevirapine		No data on influence of renal insufficiency. Less than 20% excreted unchanged in urine. Probably no dose reduction.						
Lamivudine	5-7/15-35	150 mg bid po	D&I	150 mg bid	100-150 mg qd	25-50 mg qd	HEMO: Dose AD†; CAPD/CAVH: No data	
Oseltamivir	1-3/no data	75 mg po bid	I	75 mg q12h	75 mg qd	No data	No data	
Ribavirin	13-65/Prolonged	Use with caution in patients with creatinine clearance <10 ml/min.						
Rimantadine		100 mg bid po	I	100 mg bid	100 mg qd-bid	100 mg qd recommended	HEMO/CAPD: No data	Use with caution, little data
Ritonavir & Saquinavir, SGC		Negligible renal clearance. At present, no patient data — Negligible renal clearance <10 ml/min.						
Stavudine, po	1-1.4/5.5-8	30-40 mg q12h	D&I	100%	50% q12-24h	50% q24h	HEMO: Dose AD†; CAPD: No data	CAVH: Dose for CrCl 10-50
Valacyclovir	2.5/3.3	1.0 gm q8h	D&I	1.0 gm q8h	1.0 gm q12-24h	0.5 gm q24h	HEMO: Dose AD†; CAPD: Dose for CrCl <10	CAVH: No data. Dose for CrCl 10-50
Zalcitabine	2.0/>8	0.75 mg q8h	D&I	0.75 mg q8h	0.75 mg q12h	0.75 mg q24h	HEMO: Dose AD†; CAPD: No data	CAVH: Dose for CrCl 10-50
Zidovudine	1.1-1.4/1.4-3	200 mg q8h or 300 mg q12h	D&I	200 mg q8h or 300 mg q12h	200 mg q8h or 300 mg q12h	100 mg q8h	HEMO: Dose for CrCl <10; CAPD: Dose for CrCl <10	CAVH: 100 mg q8h

† **AD** = Give dose as for CrCl <10 ml/min after dialysis.
§ Dosages are for life-threatening infections; * **D** = dosage reduction, **I** = interval extension; ** Per cent refers to % change from dose for normal renal function.
Abbreviations: HEMO = hemodialysis; **CAPD** = chronic ambulatory peritoneal dialysis; **ESRD** = endstage renal disease; **NUS** = not available in the U.S.

TABLE 18: ANTIBACTERIALS AND HEPATIC DISEASE*

The following alphabetical list indicates antibacterials excreted/metabolized by the liver wherein a dosage adjustment may be indicated in the presence of hepatic disease. Space precludes details; consult the PDR or package inserts for details. List is **not** all-inclusive:

Amprenavir	Efavirenz	Rifabutin
Cefoperazone	Indinavir	Rifampin
Ceftriaxone	Isoniazid	Rimantadine
Chloramphenicol	Metronidazole	Trovafloxacin
Clindamycin	Nafcillin	

Drug info #93, American Hospital Formulary Service Am. Soc. Hosp. Pharm., Bethesda, MD, 1993

TABLE 19: TREATMENT OF CAPD PERITONITIS[1]
Route of administration is intraperitoneal unless otherwise indicated*

DRUG	INTERMITTENT DOSING (Drugs added to 1 bag/day unless indicated)	CONTINUOUS DOSING (mg/L unless indicated)
Aminoglycosides		
Amikacin	2 mg/kg	LD 25, MD 12
Gentamicin/netilmicin/tobramycin	0.6 mg/kg	LD 8, MD 4
Carbapenems		
Imipenem/cilastatin	1 gm bid	LD 500, MD 200
Cephalosporins		
Cefazolin	15 mg/kg	LD 500, MD 125
Cefoxitin	ND	LD 200, MD 100
Cefuroxime	400 mg po or IV/d.	LD 200, MD 100–200
Cefotaxime	2000 mg	LD 500, MD 250
Ceftazidime/ceftizoxime/ceftriaxone	1000 mg	LD 250, MD 125
Penicillins		
Aztreonam	1000 mg	LD 1000, MD 250
Mezlocillin	3000 mg IV bid	LD 3 gm IV, MD 250
Piperacillin	4000 mg IV bid	LD 4 gm IV, MD 250
Ticarcillin	2000 mg IV bid	LD 1–2 gm IV, MD 125
Ampicillin	ND	MD 125 or 250–500 mg po bid
Ampicillin/sulbactam	2 gm q12h	LD 1000, MD 100
Nafcillin	ND	250–500 mg po q12h
Oxacillin	ND	MD 125
Quinolones		
Ciprofloxacin	500 mg po bid	Not recommended
Ofloxacin	400 mg po, then 200 mg po/d.	Not recommended
Other Antibacterials		
Clindamycin	ND	LD 300, MD 150
Erythromycin	500 mg po qid	LD ND, MD 150
Metronidazole	500 mg po/IV tid	ND
Minocycline	100 mg po bid	NA
Rifampin	450–600 mg po/d. or 150 mg IP 3–4 d.	NA
Vancomycin	15–30 mg/kg q5–7 d.	LD 1000, MD 25
Antifungals		
Amphotericin B	NA	1.5
Flucytosine	1 gm po/d.	50/d.
Fluconazole	ND	ND

[1] Adapted from Peritoneal Dialysis International 16:557, 1996, which also includes treatment algorithms.

* OK to mix drugs in dialysis fluid except for aminoglycosides and penicillins.

Abbreviations: LD = loading dose; **MD** = maintenance dose; **NA** = not applicable; **ND** = no data ·

TABLE 20A: RECOMMENDED CHILDHOOD IMMUNIZATION SCHEDULE: UNITED STATES, January-December 1997 (Ref.: MMWR 46:35, 1997)

Vaccines are listed under the routinely recommended ages. Bars ☐ indicate range of acceptable ages for vaccination. Shaded bars ▨ indicate catch-up vaccination: at 11-12 years of age, Hepatitis B vaccine should be administered to previously vaccinated, and Varicella Virus vaccine should be administered to unvaccinated children who lack a reliable history of chickenpox. (For use of vaccine in the immunocompromised host, see CMR 11:1, 1998).

Vaccine ▼ Age ►	Birth	1 mo.	2 mos.	4 mos.	6 mos.	12 mos.	15 mos.	18 mos.	4-6 yrs.	11-12 yrs.	14-16 yrs.
Hepatitis B[1]	Hep B-1	Hep B-1								Hep B	
			Hep B-2	Hep B-2							
					Hep B-3	Hep B-3	Hep B-3				
Diphtheria, Tetanus, Pertussis[2]			DTaP or DTP	DTaP or DTP	DTaP or DTP		DTaP or DTP	DTaP or DTP	DTaP or DTP	Td	
H. Influenzae type b			Hib	Hib	Hib	Hib	Hib				
Polio[3]			Polio[3]	Polio		Polio[3]	Polio[3]	Polio[3]	Polio		
Measles, Mumps, Rubella[4]						MMR	MMR		MMR[4]	MMR[4] or MMR[4]	
Varicella[5]						Var	Var	Var		Var[5]	

Approved by the Advisory Committee on Immunization Practices (ACIP), the American Academy of Pediatrics (AAP), and the American Academy of Family Physicians (AAFP)

Hep B Vaccination Detail (within 12 hrs of birth)

Hep B Status of Mother	Vaccine:	Age 2nd Dose	Age 3rd Dose	HBIG
HBsAg Negative	Merck (Recombivax) 2.5 µg or SKB (Engerix-B) 10 µg	≥1 mo. later	6-18 mos.	None
HBsAg Positive	Merck (Recombivax) 5.0 µg or SKB (Engerix-B) 10 µg	1-2 mos.	6 mos.	0.5 ml within 12 hrs of birth
Unknown	Merck (Recombivax) 5.0 µg or SKB (Engerix-B) 10 µg	1-2 mos.	6 mos.	Depends on results of mother's HBsAg test; if pos, give HBIG before 1 wk of age

1 Infants and Hepatitis B

2 DTaP (diphtheria and tetanus toxoids and acellular pertussis vaccine) preferred to whole-cell DTP vaccine, but whole-cell DTP an acceptable alternative. The 4th dose of DTaP may be administered as early as 12 mos. of age, provided 6 mos. have elapsed since the 3rd dose, and if the child is considered unlikely to return at 15-18 mos. of age. Td (tetanus and diphtheria toxoids, adsorbed, for adult use) is recommended at 11-12 yrs of age if at least 5 yrs have elapsed since the last dose of DTP, DTaP, or DT (Reference: MMWR 46(RR-7), 1997).

3 Two poliovirus vaccines are currently licensed in the U.S.: inactivated poliovirus vaccine (IPV) and oral poliovirus vaccine (OPV). However, for routine immunization IPV is preferred. OPV is no longer recommended except in special circumstances (e.g., a child whose parents do not accept the recommended number of injections or who will be traveling to areas with endemic polio. OPV remains vaccine of choice for mass vaccinations to control outbreaks of wild poliovirus (MMWR 47:1017, 1998).

4 The 2nd dose of MMR is routinely recommended at 4-6 yrs of age or at 11-12 yrs of age, but may be administered during any visit, provided at least 1 mo. has elapsed since receipt of the 1st dose, and that both doses are administered at or after 12 mos. of age.

5 Susceptible children may receive varicella vaccine (Var) during any visit after the 1st birthday, and unvaccinated persons who lack a reliable history of chickenpox should be vaccinated during the 11-12 year-old visit. Susceptible persons ≥13 yrs of age should receive 2 doses, at least 1 mo. apart.

TABLE 20B: ADULT IMMUNIZATION IN THE UNITED STATES[1] (Travelers: see Med Letter 38:17, 1996)

AGE GROUP (years)	VACCINE/TOXOID						
	Td[2]	Measles	Mumps	Rubella	Influenza	Pneumococcal	Hepatitis B[4]
18-24	x	x	x	x			Individuals at ↑ risk regardless of age. See Table 15, page 114 for post-exposure prophylaxis
25-64	x	x[3]	x	x			
≥ 65	x				x	x	

1 From *Guide for Adult Immunization*, 3rd Ed., Am Coll Physicians, 1994. Also see AnIM 12:35, 1996, and IDCP 5:490, 1996.

2 Td = tetanus + diphtheria toxoids, adsorbed, for adult use (contains 5 Fl units tetanus + 2 Fl units diphtheria vs childhood vaccine, which contains 5 Fl u tetanus + 12.5 Fl u diphtheria)

3 Measles vaccine indicated for persons born in 1957 or later. 9% hospital workers born before 1957 are not immune; serotest and immunize especially during outbreaks.

4 Screen all pregnant women for HBsAg (give HBIG and vaccine to infants born to HBsAg-positive mothers). Those at ↑ exposure risk: homosexual males, injecting drug users, multiple partner heterosexual exposure, other sexually transmitted diseases, household and sexual contacts of HBV carriers, health care and public safety workers with exposure to blood, residents and staff of institutions for retarded, hemodialysis patients, recipients of Factor VII or IX concentrates, morticians.

TABLE 20B (2)

ADMINISTRATION SCHEDULE FOR ABOVE PLUS OTHER SELECTED VACCINES[§]

Hepatitis A (Havrix, Vaqta): 1.0 ml IM & repeat in 6–12 mos. Antibodies detectable >15 days; use immune serum globulin 0.02 ml/kg IM for immediate protection. **Indications**: Populations at ↑ risk for HAV infection or the adverse consequences of infection [e.g., travelers to endemic areas, children (≥2 yrs of age) in communities that have high rates of hepatitis A, including U.S. states with high incidence *(NEJM 340:644, 1999)*, men who have sex with men, illegal-drug users, persons with occupational risk for infection, persons who have chronic liver disease or clotting factor disorders] *(Med Ltr 37:51, 1995; IDCP 5:122, 1996; MMWR 45:1, 1996)*. Useful for secondary prevention *(Ln 353:1136, 1999) (see Table 15)*.

Hepatitis B (Engerix B, Recombivax HB): 3 doses; initial, 1 month later, 6 months after 1st. Give IM in deltoid (not in buttocks), use 1½-inch needle; give SC only in pts at risk of bleeding (hemophiliacs). (Seroprotection associated with titers ≥10 mIU/ml.)

Influenza (killed virus): One dose (0.5 ml) IM. Annual reimmunization with current vaccine recommended.

Lyme disease: 3 doses IM in deltoid: initial, 1 month & 12 months later (0.5 ml; 30 μg). Only for persons 15–70 years old who reside, work or recreate in areas of high or moderate risk *(MMWR 48:RR-7, 1999; EID 5:321, 1999)*.

Measles (Attenuvax) (live virus vaccine): Unless contraindicated,[§] one dose (0.5 ml) sc preferably in outer aspect upper arm. Booster not required. Severely immunocompromised patients exposed to measles should receive immunoglobulin prophylaxis regardless of vaccination status because they may not be protected by the vaccine *(MMWR 47:27, 1998)*.

Measles + Rubella + Mumps (MMR) (live virus): Unless contraindicated[§] (do not give to pregnant women), one dose (0.5 ml) sc as with measles. Booster not required.

Pneumococcal (Pneumovax 23, Pnu-Immune 23) (pure antigens, 23): One dose (0.5 ml) sc. For adults—revaccination x1 after 5 yrs: (a) Immunocompetent pts with anatomic/functional asplenia or are **now** >age 65 and (b) immunocompromised persons due to HIV, malignancy, meds, or nephrotic syndrome *[MMWR 46(RR-8), 1997]*.

Rotavirus: Vaccine licensed in U.S. in August 1998 and routine immunization of infants recommended by ACIP. However, because of reports of intussusception among vaccine recipients, CDC has recommended suspending routine rotavirus vaccination pending further review *(MMWR 48:577, 1999)*.

Td (toxoids, not live): Primary: Two doses IM at least 4 wks apart, 3rd dose 6–12 mos after 2nd. Booster every 10 yrs

Typhoid (Typhim Vi): Single IM dose of 25 μg yields 95% seroconversion. Minimal side-effects. For travelers & lab workers.

Varicella (Varivax): 0.5 ml sc and repeat 4–8 wks later. For susceptible adolescents/adults who are: (1) health care worker, (2) susceptible household contact of immunocompromised person, (3) works in schools/day care centers, (4) college student/military, (5) non-pregnant woman of child-bearing age.

§ *Review package insert for specific product being administered.*

TABLE 20C/1: ANTI-TETANUS PROPHYLAXIS, WOUND CLASSIFICATION, IMMUNIZATION

WOUND CLASSIFICATION			IMMUNIZATION SCHEDULE				
Clinical Features	Tetanus Prone	Non-Tetanus Prone	History of Tetanus Immunization	Dirty, Tetanus-Prone Wound		Clean, Non-Tetanus Prone Wound	
				TD[1,2]	TIG	Td	TIG
Age of wound	> 6 hours	≤ 6 hours	Unknown or < 3 doses	Yes	Yes	Yes	No
Configuration	Stellate, avulsion	Linear					
Depth	> 1 cm	≤ 1 cm	3 or more doses	No[3]	No	No[4]	No
Mechanism of injury	Missile, crush, burn, frostbite	Sharp surface (glass, knife)					
Devitalized tissue	Present	Absent					
Contaminants (dirt, saliva, etc.)	Present	Absent					

[1] Td = Tetanus & diphtheria toxoids adsorbed (adult)
TIG = Tetanus immune globulin (human)
[2] Yes if wound >24 hours old.
For children <7 years, DPT (DT if pertussis vaccine contraindicated).
For persons ≥7 years, Td preferred to tetanus toxoid alone.
[3] Yes if >5 years since last booster
[4] Yes if >10 years since last booster

(From ACS Bull. 69:22,23, 1984, No. 10)   *(From MMWR 39:37, 1990; MMWR 46(SS-2):15, 1997)*

TABLE 20C/2: RABIES POST-EXPOSURE PROPHYLAXIS[1]. All wounds should be cleaned immediately and thoroughly with soap and water. This has been shown to protect 90% of experimental animals!

Post-Exposure Prophylaxis Guide, United States, 1991

Animal Type	Evaluation and Disposition of Animal	Recommendations for Prophylaxis
Dogs, cats	Healthy and available for 10-day observation	Don't start unless animal develops sx, then immediately begin HRIG + HDCV or RVA
	Rabid or suspected rabid	Immediate vaccination
	Unknown (escaped)	Consult public health officials
Skunks, raccoons, bats,* foxes, most carnivores	Regard as rabid	Immediate vaccination
Livestock, rodents, rabbits; includes hares, squirrels,, hamsters, guinea pigs, gerbils, chipmunks, rats, mice		Almost never require anti-rabies rx

* Most recent cases of human rabies in U.S. due to contact (not bites) with silver-haired bats or rarely big brown bats *(MMWR 46:770, 1997; AIM 128:922, 1998)*

Post-Exposure Rabies Immunization Schedule (Unvaccinated Persons)

Immunizing Product	Regimen
HRIG[2]	20 IU/kg, if feasible infiltrate ½ of dose around the wound(s), the rest IM in gluteal area. Not in same syringe as vaccine.[3]
Vaccine: HDCV or RVA or PCEC[2] *(Med Lett 40:64, 1998)*	1.0 ml IM in deltoid area (only acceptable site in adults and older children; younger children, outer aspect of thigh) (never in gluteal area). Days 0, 3, 7, 14, 28

[1] From *Morb Mort Wkly Rpt 40:RR-3, 1991 (March 22)*
[2] **HRIG** = Human rabies immune globulin (BayRab, Imogam Rabies); **HDCV** = human diploid cell vaccine, rabies (inactivated) (Imovax Rabies); **RVA** = rabies vaccine absorbed (inactivated), (liquid) (should not be used intradermally); **PCEC** = purified chick embryo cell culture vaccine (RabAvert) *(MMWR 47:12, 1998)*
[3] In most reported post-exposure treatment failures, only identified deficiency was failure to infiltrate wound(s) with HRIG *(CID 22:228, 1996)*. However, several failures reported from SE Asia in patients in whom WHO protocol followed *(CID 28:143, 1999)*.

TABLE 21: ANTI-INFECTIVE DRUG-DRUG INTERACTIONS
Significance/Certainty: ± = theory/anecdotal; + = of probable importance; ++ = of definite importance

ANTI-INFECTIVE AGENT (A)	OTHER DRUG (B)	EFFECT	SIGNIFICANCE/ CERTAINTY
Acyclovir (Zovirax)	Nephrotoxic drugs	Crystalluria of A may aggravate	+
Amantadine (Symmetrel)	Alcohol	↑ CNS effects	+
	Anticholinergic and anti-Parkinson agents (ex. Artane, scopolamine)	↑ effect of B: dry mouth, ataxia, blurred vision, slurred speech, toxic psychosis	+
	Trimethoprim	↑ levels of A & B	+
	Digoxin	↑ levels of B	±
Aminoglycosides— parenteral (amikacin, gentamicin, kanamycin, netilmicin, sisomicin, streptomycin, tobramycin) NOTE: Capreomycin is an aminoglycoside, used as alternative drug to treat mycobacterial infections.	Amphotericin B	↑ nephrotoxicity	++
	Cis platinum (Platinol)	↑ nephro & ototoxicity	+
	Cyclosporine	↑ nephrotoxicity	+
	Neuromuscular blocking agents	↑ apnea or respiratory paralysis	+
	Loop diuretics (e.g., furosemide)	↑ ototoxicity	++
	"Noise"	↑ ototoxicity	+
	NSAIDs	↑ nephrotoxicity	+
	Non-polarizing muscle relaxants	↑ apnea	+
	Radiographic contrast	↑ nephrotoxicity	+
	Vancomycin	↑ nephrotoxicity	+
Aminoglycosides—oral (kanamycin, neomycin)	Oral anticoagulants (dicumarol, phenindione, warfarin)	↑ prothrombin time	+
Amphotericin B and ampho B lipid formulations	Antineoplastic drugs	↑ nephrotoxicity risk	+
	Corticosteroids & ACTH	May potentiate hypokalemia	+
	Digitalis	↑ toxicity of B if K⁺ ↓	+
	Nephrotoxic drugs: aminoglycosides, cidofovir, cyclosporin, foscarnet, pentamidine	↑ nephrotoxicity of A	++
Ampicillin, amoxicillin	Allopurinol	↑ frequency of rash	+
Amprenavir	Rifabutin	↑ levels of B (↓ dose by 50%)	++
	Rifampin	↓ levels of A	++
	Antiretrovirals—see Table 21B		
Atovaquone	Rifampin (perhaps rifabutin)	↓ serum levels of A; ↑ levels of B	+

Azole Antifungal Agents[1] *(Flu = fluconazole, Itr = itraconazole, Ket = ketoconazole, + = occurs, NRS = not reported but not studied)*

Flu	Itr	Ket			
+	NRS	NRS	Amitriptyline	↑ levels of B	+
+	+	+	Antihistaminics, non-sedating[2]	↑ levels of B (cardiac arrhythmias)	++
−	+	−	Carbamazepine	↓ levels of A	+
+	**+**	**+**	**Cisapride**	**↑ levels of B (arrhythmias,↑ Q-T interval)**	**++**
+	+	+	Cyclosporine, tacrolimus	↑ levels of B, ↑ risk of nephrotoxicity	+
NRS	+	+	Didanosine	↓ absorption of A	+
−	+	+	H₂ blockers, antacids, sucralfate	↓ absorption of A	+
+	+	+	Hydantoins (phenytoin, Dilantin)	↑ levels of B, ↓ levels of A	++
−	+	+	Isoniazid	↓ levels of A	+
NRS	+	NRS	Lovastatin/simvastatin	Rhabdomyolysis reported	+
+	+	+	Midazolam/triazolam, po	↑ levels of B	++
+	+	+	Oral anticoagulants	↑ effect of B	++
+	+	NRS	Oral hypoglycemics	↑ levels of B	++
−	+	+	Proton pump inhibitors	↓ absorption of A	+
+	+	+	Rifampin/rifabutin	↑ levels of B, ↓ serum levels of A	+
+	NRS	+	Tacrolimus	↑ levels of B with toxicity	++
+	+	+	Theophyllines	↑ levels of B	+
+	−	NRS	Zidovudine	↑ levels of B	+
Cephalosporins with methyltetrathiozole-thiol side-chain[3]	Oral anticoagulants (dicumarol, warfarin), heparin, thrombolytic agents, platelet aggregation inhibitors	↑ effects of B, bleeding	+
Cefoperazone (Cefobid) Cefamandole (Mandol)	Alcohol	Disulfiram-like reaction (tachycardia, flushing, diarrhea)	+

[1] Major interactions given; unusual or minor interactions manifest as toxicity of non-azole drug due to ↑ serum levels: Caffeine (Flu), digoxin (Itr), felodipine (Itr), fluoxetine (Itr), indinavir (Ket), lovastatin/simvastatin (Ket), quinidine (Ket), tricyclics (Flu), vincristine (Itr), and ↓ effectiveness of oral contraceptives.

[2] Antihistaminics, non-sedating: astemizole, terfenadine, loratadine (less or no azole interactions)

[3] Cefamandole, cefotetan, cefmetazole,ᴺᵁˢ cefoperazone

TABLE 21 (2)

ANTI-INFECTIVE AGENT (A)	OTHER DRUG (B)	EFFECT	SIGNIFICANCE/ CERTAINTY
Chloramphenicol	Hydantoins	↑ toxicity of B, nystagmus, ataxia	++
	Iron salts, Vitamin B12	↓ response to B	++
	Oral anticoagulants	↑ prothrombin time	+
	Sulfonylureas	↑ effect of B, hypoglycemia	+
Clindamycin (Cleocin)	Kaolin	↓ absorption of A	+
	Muscle relaxants, e.g., atracurium, baclofen, diazepam	↑ frequency/duration of respiratory paralysis	+
	Erythromycin	Mutual antagonism	+
Cycloserine	Ethanol	↑ frequency of seizures	+
	INH, ethionamide	↑ frequency of drowsiness/dizziness	+
Dapsone	Didanosine	↓ absorption of A	+
	Oral contraceptives	↓ effectiveness of B	+
	Pyrimethamine	↑ in marrow toxicity	+
	Rifampin/Rifabutin	↓ serum levels of A	+
	Trimethoprim	↑ levels of A & B (methemoglobinemia)	+
	Zidovudine	May ↑ marrow toxicity	+
Delavirdine (Rescriptor)	Alprazolam, midazolam, triazolam	↑ levels of B	++
	Astemizole, terfenadine	↑ levels of B	++
	Cisapride	↑ levels of B	++
	Clarithromycin	↑ levels of B	++
	Dapsone	↑ levels of B	++
	Dihydropyridine Ca^{++} channel blockers	↑ levels of B	++
	Ergot alkaloids	↑ levels of B	++
	Protease inhibitors	↑ levels of B *(see Table 21B)*	++
	Quinidine, rifamycins	↑ levels of B	++
	Warfarin	↑ levels of B	++
Didanosine (ddI) (Videx)	Cisplatin, dapsone, INH, metronidazole, nitrofurantoin, stavudine, vincristine, zalcitabine	↑ risk of peripheral neuropathy	+
	Ethanol, lamivudine, pentamidine	↑ risk of pancreatitis	+
	Fluoroquinolones	↓ absorption 2° to chelation	+
	Low pH drug solubility: dapsone, indinavir, itra/ketoconazole, pyrimethamine, rifampin, trimethoprim	↓ absorption	+
Doxycycline	Aluminum, bismuth, iron, Mg^{++}	↓ absorption of A	+
	Barbiturates, hydantoins	↓ serum t/2 of A	+
	Carbamazepine (Tegretol)	↓ serum t/2 of A	+
	Digoxin	↑ serum levels of B	+
Efavirenz (Sustiva)	Antiretrovirals	*See Table 21B*	
	Rifampin	↓ levels of A	+
Ethambutol (Myambutol)	Aluminum salts (includes didanosine buffer)	↓ absorption of A & B	+

Fluoroquinolones (**Cipro** = ciprofloxacin; **Gati** = gatifloxacin; **Levo** = levofloxacin; **Lome** = lomefloxacin; **Moxi** = moxifloxacin **Norflox** = norfloxacin; **Oflox** = ofloxacin; **Spar** = sparfloxacin; **Trova** = trovafloxacin)

Cipro	Gati	Levo	Lome	Moxi	Norflox	Oflox	Spar	Trova	OTHER DRUG (B)	EFFECT	SIG.
				+*			+		Antiarrhythmics (*procainamide, amiodarone)	↑ Q-T interval (torsade)	++
+							+		Insulin, oral hypoglycemics	↑ & ↓ blood sugar	+
+							+	+	Caffeine	↑ levels of B	+
+		+				+	+		Cimetidine	↑ levels of A	+
+		+				+	+	+	Cyclosporine	↑ levels of B	±
+	+	+	+		+	+	+	+	Didanosine	↓ absorption of A	++
+	+	+	+	+	+	+	+	+	**Cations: Al^{+++}, Ca^{++}[1], Fe^{++}, Mg^{++}, Zn^{++} (antacids, vitamins, dairy products), citrate/citric acid**	↓ absorption of A (some variability between drugs)	++
+									Foscarnet	↑ risk of seizures	+
+		+	+			+	+	+	**NSAIDs**	↑ risk CNS stimulation/seizures	++
+									Phenytoin	↑ or ↓ levels of B	+
+		+				+	+		Probenecid	↓ renal clearance of A	+
+	+	+	+		+	+	+	+	Sucralfate	↓ absorption of A	++
+							+		Theophylline	↑ levels of B	++
+		+	+			+	+		Warfarin	↑ prothrombin time	+

[1] Neither gati nor moxi interacts with Ca^{++}

TABLE 21 (3)

ANTI-INFECTIVE AGENT (A)	OTHER DRUG (B)	EFFECT	SIGNIFICANCE/ CERTAINTY
Foscarnet (Foscavir)	Ciprofloxacin	↑ risk of seizures	+
	Nephrotoxic drugs: aminoglyco-sides, ampho B, cis-platinum, cyclosporine	↑ risk of nephrotoxicity	+
	Pentamidine IV	↑ risk of severe hypocalcemia	++
Ganciclovir (Cytovene)	Imipenem	↑ risk of seizures reported	+
	Probenecid	↑ levels of A	+
	Zidovudine	↓ levels of A, ↑ levels of B	+
Gentamicin	See Aminoglycosides—parenteral		
Indinavir	See protease inhibitors and Table 21B		
Isoniazid	Alcohol, rifampin	↑ risk of hepatic injury	+
	Aluminum salts	↓ absorption (take fasting)	+
	Carbamazepine, phenytoin	↑ levels of B with nausea, vomiting, nystagmus, ataxia	++
	Itraconazole, ketoconazole	↓ levels of B	+
	Oral hypoglycemics	↓ effects of B	+

Macrolides (**Ery** = erythromycin, **Azi** = azithromycin, **Clr** = clarithromycin; **Dir** = dirithromycin, **+** = occurs, **0** = does not occur; **NRS** = not reported but not studied)

Ery	Dir	Azi	Clr			
+	NRS	NRS	+	Carbamazepine	↑ serum levels of B, nystagmus, nausea, vomiting, ataxia	++ (avoid with erythro)
+			+	Cimetidine, ritonavir	↑ levels of A	+
+	NRS	NRS	+	**Cisapride**	**↑ Q-T interval; ↑ risk arrhythmias**	++
+		NRS	NRS	Clozapine	↑ serum levels of B, CNS toxicity	+
+		NRS	NRS	Corticosteroids	↑ effects of B	+
+	+	+	+	Cyclosporine	↑ serum levels of B with toxicity	+
+	NRS	+	+	Digoxin, digitoxin	↑ serum levels of B (10% of cases)	+
			+	Efavirenz	↓ levels of A	++
			+	Ergot alkaloids	↑ levels of B	++
+		NRS		Midazolam, triazolam	↑ levels of B, ↑ sedative effects	+
+			+	Phenytoin	↑ levels of B	+
+	+	+	+	Pimozide	↑ Q-T interval	++
+			+	Rifampin, rifabutin	↓ levels of A	+
+			+	Tacrolimus	↑ levels of B	++
+	0	0	+	**Terfenadine, astemizole**	↑ Q-T interval; ↑ risk of arrhythmias	++
+	0	0	+	Theophyllines	↑ serum levels of B with nausea, vomiting, seizures, apnea	++
+	NRS	NRS	+	Triazolam	↑ levels of B	+
+		NRS	+	Valproic acid	↑ levels of B	+
+	NRS	0	+	Warfarin	May ↑ prothrombin time	+
NRS		0	+	Zidovudine	↓ levels of B	+
Mefloquine				ß-adrenergic blockers, calcium channel blockers, quinidine, quinine	↑ arrhythmias	+
				Divalproex, valproic acid	↓ level of B with seizures	++
Methenamine mandelate or hippurate				Acetazolamide, sodium bicarbonate, thiazide diuretics	↓ antibacterial effect 2° to ↑ urine pH	++
Metronidazole				**Alcohol**	Disulfiram-like reaction	+
				Disulfiram (Antabuse)	Acute toxic psychosis	+
				Oral anticoagulants	↑ anticoagulant effect	++
				Phenobarbital, hydantoins	↑ metabolism of A with ↓ effectiveness	+
Nelfinavir				See protease inhibitors and Table 21B		
Nevirapine (Viramune)				Opiates	↓ levels of B	++
				Protease inhibitors	See Table 21B	
Nitrofurantoin				Antacids	↓ absorption of A	+
Pentamidine, IV				Amphotericin B	↑ risk of nephrotoxicity	+
				Foscarnet	↑ risk of hypocalcemia	+
				Pancreatitis-associated drugs, e.g., alcohol, valproic acid	↑ risk of pancreatitis	+
Piperacillin				Cefoxitin	Antagonism vs pseudomonas	++
Piperazine				Chlorpromazine	Convulsions (occ. fatal)	++
Primaquine				Chloroquine, dapsone, INH, probenecid, quinine, sulfonamides, TMP/SMX, others	↑ risk of hemolysis in G6PD-deficient patients	++

TABLE 21 (4)

Protease Inhibitors—Anti-HIV Drugs. (**Ampren** = amprenavir, **Indin** = indinavir; **Nelfin** = nelfinavir; **Riton** = ritonavir; **Saquin** = saquinavir). For interactions with antiretrovirals, see Table 21B, p. 134
Only a partial list—check package insert

Ampren	Indin	Nelfin	Riton	Saquin	OTHER DRUG (B)	EFFECT	SIGNIFICANCE/CERTAINTY
					Analgesics:		
			+		1. Alfentanil, fentanyl, hydrocodone, tramadol	↑ levels of B	+
			+		2. Codeine, hydromorphone, morphine	↓ levels of B	+
			+		**Anti-arrhythmics: amiodarone, lidocaine, mexiletine**	↑ levels of B	+
		+	+	+	**Anticonvulsants: carbamazepine, clonazepam, phenytoin, phenobarbital**	↓ levels of A, ↑ levels of B	++
			+		Antidepressants, all tricyclic	↑ levels of B	+
			+		Antidepressants, all other	↑ levels of B	+
			+		**Antihistamine:** Loratadine *(see below)*	↑ levels of B	++
	+	+	+	+	**Astemizole/terfenadine**	↑ levels of B—do not use	++
	+	+	+		**Benzodiazepines**	↑ levels of B—do not use	++
			+		Beta blockers: Metoprolol, pindolol, propranolol, timolol	↑ levels of B	+
			+		Calcium channel blockers (all)	↑ levels of B	++
+		+	+	+	**Cisapride**	↑ levels of B—do not use	++
		+	+		Contraceptives, oral	↓ levels of B	++
			+	+	Corticosteroids: prednisone, dexamethasone	↓ levels of A, ↑ levels of B	+
			+		Cyclosporine	↓ levels of B	+
			+		Diazepam and others	↑ level of B—do not use	++
+	+	+	+	+	Erythromycin, clarithromycin	levels of A & B	+
	+	+		+	Grapefruit juice (>200 ml/day)	↓ indinavir & ↑ saquinavir levels	++
+	+	+		+	Ketoconazole, itraconazole	↑ levels of A	+
+	+	+	+	+	Lipid-lowering drugs (statins)	↑ levels of B → hypolipidemia	++ (avoid)
			+		Metronidazole	Poss. disulfiram reaction, alcohol	+
+	+	+	+	+	Rifampin, rifabutin	↓ levels of A, ↑ levels of B	++
+	+	+	+	+	Sildenafil (Viagra)	Varies, some ↑ & some ↓ levels of B	++
			+		Theophylline	↓ levels of B	+
			+		Warfarin	↑ levels of B	+
Pyrazinamide					INH, rifampin	May ↑ risk of hepatotoxicity	±
Pyrimethamine					Lorazepam	↑ risk of hepatotoxicity	+
					Sulfonamides, TMP/SMX	↑ risk of marrow suppression	+
					Zidovudine	↑ risk of marrow suppression	+
Quinine					Digoxin	↑ digoxin levels; ↑ toxicity	++
					Mefloquine	↑ arrhythmias	+
					Oral anticoagulants	↑ prothrombin time	++
Rifamycins (rifampin, rifabutin) *See footnote for less severe or less common interactions*[1]					Al OH, ketoconazole, PZA	↓ levels of A	+
					Beta adrenergic blockers (metoprolol, propranolol)	↓ effect of B	+
					Clarithromycin	↑ levels of A[2], ↓ levels of B	++
					Corticosteroids	↑ replacement requirement of B	++
					Cyclosporine	↓ effect of B	++
					Delavirdine	↑ levels of A, ↓ levels of B—avoid	++
					Disopyramide	↓ levels of B	++
					Fluconazole	↑ levels of A[2]	+
					Amprenavir, indinavir, nelfinavir, ritonavir	↑ levels of A (↓ dose of A), ↓ levels of B	++
					INH	Converts INH to toxic hydrazine	++
					Itraconazole[2], ketoconazole	↓ levels of B, ↑ levels of A[2]	++
					Methadone	↓ serum levels (withdrawal)	+
					Nevirapine	↓ levels of B—avoid	++
					Oral anticoagulants	Suboptimal anticoagulation	++

[1] The following is a partial list of drugs with rifampin-induced ↑ metabolism and hence lower than anticipated serum levels: ACE inhibitors, dapsone, diazepam, digoxin, diltiazem, doxycycline, fluconazole, fluvastatin, haloperidol, nifedipine, progestins, triazolam, tricyclics, zidovudine

[2] Up to 4 weeks may be required after RIF discontinued to achieve detectable serum itra levels; ↑ levels associated with uveitis or polymyolysis

TABLE 21 (5)

ANTI-INFECTIVE AGENT (A)	OTHER DRUG (B)	EFFECT	SIGNIFICANCE/ CERTAINTY
Rifamycins (rifampin, rifabutin) *(continued) See footnote on page 132 for less severe or less common interactions*	Oral contraceptives	↓ effectiveness; spotting, pregnancy	+
	Phenytoin	↓ levels of B	+
	Quinidine	↓ effect of B	+
	Sulfonylureas	↓ hypoglycemic effect	+
	Tacrolimus	↓ levels of B	+ +
	Theophylline	↓ levels of B	+
	TMP/SMX	↑ levels of A	+
	Tocainide	↓ effect of B	+
Rimantadine	*See Amantadine*		
Ritonavir	*See protease inhibitors and Table 21B*		
Saquinavir	*See protease inhibitors and Table 21B*		
Stavudine	Dapsone, INH	May ↑ risk of peripheral neuropathy	±
Sulfonamides	Cyclosporine	↓ cyclosporine levels	+
	Methotrexate	↑ antifolate activity	+
	Oral anticoagulants	↑ prothrombin time; bleeding	+
	Phenytoin	↑ levels of B; nystagmus, ataxia	+
	Sulfonylureas	↑ hypoglycemic effect	+
Terbinafine	Cimetidine	↑ levels of A	+
	Phenobarbital, rifampin	↓ levels of A	+
Tetracyclines	*See Doxycycline, plus:*		
	Digoxin	↑ toxicity of B (may persist several months—up to 10% pts)	+ +
	Methoxyflurane	↑ toxicity; polyuria, renal failure	+
	Sucralfate	↓ absorption of A (separate by ≥2 hrs)	+
Thiabendazole	Theophyllines	↑ serum theophylline, nausea	+
Tobramycin	*See Aminoglycosides*		
Trimethoprim	Amantadine, dapsone, digoxin, methotrexate, procainamide, zidovudine	↑ serum levels of B	+ +
	Potassium-sparing diuretics	↑ serum K⁺	+ +
	Thiazide diuretics	↓ serum Na⁺	+
Trimethoprim/Sulfa- methoxazole	Azathioprine	Reports of leucopenia	+
	Cyclosporine	↓ levels of B, ↑ serum creatinine	+
	Loperamide	↑ levels of B	+
	Methotrexate	Enhanced marrow suppression	+ +
	Oral contraceptives, pimozide, and 6-mercaptopurine	↓ effect of B	+
	Phenytoin	↑ levels of B	+
	Rifampin	↑ levels of B	+
	Warfarin	↑ activity of B	+
Vancomycin	Aminoglycosides	↑ frequency of nephrotoxicity	+ +
Zalcitabine (ddC) (HIVID)	Valproic acid, pentamidine (IV), alcohol, lamivudine	↑ pancreatitis risk	+
	Cisplatin, INH, metronidazole, vincristine, nitrofurantoin, d4T, dapsone	↑ risk of peripheral neuropathy	+
Zidovudine (ZDV) (Retrovir)	Atovaquone, fluconazole, metha-done	↑ levels of A	+
	Clarithromycin	↓ levels of A	±
	Indomethacin	↑ levels of ZDV toxic metabolite	+
	Nelfinavir	↓ levels of A	+ +
	Probenecid, TMP/SMX	↑ levels of A	+
	Ribavirin	**↓ levels of A—avoid**	+ +
	Rifampin/rifabutin	↓ levels of A	+ +

TABLE 21B: DRUG-DRUG INTERACTIONS BETWEEN ANTIRETROVIRALS (*1 = Investigational)

NAME (Abbreviation, Trade Name)	Amprenavir (APV, Agenerase)	Indinavir (IDV, Crixivan)	Nelfinavir (NFV, Viracept)	Ritonavir (RTV, Norvir)	Saquinavir—soft gel (SQV, Fortovase)	Efavirenz (EFZ, Sustiva)	Delavirdine (DLV, Rescriptor)	Nevirapine (NVP, Viramune)
Amprenavir (APV, Agenerase)		Levels: APV ↑; IDV ↓. Dosage change: no data	Levels: APV ↓; NFV ↑. Usual dosage	No data	No interaction	APV levels ↓. Dosage change: no data	No data	No data
Indinavir (IDV, Crixivan)	Levels: APV ↑; IDV ↓. Dosage change: no data		Levels: NFV ↑ 2x; IDV ↑ 50%. Dose: 400 mg of each bid **(I)***	Levels: IDV ↑s RTV; RTV ↑s IDV	SQV ↑ 4–7x; no effect IDV. Antiviral antagonism. **Do not combine**	IDV levels ↓; ↑ IDV dose: 1000 mg q8h	IDV levels ↑ 2x. No change DLV. Dose of IDV: 400–600 mg q8h	NVP levels ↑ 2x; IDV ↓ 10–30%. Dose of IDV: 1000 mg q8h
Nelfinavir (NFV, Viracept)	No data	Levels: NFV ↑ 2x; IDV ↑ 50%. Dose: 400 mg of each bid **(I)***		NFV levels ↑ 2x; no effect RTV. Dosage: (RTV 400 mg bid + NFV 500–750 mg bid) —I*	SQV levels ↑ 3–5x; no effect NFV. Usual dosage.	NFV levels ↑: no effect EFZ. Usual dosage	DLV levels ↓ 50%. Usual dosage	Standard dose of both
Ritonavir (RTV, Norvir)	No data	Levels: IDV ↑s RTV RTV ↑s IDV	NFV levels ↑ 2x; no effect RTV. Dosage: (RTV 400 mg bid + NFV 500–750 mg bid) —I*		SQV levels ↑ 20x, RTV no effect. Dosage: 400 mg of each bid	Modest ↑ levels of both drugs. Usual dosage	RTV levels ↑ 70%. Dosage: Consider ↓ RTV to 400 mg bid	No interaction
Saquinavir—soft gel (SQV, Fortovase)	No interaction	Levels: SQV ↑ 4–7x; no effect IDV. Antiviral antagonism. **Do not combine**	SQV levels ↑ 3–5x; no effect NFV. Usual dosage	SQV levels ↑ 20x, RTV no effect. Dosage: 400 mg of each bid		↓ levels of SQV. **Do not combine**	SQV levels ↑ 5x. Dose: SQV 800 mg tid + DLV standard	SQV levels ↓ 25%. **Avoid combination**
Efavirenz (EFZ, Sustiva)	APV levels ↓. Dosage change: no data	IDV levels ↓; ↑ IDV dose: 1000 mg q8h	NFV levels ↑: no effect EFZ. Usual dosage	Modest ↑ levels of both drugs. Usual dosage	↓ levels of SQV. **Do not combine**		No data	No data
Delavirdine (DLV, Rescriptor)	No data	IDV levels ↑ 2x; no change DLV. Dose IDV: 400–600 mg q8h	DLV levels ↓ 50%. Usual dosage	RTV levels ↑ 70%. Dosage: Consider ↓ RTV to 400 mg bid	SQV levels ↑ 5x. Dose: SQV 800 mg bid + DLV standard	No data		**Do not use together**
Nevirapine (NVP, Viramune)	No data	NVP levels ↑ 2x; IDV ↓ 10–30%. Dose of IDV: 1000 mg q8h	Standard dose of both	No interaction	SQV levels ↓ 25%. **Avoid combination**	No data	**Do not use together**	

TABLE 22
LIST OF GENERIC AND COMMON TRADE NAMES

GENERIC NAME: TRADE NAMES	GENERIC NAME: TRADE NAMES	GENERIC NAME: TRADE NAMES
Abacavir: Ziagen	Doxycycline: Vibramycin	Ofloxacin: Floxin
Acyclovir: Zovirax	Efavirenz: Sustiva	Oseltamivir: Tamiflu
Albendazole: Albenza	Erythromycin(s): Ilotycin	Oxacillin: Prostaphlin
Amantadine: Symmetrel	*Ethyl succinate:* Pediamycin *Glucoheptonate:* Erythrocin	Palivizumab: Synagis
Amikacin: Amikin	*Estolate:* Ilosone	Paromomycin: Humatin
Amoxicillin: Amoxil, Polymox	Erythro/sulfisoxazole: Pediazole	Pefloxacin: Peflacine
Amoxicillin/clavulanate: Augmentin	Ethambutol: Myambutol	Penicillin G
Amphotericin B: Fungizone	Ethionamide: Trecator	crystalline-sodium: Crystapen
Ampho B-liposomal: AmBisome	Famciclovir: Famvir	procaine: Duracillin
Ampho B-cholesteryl complex: Amphotec	Fluconazole: Diflucan	benzathine: Bicillin
	Flucytosine: Ancobon	Penicillin V: Pen-Vee K
Ampho B-lipid complex: Abelcet	Foscarnet: Foscavir	Pentamidine: NebuPent, Pentam 300
Ampicillin: Omnipen, Polycillin	Fosfomycin: Monurol	Piperacillin: Pipracil
Ampicillin/sulbactam: Unasyn	Furazolidone: Furoxone	Piperacillin/tazobactam: Zosyn
Amprenavir: Agenerase	Ganciclovir: Cytovene	Piperazine: Antepar
Atovaquone: Mepron	Gatifloxacin: Tequin	Podophyllotoxin: Condylox
Atovaquone + proguanil: Malarone	Gentamicin: Garamycin	Praziquantel: Biltricide
Azithromycin: Zithromax	Griseofulvin: Fulvicin	Primaquine: Primachine
Aztreonam: Azactam	Halofantrine: Halfan	Proguanil: Paludrine
Cefaclor: Ceclor, Ceclor CD	Idoxuridine: Dendrid, Stoxil	Pyrantel pamoate: Antiminth
Cefadroxil: Duricef	INH + RIF: Rifamate	Pyrimethamine: Daraprim
Cefamandole: Mandol	INH + RIF + PZA: Rifater	Pyrimethamine/sulfadoxine: Fansidar
Cefazolin: Ancef, Kefzol	Interferon + ribavirin: Rebetron	Quinupristin/dalfopristin: Synercid
Cefdinir: Omnicef	Imipenem + cilastatin: Primaxin	Ribavirin: Virazole
Cefepime: Maxipime	Imiquimod: Aldara	Rifabutin: Mycobutin
Cefixime: Suprax	Indinavir: Crixivan	Rifampin: Rifadin, Rimactane
Cefoperazone: Cefobid	Itraconazole: Sporanox	Rifapentine: Priftin
Cefotaxime: Claforan	Ivermectin: Stromectol	Rimantadine: Flumadine
Cefotetan: Cefotan	Kanamycin: Kantrex	Ritonavir: Norvir
Cefoxitin: Mefoxin	Ketoconazole: Nizoral	Saquinavir: Invirase, Fortovase
Cefpodoxime proxetil: Vantin	Lamivudine: Epivir, Epivir-HBV	Sparfloxacin: Zagam
Cefprozil: Cefzil	Levofloxacin: Levaquin	Spectinomycin: Trobicin
Ceftazidime: Fortaz, Tazicef, Tazidime	Linezolid: Zyvox	Stavudine: Zerit
Ceftibuten: Cedax	Lomefloxacin: Maxaquin	Stibogluconate: Pentostam
Ceftizoxime: Cefizox	Loracarbef: Lorabid	Stibophen: Fuadin
Ceftriaxone: Rocephin	Mafenide: Sulfamylon	Silver sulfadiazine: Silvadene
Cefuroxime: Zinacef, Kefurox	Mebendazole: Vermox	Sulfamethoxazole: Gantanol
Cefuroxime axetil: Ceftin	Mefloquine: Lariam	Sulfasalazine: Azulfidine
Cephalexin: Keflex	Meropenem: Merrem	Sulfisoxazole: Gantrisin
Cephapirin: Cefadyl	Mesalamine: Asacol, Pentasa	Terbinafine: Lamisil
Cephradine: Anspor, Velosef	Methenamine hippurate: Hiprex	Thalidomide: Thalomid
Chloroquine: Aralen	Methenamine mandel.: Mandelamine	Thiabendazole: Mintezol
Cidofovir: Vistide	Metronidazole: Flagyl	Ticarcillin: Ticar
Ciprofloxacin: Cipro	Mezlocillin: Mezlin	Tobramycin: Nebcin
Clarithromycin: Biaxin, Biaxin XL	Minocycline: Minocin	Tretinoin: Retin A
Clindamycin: Cleocin	Moxifloxacin: Avelox	Trifluridine: Viroptic
Clofazimine: Lamprene	Mupirocin: Bactroban	Trimethoprim: Proloprim, Trimpex
Clotrimazole: Lotrimin, Mycelex	Nafcillin: Unipen	Trimethoprim/sulfamethoxazole: Bactrim, Septra
Cloxacillin: Tegopen	Nelfinavir: Viracept	Trimetrexate: Neutrexin
Cycloserine: Seromycin	Neomycin: Mycifradin	Trovafloxacin/alatrofloxacin: Trovan
Delavirdine: Rescriptor	Netilmicin: Netromycin	Valacyclovir: Valtrex
Dicloxacillin: Dynapen	Nevirapine: Viramune	Vancomycin: Vancocin
Didanosine: Videx	Niclosamide: Yomesan	Zalcitabine: HIVID
Diethylcarbamazine: Hetrazan	Nitrofurantoin: Macrobid, Macrodantin	Zanamivir: Relenza
Diloxanide furoate: Furamide	Norfloxacin: Noroxin	Zidovudine (ZDV): Retrovir
Dirithromycin: Dynabac	Nystatin: Mycostatin	Zidovudine + 3TC: Combivir

TABLE 22 (2)
LIST OF COMMON TRADE AND GENERIC NAMES

TRADE NAME: GENERIC NAME	TRADE NAME: GENERIC NAME	TRADE NAME: GENERIC NAME
Abelcet: Ampho B-lipid complex	Halfan: Halofantrine	Rebetron: Interferon + ribavirin
Achromycin: Tetracycline	Herplex: Idoxuridine	Relenza: Zanamivir
Agenerase: Amprenavir	Hiprex: Methenamine hippurate	Rescriptor: Delavirdine
Albenza: Albendazole	HIVID: Zalcitabine	Retin A: Tretinoin
Aldara: Imiquimod	Humatin: Paromomycin	Retrovir: Zidovudine (ZDV)
AmBisome: Ampho B-liposomal	Ilosone: Erythromycin estolate	Rifadin: Rifampin
Amikin: Amikacin	Ilotycin: Erythromycin	Rifamate: INH + RIF
Amoxil: Amoxicillin	Invirase: Saquinavir	Rifater: INH + RIF + PZA
Amphotec: Ampho B-cholesteryl complex	Kantrex: Kanamycin	Rimactane: Rifampin
	Keflex: Cephalexin	Rocephin: Ceftriaxone
Ancef: Cefazolin	Kefurox: Cefuroxime	Septra: Trimethoprim/sulfamethoxazole
Ancobon: Flucytosine	Lamisil: Terbinafine	
Anspor: Cephradine	Lamprene: Clofazimine	Seromycin: Cycloserine
Antepar: Piperazine	Lariam: Mefloquine	Silvadene: Silver sulfadiazine
Antiminth: Pyrantel pamoate	Levaquin: Levofloxacin	Sporanox: Itraconazole
Aralen: Chloroquine	Lorabid: Loracarbef	Stoxil: Idoxuridine
Asacol: Mesalamine	Lotrimin: Clotrimazole	Stromectol: Ivermectin
Augmentin: Amoxicillin clavulanate	Macrodantin, Macrobid: Nitrofurantoin	Sulfamylon: Mafenide
Avelox: Moxifloxacin	Malarone: Atovaquone + proguanil	Suprax: Cefixime
Azactam: Aztreonam	Mandelamine: Methenamine mandel.	Sustiva: Efavirenz
Azulfidine: Sulfasalazine	Mandol: Cefamandole	Symmetrel: Amantadine
Bactroban: Mupirocin	Maxaquin: Lomefloxacin	Synagis: Palivizumab
Bactrim: Trimethoprim/ sulfamethoxazole	Maxipime: Cefepime	Synercid: Quinupristin/dalfopristin
	Mefoxin: Cefoxitin	Tamiflu: Oseltamivir
Biaxin, Biaxin XL: Clarithromycin	Mepron: Atovaquone	Tazicef: Ceftazidime
Biltricide: Praziquantel	Merrem: Meropenem	Tegopen: Cloxacillin
Ceclor, Ceclor CD: Cefaclor	Mezlin: Mezlocillin	Tequin: Gatifloxacin
Cedax: Ceftibuten	Minocin: Minocycline	Thalomid: Thalidomide
Cefadyl: Cephapirin	Mintezol: Thiabendazole	Ticar: Ticarcillin
Cefizox: Ceftizoxime	Monocid: Cefonicid	Timentin: Ticarcillin-clavulanic acid
Cefobid: Cefoperazone	Monurol: Fosfomycin	Tinactin: Tolnaftate
Cefotan: Cefotetan	Myambutol: Ethambutol	Trecator SC: Ethionamide
Ceftin: Cefuroxime axetil	Mycobutin: Rifabutin	Trobicin: Spectinomycin
Cefzil: Cefprozil	Mycostatin: Nystatin	Trovan: Trovafloxacin/alatrofloxacin
Cipro: Ciprofloxacin	Nafcil: Nafcillin	Unasyn: Ampicillin/sulbactam
Claforan: Cefotaxime	Nebcin: Tobramycin	Unipen: Nafcillin
Combivir: ZDV + 3TC	NebuPent: Pentamidine	Valtrex: Valacyclovir
Crixivan: Indinavir	Netromycin: Netilmicin	Vancocin: Vancomycin
Cytovene: Ganciclovir	Neutrexin: Trimetrexate	Vantin: Cefpodoxime proxetil
Daraprim: Pyrimethamine	Nizoral: Ketoconazole	Velosef: Cephradine
Diflucan: Fluconazole	Noroxin: Norfloxacin	Vermox: Mebendazole
Duricef: Cefadroxil	Norvir: Ritonavir	Vibramycin: Doxycycline
Dynapen: Dicloxacillin	Omnicef: Cefdinir	Videx: Didanosine
Epivir, Epivir-HBV: Lamivudine	Omnipen: Ampicillin	Viracept: Nelfinavir
Famvir: Famciclovir	Pediamycin: Erythro. ethyl succinate	Viramune: Nevirapine
Fansidar: Pyrimethamine + sulfadoxine	Pediazole: Erythro. ethyl succinate + sulfisoxazole	Virazole: Ribavirin
Flagyl: Metronidazole	Peflacine: Pefloxacin	Vistide: Cidofovir
Floxin: Ofloxacin	Pen Vee K: Penicillin V	Zagam: Sparfloxacin
Flumadine: Rimantadine	Pentam 300: Pentamidine	Zerit: Stavudine
Fortaz: Ceftazidime	Pentasa: Mesalamine	Ziagen: Abacavir
Fortovase: Saquinavir	Pipracil: Piperacillin	Zinacef: Cefuroxime
Fulvicin: Griseofulvin	Polycillin: Ampicillin	Zithromax: Azithromycin
Fungizone: Amphotericin B	Polymox: Amoxicillin	Zovirax: Acyclovir
Furadantin: Nitrofurantoin	Priftin: Rifapentine	Zosyn: Piperacillin/tazobactam
Furoxone: Furazolidone	Primaxin: Imipenem + cilastatin	Zyvox: Linezolid
Gantanol: Sulfamethoxazole	Proloprim: Trimethoprim	
Gantrisin: Sulfisoxazole	Prostaphlin: Oxacillin	
Garamycin: Gentamicin		

Bold numbers indicate major considerations. Recommendations in Table 1 not indexed; antibiotic selection often depends on modifying circumstances and alternative agents.

Bold numbers indicate major considerations. Recommendations in Table 1 not indexed; antibiotic selection often depends on modifying circumstances and alternative agents.

Bold numbers indicate major considerations. Recommendations in Table 1 not indexed; antibiotic selection often depends on modifying circumstances and alternative agents.

Bold numbers indicate major considerations. Recommendations in Table 1 not indexed; antibiotic selection often depends on modifying circumstances and alternative agents.

Bold numbers indicate major considerations. Recommendations in Table 1 not indexed; antibiotic selection often depends on modifying circumstances and alternative agents.

Bold numbers indicate major considerations. Recommendations in Table 1 not indexed; antibiotic selection often depends on modifying circumstances and alternative agents.